Atlas of
INFECTIOUS DISEASES

Volume IV

UPPER RESPIRATORY AND
HEAD AND NECK INFECTIONS

Atlas of
INFECTIOUS DISEASES

Volume IV

UPPER RESPIRATORY AND HEAD AND NECK INFECTIONS

Editor-in-Chief

Gerald L. Mandell, MD

Professor of Medicine
Owen R. Cheatham Professor of the Sciences
Chief, Division of Infectious Diseases
University of Virginia Health Sciences Center
Charlottesville, Virginia

Editor

Itzhak Brook, MD

Professor, Department of Pediatrics
Georgetown University School of Medicine
Washington, DC
Senior Investigator, Naval Medical Research Institute
Bethesda, Maryland

**Churchill
Livingstone**

DEVELOPED BY CURRENT MEDICINE, INC.
PHILADELPHIA

CURRENT MEDICINE
400 MARKET STREET, SUITE 700
PHILADELPHIA, PA 19106

Library of Congress Cataloging-in-Publication Data

Library of Congress Cataloging-in-Publication Data
Upper respiratory and head and neck infections/editor-in-chief,
Gerald L. Mandell; editor, Itzhak Brook.
      p. cm.–(Atlas of infectious diseases; v. 4)
  Includes bibliographical references and index.
  ISBN 0-443-07710-X (hard cover)
   1. Head–Infections–Atlases. 2. Neck–Infections–Atlases.
I. Mandell, Gerald L. II. Brook, Itzhak. III. Series.
   [DNLM: 1. Respiratory Tract Infections–atlases.
2. Otorhinolaryngologic Diseases–atlases. 3. Eye Infections–atlases. 4.
Neck–pathology–atlases. WF 17 U68 1995]
RC936.U67 1995
617.5'1–dc20
DNLM/DLC
for Library of Congress   95-1977
                                                 CIP

Development Editor:	**Lee Tevebaugh**
Editorial Assistant:	**Jabin White**
Art Director:	**Paul Fennessy**
Design and Layout:	**Patrick Whelan**
Illustration Director:	**Ann Saydlowski**
Illustrators:	**Liz Carrozza, Wendy Jackelow, Beth Starkey, Lisa Weischedel, and Gary Welch**
Production:	**David Myers and Wendy Feinstein**
Typesetting Director:	**Colleen Ward**
Managing Editor:	**Lori J. Bainbridge**

Printed in Hong Kong by Paramount Printing Group Limited.

10 9 8 7 6 5 4 3 2 1

PREFACE

The diagnosis and management of patients with infectious diseases are based in large part on visual clues. Skin and mucous membrane lesions, eye findings, imaging studies, Gram stains, culture plates, insect vectors, preparations of blood, urine, pus cerebrospinal fluid, and biopsy specimens are studied to establish the proper diagnosis and to choose the most effective therapy. The *Atlas of Infectious Diseases* will be a modern, complete collection of these images. Current Medicine, with its capability of superb color reproduction and its state-of-the-art computer imaging facilities, is the ideal publisher for the atlas. Infectious diseases physicians, scientists, microbiologists, and pathologists frequently teach other healthcare professionals, and this comprehensive atlas with available slides is an effective teaching tool.

Dr. Itzhak Brook has extensive experience and expertise in all aspects of upper respiratory and head and neck infections. He has focused a group of expert clinicians and scientists on this topic and produced an outstanding atlas volume, which will be utilized frequently as a diagnostic and teaching tool.

Gerald L. Mandell, MD
Professor of Medicine
Owen R. Cheatham Professor of the Sciences
Chief, Division of Infectious Diseases
University of Virginia Health Sciences Center
Charlottesville, Virginia

CONTRIBUTORS

Stephen G. Baum, MD
Chairman, Department of Medicine
Beth Israel Medical Center
Professor, The Albert Einstein College of Medicine
New York, New York

James N. Endicott, MD
Professor of Surgery
Division of Otolaryngology
University of South Florida
Tampa, Florida

Theodore W. Fetter, MD
Clinical Assistant Professor of Surgery (Otolaryngology)
Uniformed Services, University of the Health Sciences
Bethesda, Maryland
Clinical Assistant Professor of Otolaryngology
Georgetown University Medical School
Washington, DC

Marlin E. Gher, Jr, DDS, MEd
Former Chairman of Periodontics & Director of the
  Graduate Program in Periodontics
Naval Dental School
Bethesda, Maryland
Specialty Advisor for Periodontics
Bureau of Medicine & Surgery
Carlsbad, California

Kenneth M. Grundfast, MD, FACS, FAAP
Vice-Chairman, Department of Otolaryngology
Director of Ear and Hearing Disorders Clinic
Children's National Medical Center
Washington, DC

Rande H. Lazar, MD, FICS
Director, Pediatric Otolaryngology Fellowship Training
LeBonheur Children's Medical Center
Memphis, Tennessee

Andrew M. Margileth, MD, FAAP, FACP
Clinical Professor of Pediatrics
University of Virginia Medical Center
Charlottesville, Virginia

Moses Nussbaum, MD
Chairman, Department of Surgery
Beth Israel Medical Center
Professor, The Albert Einstein College of Medicine
New York, New York

George Quintero, DDS
Private Practice
Atlanta, Georgia

Janet Seper, MD
Resident
Division of Otolaryngology
University of South Florida
Tampa, Florida

Harris R. Stutman, MD
Director, Pediatric Infectious Disease
Memorial Miller Children's Hospital
Associate Professor of Pediatrics
University of California, Irvine
Long Beach, California

Debra A. Tristram, MD
Children's Hospital of Buffalo
Division of Infectious Diseases
Assistant Professor of of Pediatrics
Department of Pediatrics
State University of New York at Buffalo
Buffalo, New York

Ellen R. Wald, MD
Professor of Pediatrics & Otolaryngology
University of Pittsburgh School of Medicine
Division Chief, Infectious Diseases
Children's Hospital of Pittsburgh
Pittsburgh, Pennsylvania

Ayal Willner, MD
Associate, Department of Otolaryngology
Children's National Medical Center
Assistant Professor of Otolaryngology & Pediatrics
George Washington University School of Medicine
Washington, DC

CONTENTS

CHAPTER 1

Eye and Orbit Infections

Ellen R. Wald

ANATOMY OF THE ORBIT

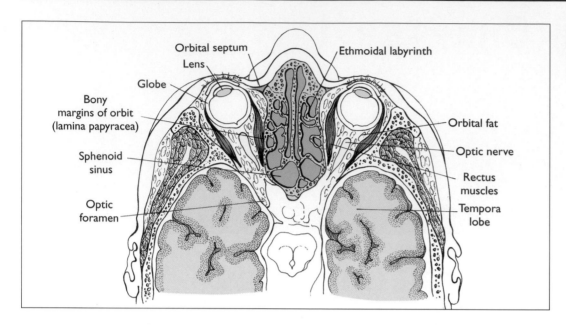

FIGURE 1-1 Anatomy of the eye and surrounding structures. The relationship between the paranasal sinuses and orbit is delineated.

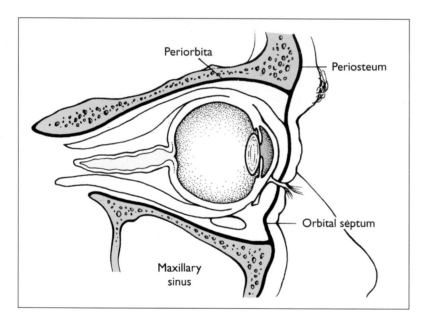

FIGURE 1-2 Anatomy of the orbital septum. The position of the septum, a connective tissue reflection of periosteum occurring within the upper and lower lids, is shown. Swelling of the lid and face anterior to the septum constitutes an example of a disorder known as *preseptal cellulitis*. Infections of the conjunctiva, eyelid, eyelashes, skin, lacrimal duct, and lacrimal gland are all preseptal in location. (*From* Wald ER: Acute and chronic sinusitis: Diagnosis and management. *Pediatr Rev* 1985, 7:150–157; with permission.)

PRESEPTAL CELLULITIS

Infections of the Conjunctiva and Lid Structures

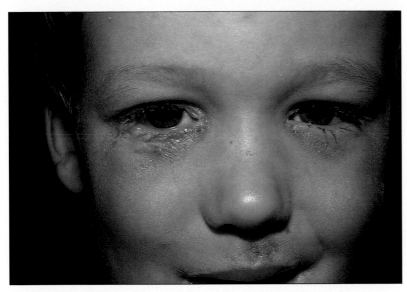

FIGURE 1-3 Conjunctivitis. Conjunctivitis is probably the most common eye infection to present to the practitioner. Beyond the neonatal period, the causes of conjunctivitis are usually bacterial or viral. In either case, the diagnosis is usually apparent at a glance. The lids are thickened and crusted. Occasionally, the eyes are matted shut in the morning. This case shows an example of conjunctivitis caused by *Haemophilus influenzae*. Conjunctivitis is one cause of preseptal cellulitis.

Etiology of conjunctivitis

Etiology	Other site of infection	Treatment
Infants and children		
Haemophilus influenzae	Otitis media	Topical/oral*
Streptococcus pneumoniae	Otitis media	Topical/oral
Adenovirus	Pharyngitis	Symptomatic
Enterovirus	Pharyngitis	Symptomatic
Adolescents and adults		
Adenovirus	Pharyngitis	Symptomatic
Neisseria gonorrhoeae	Urethritis	Ceftriaxone, cefixime
Chlamydia trachomatis	Urethritis	Doxycycline, erythromycin, azithromycin

*Topical treatment is with polymyxin B-bacitracin or sodium sulfac-etamide. Oral treatment is with amoxicillin-potassium clavulate.

FIGURE 1-4 Etiology of conjunctivitis. When conjunctivitis is associated with otitis media, the usual cause is bacterial: *Haemophilus influenzae* (nontypeable) in 80% of cases and *Streptococcus pneumoniae* in 20%. When conjunctivitis is associated with pharyngitis, the usual etiology is adenovirus.

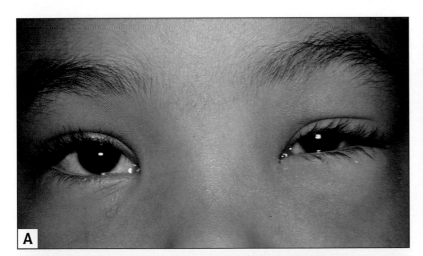

A

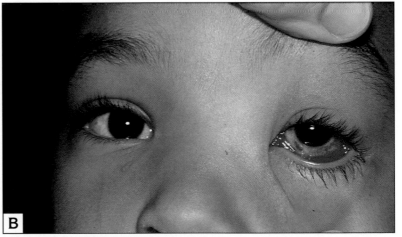

B

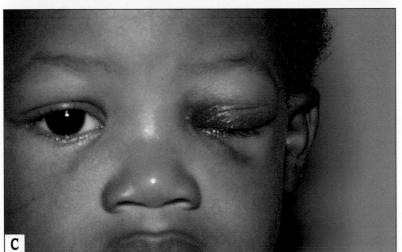

C

FIGURE 1-5 Hemorrhagic conjunctivitis. **A,** In this case of conjunctivitis, the lids are not thickened and crusted but diffusely swollen. **B,** When the lid is retracted, the diagnosis of hemorrhagic conjunctivitis is apparent. Adenovirus 19 was cultured from the swab of the conjunctiva. **C,** A child with hemorrhagic conjunctivitis caused by adenovirus, in whom the hemorrhagic aspects extend to the cutaneous portion of the lid, is shown.

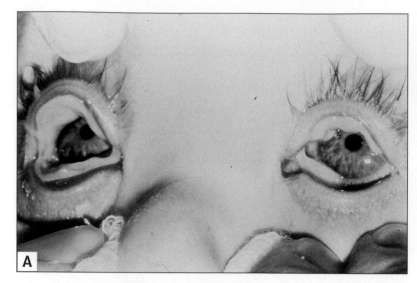

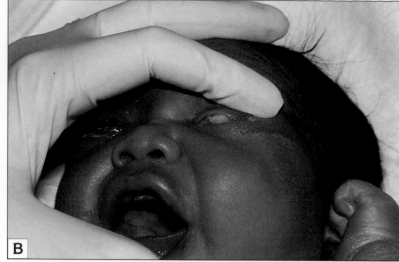

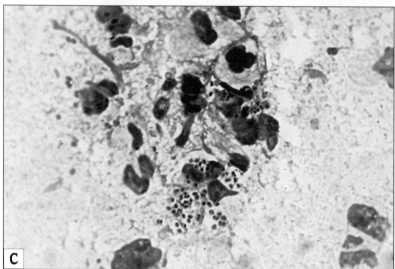

FIGURE 1-6 Ophthalmia neonatorum. In the first 30 days of life, suppurative conjunctivitis occurring in infants is called *ophthalmia neonatorum*. The most common causes are *Neisseria gonorrhoeae* and *Chlamydia trachomatis*, which are clinically indistinguishable from each other. Each is transmitted from mother to child at the time of birth. **A**, *N. gonorrhoeae* usually causes symptoms in the first week of life. **B**, *C. trachomatis* causes symptoms in week 2. Occasionally, *Pseudomonas* species are the cause of ophthalmia neonatorum. Cultures should be obtained for bacterial species, particularly *N. gonorrhoeae* and *C. trachomatis*; special media are required for both. **C**, Gram stain of conjunctival exudate from a neonate with gonococcal ophthalmia shows intracellular gram-negative diplococci. (Panels 6A and 6B *from* Cheng KP, Biglan AW, Hiles DA: Pediatric ophthalmology. *In* Zitelli BJ, Davis HW (eds.): *Atlas of Pediatric Physical Diagnosis*, 2nd ed. New York: Gower Medical Publishing; 1992; with permission.)

Ophthalmia neonatorum	
Etiology	*Neisseria gonorrhoeae*
	Chlamydia trachomatis
Clinical findings	Variable severity
	Etiologies clinically indistinguishable
	Different time of onset
Diagnosis	Culture of scraping
Treatment	Ceftriaxone parentally (*Neisseria*)
	Erythromycin orally (*Chlamydia*)

FIGURE 1-7 Characteristics of ophthalmia neonatorum. Although, clinically, infections due to the two agents are indistinguishable, infection with *Neisseria gonorrhoeae* presents in neonates at age 2–5 days, whereas that with *Chlamydia trachomatis* is observed between 7 and 21 days of age. Treatment of neonatal ophthalmia should be undertaken promptly to avoid complications. If untreated, *N. gonorrhoeae* may cause corneal perforation and endophthalmitis. Untreated *C. trachomatis* infection may result in chronic infection.

Features that distinguish bacterial from viral and chlamydial conjunctivitis

Feature	Bacterial	Viral	Chlamydial
Conjunctival injection	Moderately severe	Minimal	Absent or minimal
Exudate	Moderate to profuse (poly-morphonuclear)	Minimal (usually mononuclear)	Minimal in adults, copious in newborns
Sticking of lids on awakening	Yes	No	Absent in adults, present in newborns
Papillae (palpebral conjunctiva)	Present	Usually absent	May be present
Follicles (palpebral conjunctiva)	Usually absent	Present	Present in adults, absent in newborns
Preauricular lymphadenopathy	Absent	Present	Present in adults, absent in newborns
Response to antibiotic therapy	Yes	No	Yes
Duration of untreated disease	Up to several weeks	Several weeks	Persistent

FIGURE 1-8 Features that distinguish bacterial, viral, and chlamydial conjunctivitis. (*From* Baum J, Barza M: Infections of the eye and adjacent sinuses. *In* Gorbach S, Bartlett J, Blacklow NR (eds.): *Infectious Diseases.* Philadelphia: W.B. Saunders; 1992:1137; with permission.)

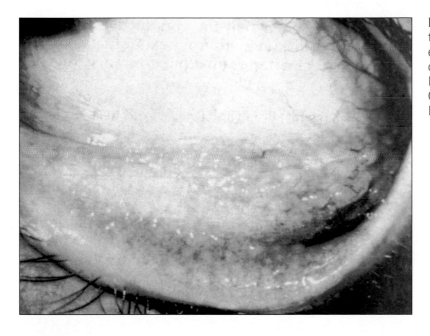

FIGURE 1-9 Inclusion (chlamydial) conjunctivitis. Inclusion conjunctivitis in adults is a common sexually transmitted infection of the eye in the United States. Large follicles on the inferior palpebral conjunctiva are typically seen in adults, but not in infants. (*From* Baum J, Barza M: Infections of the eye and adjacent sinuses. *In* Gorbach S, Bartlett J, Blacklow NR (eds.): *Infectious Diseases.* Philadelphia: W.B. Saunders; 1992:1138; with permission.)

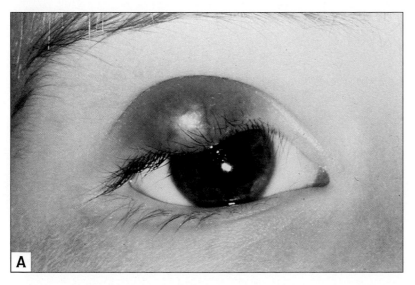

FIGURE 1-10 Hordeolum. **A,** An external hordeolum, or stye, is a bacterial infection of a hair follicle or sebaceous gland. The stye usually points to the lid margin and is easily identifiable by its localized erythematous or pustular appearance. (*continued*)

A

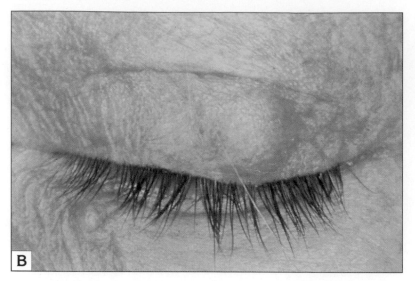

B

FIGURE 1-10 (*continued*) **B,** Occasionally, an internal hordeolum may be seen, which points to the conjunctival surface. It may cause a localized bulge, as shown in this example, or a more diffuse swelling. In the latter instance, the clinician may suspect a more serious cause of the eyelid swelling. The diagnosis can be clarified by everting the lid; in an internal hordeolum, a pustule pointing toward the conjunctiva can be seen. (*From* Cheng KP, Biglan AW, Hiles DA: Pediatric ophthalmology. *In* Zitelli BG, Davis HW (eds.): *Atlas of Pediatric Physical Diagnosis*, 2nd ed. New York: Gower Medical Publishing; 1992; with permission.)

Infections of the Lacrima

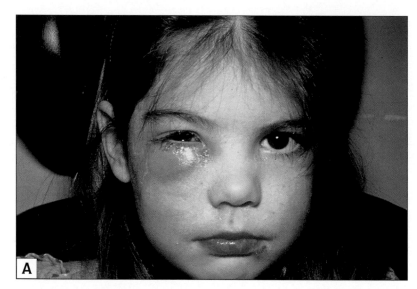

A

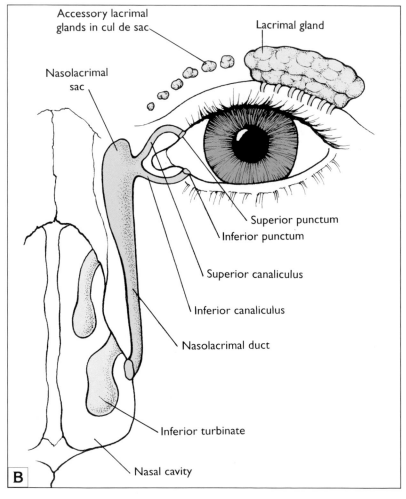

B

FIGURE 1-11 Dacryocystitis. **A,** This child had an upper respiratory tract infection for 3–4 days and then developed fever and an erythematous area beneath the medial canthus. This area is indurated, warm to touch, and exquisitely tender. This is an example of dacryocystitis, a bacterial infection of the lacrimal sac and duct. These infections are rare, although they can occur at any age as a complication of a viral upper respiratory tract infection. **B,** The lacrimal secretory and collecting system is diagrammed.

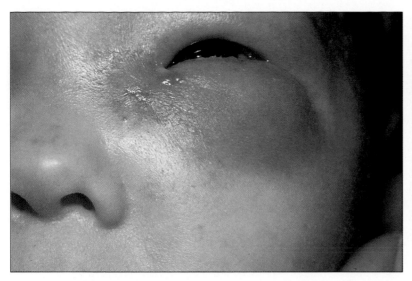

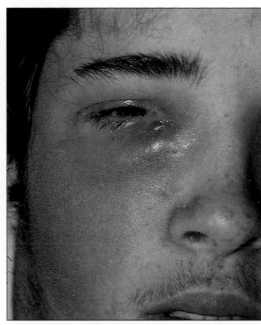

FIGURE 1-13
Dacryocystitis in a 16-year-old boy. The usual cause of dacryocystitis is *Staphylococcus aureus*. Treatment is with the parenteral administration of nafcillin. Surgery is rarely necessary, as medical therapy is usually successful. Occasionally, the lacrimal duct must be probed after the acute infection has resolved.

FIGURE 1-12 Dacryocystitis in a 2-week-old neonate. The purulent material spontaneously decompressed, leaving a nearly normal appearance on the following day.

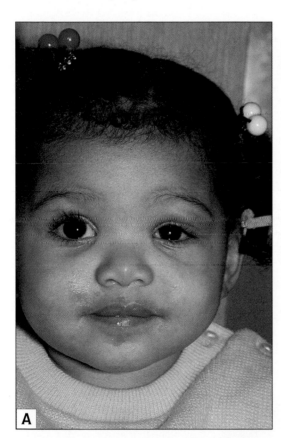

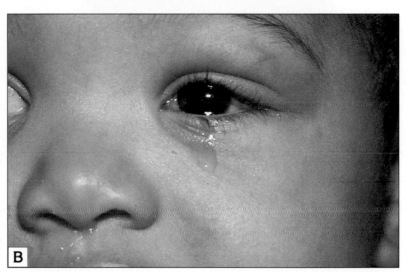

FIGURE 1-14 Dacryoadenitis. **A**, A 2-year-old girl, who had a viral upper respiratory tract infection for the preceding 5 days, developed swelling and erythema above the lateral portion of her upper lid. The swelling was painless and occurred during the fourth day of amoxicillin therapy, which was prescribed for the treatment of a right-sided otitis media. No additional treatment was instituted. The swelling resolved spontaneously over the next 2 days. This child had dacryoadenitis, or inflammation of the lacrimal gland. **B**, The location of the swelling, above the lateral portion of the upper lid, is the key to the diagnosis.

Etiology of dacryoadenitis	
Viral	Mumps virus
	Epstein-Barr virus
Bacterial	*Staphylococcus aureus*
	Streptococcus pyogenes
	Neisseria gonorrhoeae
	Mycobacterium tuberculosis
	Treponema pallidum

FIGURE 1-15 Etiology of dacryoadenitis. Dacryoadenitis is usually viral in etiology, with mumps and Epstein-Barr virus being known causes. When dacryoadenitis is caused by bacterial agents, it results in a very tender swelling. Treatment for dacryoadenitis is usually empiric because material for culture is not readily available.

Cutaneous Infections of the Eyelid and Periorbital Area

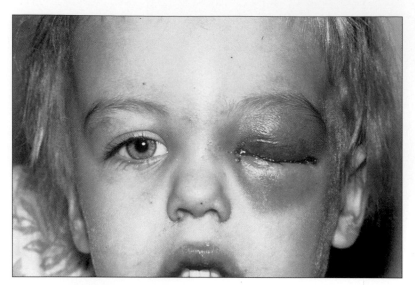

FIGURE 1-16 Streptococcal bacterial cellulitis secondary to orbital trauma. A 2-year-old boy had nasal discharge, nasal congestion, and low-grade fever for about 10 days. The morning before presentation, he fell and sustained a 7-mm laceration just lateral to his left eye. Despite careful cleansing of the area, he developed dramatic periorbital swelling and erythema over the next 24–36 hours. His 9-year-old brother had had a "strep" throat the preceding week. Group A streptococcus was recovered from the culture of the wound. Bacterial cellulitis secondary to trauma is usually due to *Staphylococcus aureus* or *Streptococcus pyogenes* (group A streptococcus). Parenteral therapy was initiated with good response.

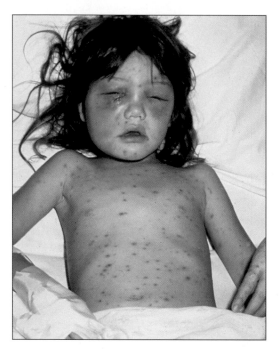

FIGURE 1-17 Streptococcal bacterial cellulitis complicating varicella. A previously healthy 8-year-old Amerasian girl developed varicella. On the fourth day of her rash, her fever spiked to 40° C (104° F), and she rapidly developed bilateral periorbital erythema and swelling and looked much sicker than she had on previous days. Both upper and lower lids were markedly erythematous, tender, and swollen. An excoriated varicella lesion was noted on her right lower lid. Extraocular eye movements were normal and there was no proptosis. Cultures of her blood and lesion grew *Streptococcus pyogenes*. (*Courtesy of* R. Moriarity, MD.)

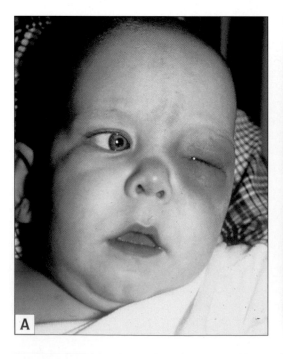
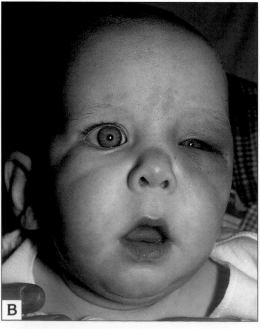

FIGURE 1-18 *Haemophilus influenzae* type b bacteremic cellulitis. A 9-month-old boy had an upper respiratory tract infection for 3 days. On the morning of admission, he had a temperature of 40° C (104° F) and a small erythematous area under the medial portion of the lower lid. **A,** Within 6 hours, the erythema and swelling progressed to involve both upper and lower lids. The area was nontender. Eversion of the lids showed the globe to be normally placed with intact extraocular movements. The blood culture was positive for *H. influenzae* type b. Parenteral antibiotics were initiated and resolution was prompt. **B,** Within 24 hours, the erythema had receded partially, and the eye was approximately 25% open. In 48 hours, the eye was nearly completely open, and the cutaneous findings had resolved. (*continued*)

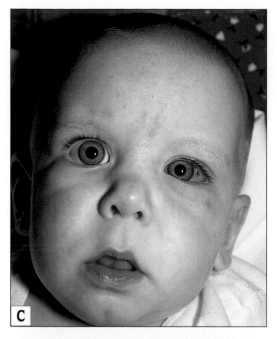

FIGURE 1-18 (*continued*) **C**, The intense erythema of the conjunctiva seen here represents hyperemia to the area of inflammation. It is seen during the evolution and resolution of the process and can be mistaken for conjunctivitis.

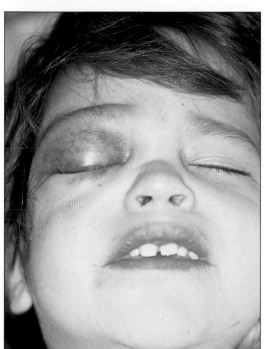

FIGURE 1-19 Bacteremic periorbital cellulitis due to *Haemophilus influenzae* type b. The etiologic agents arise from the nasopharynx and become blood-borne, seeding the meninges, lung, skeleton, or facial skin (buccal or periorbital). The usual age group affected is between 3 and 18 months. Typically, there is a prodromal upper respiratory tract infection. On the third or fourth day, there is the onset of high fever and eye swelling with erythema that progresses to lid closure very rapidly. *H. influenzae* type b is responsible for approximately 80% of cases, with *Streptococcus pneumoniae* accounting for 20%. The organism is recoverable from the blood culture or tissue aspirate (if performed). Routine immunization of infants with *H. influenzae* type b conjugate vaccines will prevent most cases of this infection.

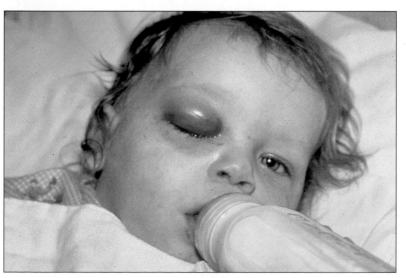

FIGURE 1-20 Bacteremic periorbital cellulitis due to *Haemophilus influenzae* type b. A previously well 7-month-old infant had several days of nasal discharge and cough. Redness and swelling developed around his right eye 1 day before he was taken to his primary care practitioner. He had not yet received any doses of the *H. influenzae* type b conjugate vaccine. Physical examination showed erythema and swelling of both lids, with a violaceous hue of the upper lid margin. Extraocular eye movements could not be assessed because of the degree of lid swelling, but a computed tomographic scan showed all of the swelling to be preseptal, *ie*, confined to the eyelid. The orbits were normal. His pretreatment blood culture grew *H. influenzae* type b. (*Courtesy of* R. Moriarity, MD.)

Keys to diagnosis of bacteremic periorbital cellulitis

Young age (< 18 mos)
High fever (> 39.4° C or 103° F)
Rapid progression to eyelid closure (within 24 hrs of onset of
  eyelid swelling)

FIGURE 1-21 Keys to diagnosis of bacteremic periorbital cellulitis. The acute onset and rapid progression of eye swelling differentiate bacteremic periorbital cellulitis from inflammatory edema.

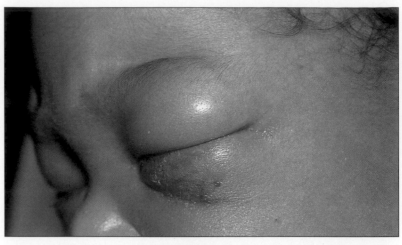

FIGURE 1-22 Bacteremic periorbital cellulitis due to group B streptococcus. In this case, group B streptococcus was recovered from the blood culture. The age group in which group B streptococci cause bacteremic periorbital cellulitis is between birth and 2–3 months.

A. Orbital complications of acute sinusitis

1. Inflammatory edema or sympathetic effusion
2. Subperiosteal abscess
3. Orbital abscess
4. Orbital cellulitis
5. Cavernous sinus thrombosis

FIGURE 1-23 Orbital complications of acute sinusitis. **A**, Although inflammatory edema or sympathetic effusion is considered by some to be an orbital complication of sinusitis, the infection, in fact, is limited to the sinus cavity. In the other examples—subperiosteal abscess, orbital abscess and cellulitis, and cavernous sinus thrombosis—the infection extends into the conal area. **B**, Diagram of the orbital complications of acute sinusitis: 1) inflammatory edema or sympathetic effusion; 2) subperiosteal abscess; 3) orbital abscess; 4) orbital cellulitis; 5) cavernous sinus thrombosis. (Chandler JR, Langenbrunner DJ, Stevens ER: The pathogenesis of orbital complications in acute sinusitis. *Laryngoscope* 1970, 80:1414.)

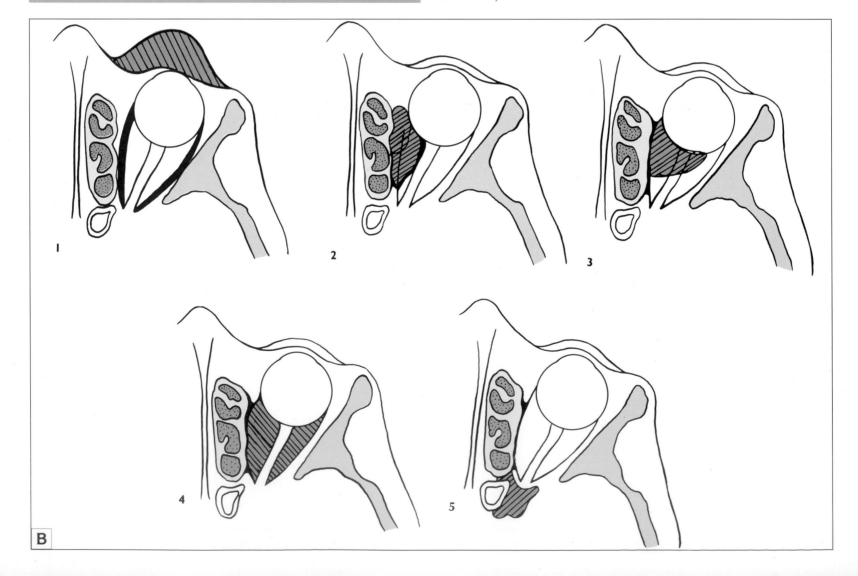

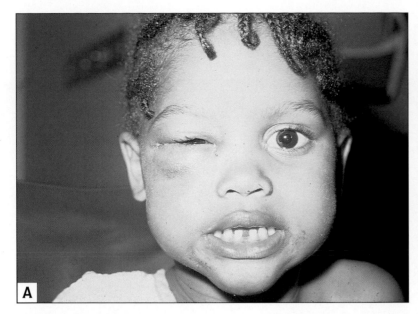
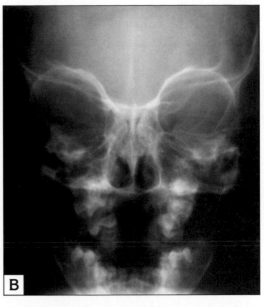

FIGURE 1-24 Inflammatory edema. **A**, A child had a viral upper respiratory tract infection for 5 days, consisting of nasal discharge, nasal congestion, and cough. The day before presentation, she had some swelling about her eye in the morning, which resolved later in the day. On the morning of presentation, she awoke and again had periorbital swelling; however, at this time, the swelling persisted. On physical examination, the patient had a low-grade fever of 38.3° C (101° F). Eversion of the lids showed the globe to be normally placed with normal extraocular movements. The diagnosis was inflammatory edema, or sympathetic effusion. (*From* Wald ER: Acute and chronic sinusitis: Diagnosis and management. *Pediatr Rev* 1985, 7:150–157; with permission.) **B**, Sinus radiographs were performed, and the anteroposterior view shows that the actual site of bacterial infection is the ethmoid sinus. Although bilateral ethmoiditis is seen radiographically, the congestion is greatest on the right. The lid and periorbital swelling represent passive venous congestion from the impedance of drainage imposed by the congested ethmoid sinuses.

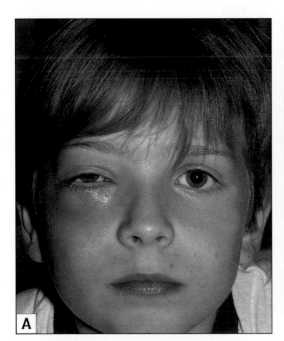
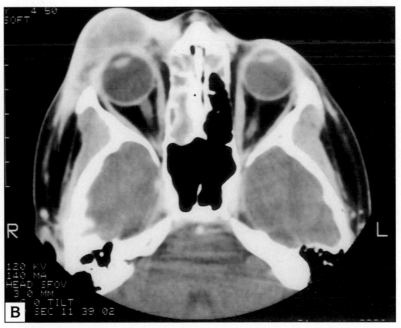

FIGURE 1-25 Inflammatory edema. **A**, A 10-year-old boy had an upper respiratory tract infection for several days with clear nasal discharge and daytime cough. The onset of eye swelling prompted a visit to his pediatrician. The globe was normally placed, and extraocular eye movements were within normal limits. The periorbital area was puffy but neither tender nor indurated. **B**, A computed tomography (CT) scan shows that the primary site of infection is the ethmoid sinus. Within the bony orbit, the muscle and globe of the eye are normal. All the swelling is in the eyelid. Accordingly, this is a case of preseptal cellulitis.

TRUE ORBITAL INFECTIONS

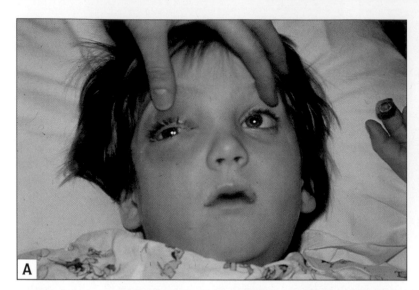

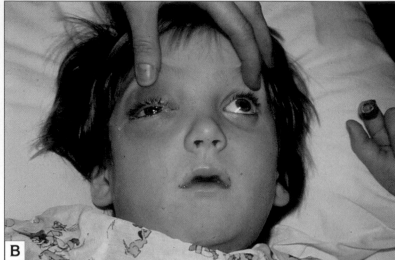

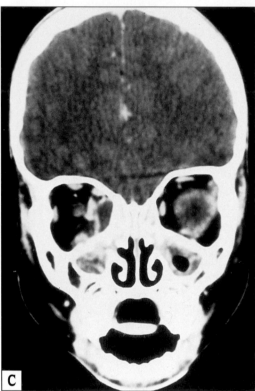

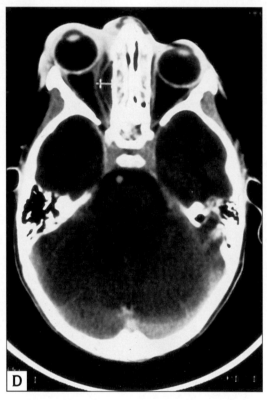

opened spontaneously. When his lids were everted manually, the globe of his right eye was anteriorly displaced (proptotic). **A**, The patient is shown moving his eyes to the right. **B**, When he is moving his eyes up, there is an impairment of upward gaze. The remaining extraocular eye movements were within normal limits. The hallmark of a true orbital infection is 1) displacement of the globe, 2) impairment of extraocular eye movements, or 3) loss of visual acuity. **C** and **D**, Computed tomography (CT) scans show that the ethmoid sinus is completely opacified. There is a subperiosteal abscess consequent to osteitis of the lateral wall of the ethmoid sinus (lamina papyracea), as evident in the axial (*panel 26C*) and coronal planes (*panel 26D*). This finding mandates surgical exploration and drainage of the abscess and the sinuses as well. There is bilateral maxillary involvement: complete opacification on the right and mucosal thickening on the left. High-dose parenteral antibiotics are indicated. Culture of the subperiosteal abscess grew *Streptococcus pneumoniae*. (Panels 26C and 26D *from* Wald ER: Rhinitis and acute and chronic sinusitis. *In* Bluestone CB, Stool SE (eds.): *Pediatric Otolaryngology*, 2nd ed. Philadelphia: W.B. Saunders; 1990:736; with permission.)

FIGURE 1-26 Subperiosteal abscess. A 6-year-old boy had an upper respiratory tract infection for 5 days. He had been complaining of eye discomfort and headache behind his eye for 12 hours. On physical examination, he was afebrile. His eyelid was swollen and could not be

Differentiation of preseptal and orbital cellulitis

Clinical signs	Preseptal	Orbital
Cutaneous findings (erythema, swelling)	Present	Present
Vision	Normal	May be impaired
Extraocular eye movements	Normal	May be impaired
Proptosis	None	Usually present
Chemosis	None	May be present

FIGURE 1-27 Differentiation of preseptal and orbital cellulitis. Anterior and lateral displacement of the globe and impairment of upward gaze are the most common findings in orbital cellulitis.

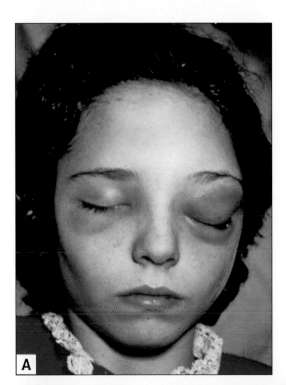

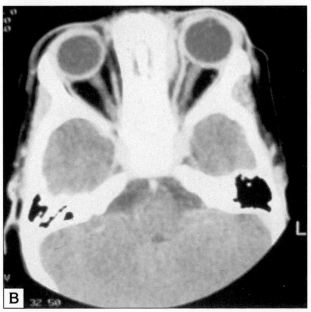

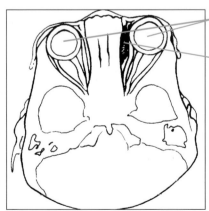

Eye

Possible pus between lateral rectus and ethmoid bone

FIGURE 1-28 Subperiosteal abscess. A 14-year-old girl had a 1-week history of nasal congestion, cough, and low-grade fever. She developed a frontal headache, bilateral eye pain, and erythema first around the left eye and then around the right for 2 days before visiting her physician. **A,** Her left eye appeared to be bulging. On physical examination, there was modest proptosis of her left globe with limitation of upward gaze of her left eye. **B,** A computed tomography scan showed a possible accumulation of pus between the left medial rectus and the left ethmoid sinus. Because the abscess was not well defined, high-dose parenteral therapy was initiated. She did very well, and surgery was not required. (*Courtesy of* R. Moriarity, MD.)

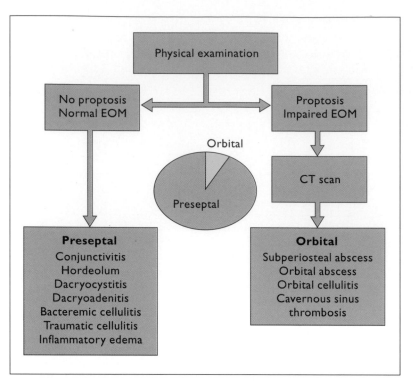

FIGURE 1-29 Differential considerations in the patient with a swollen eye. The physical findings of proptosis and extraocular eye movements (EOMs) should prompt the performance of a computed tomography scan. If a well-formed abscess is noted, surgical intervention is required. If there is no proptosis and the EOMs are normal, the practitioner must consider the differential diagnosis of a preseptal process.

Diagnosis, etiology, and treatment of preseptal cellulitis

Diagnosis	Etiology	Treatment
Conjunctivitis	Adenovirus	Symptomatic
	Enterovirus	
Hordeolum	*Staphylococcus aureus*	Ophthalmic polymyxin-bacitracin
Dacryocystitis	*Staphylococcus aureus*	Nafcillin iv
Dacryoadenitis	*Staphylococcus aureus*	Nafcillin iv
Bacteremic cellulitis	*Streptococcus pneumoniae*	Cefuroxime iv
	Haemophilus influenzae b	
Traumatic cellulitis	*Staphylococcus aureus*	Nafcillin iv
	Streptococcus pyogenes	
Inflammatory edema	*Streptococcus pneumoniae*	Cefuroxime iv
	Haemophilus influenzae	
	Moraxella catarrhalis	

iv—intravenously.

FIGURE 1-30 Diagnosis, etiology, and treatment of preseptal cellulitis.

EYE INFECTIONS

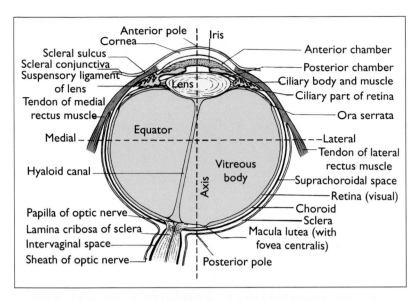

FIGURE 1-31 Anatomy of the eyeball. The globe is divided into three compartments: the anterior and posterior chambers and the vitreous cavity. Surrounding these compartments are three tissue layers that are referred to as tunics. The cornea, sclera, and limbus comprise the outer tunic. The uvea is the middle tunic, consisting of the choroid, ciliary body, and iris. The inner tunic is the retina. In endophthalmitis, there is inflammation of the inner and/or middle layers and adjacent compartments. When all three tunics are inflamed, the process is referred to as panophthalmitis.

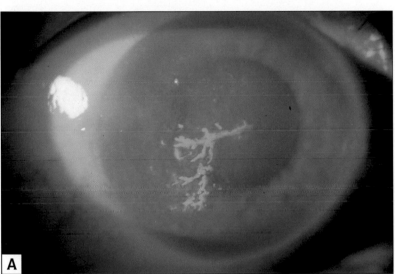

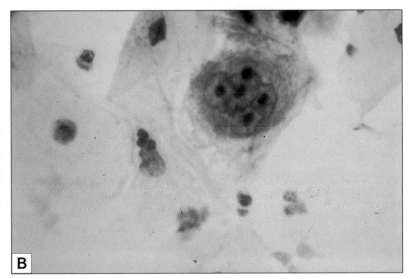

FIGURE 1-32 Keratitis. Keratitis is an inflammation of the cornea. It may be caused by bacteria, fungi, protozoa, or viruses, as in this example of Herpes simplex keratoconjunctivitis. Keratitis should be evaluated by obtaining scrapings of the conjunctiva and cornea for cytologic study, culture, and immunofluorescent staining. (Van Dyke RB, Desky AB, Daum RS: Infections of the eye and periorbital structures. *Adv Pediatr Infect Dis* 1988, 3:125–180.)

Herpes simplex often causes a typical dendritic ulcer that may be appreciated with fluorescein dye and cobalt-blue–filtered illumination. **A,** The infected area of the epithelium allows absorption of the fluorescein dye, which is excited by the blue illumination. (*Courtesy of* K. Cheng, MD.) **B,** A multinucleated giant cell is shown, as is seen in cells infected by herpes simplex or varicella-zoster virus.

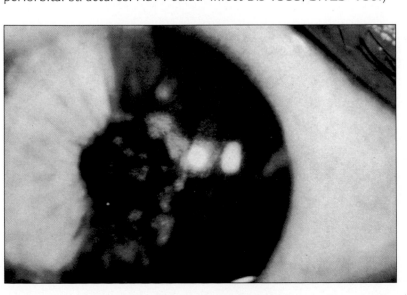

FIGURE 1-33 Viral keratoconjunctivitis. In the United States, viral conjunctivitis is more common than bacterial or chlamydial conjunctivitis. The most common viral cause is adenovirus, which usually presents clinically as epidemic keratoconjunctivitis (pictured here) or pharyngoconjunctival fever. Characteristic focal subepithelial corneal infiltrates are seen on slit-lamp examination (*From* Baum J, Barza M: Infections of the eye and adjacent sinuses. *In* Gorbach S, Bartlett J, Blacklow NR (eds.): *Infectious Diseases.* Philadelphia: W.B. Saunders; 1992:1139; with permission.)

Differentiation of conjunctivitis from keratitis or iritis

Clinical signs	Conjunctivitis	Keratitis or iritis
Vision	Normal	May be reduced
Pain	Gritty irritation	True pain
Conjunctiva	Diffuse injection	Ciliary flush
Exudate	Minimal to profuse	Usually none
Mattering of lids (dried exudate)	May be present	Absent
Photophobia	Absent	Present
Lacrimation	Usually absent	Present
Pupillary diameter	Normal	Usually small

FIGURE 1-34 Differentiation of conjunctivitis from keratitis or iritis. (*From* Baum J, Barza M: Infections of the eye and adjacent sinuses. *In* Gorbach S, Bartlett J, Blacklow NR (eds.): *Infectious Diseases*. Philadelphia: W.B. Saunders; 1992:1137; with permission.)

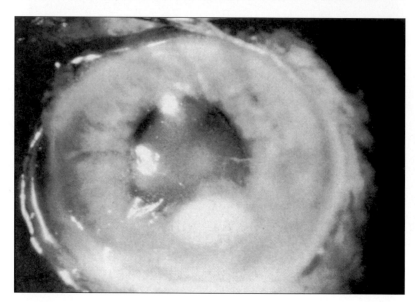

FIGURE 1-35 Bacterial keratitis. Although bacterial keratitis is less common than viral keratitis, bacterial infections are usually more fulminant and require prompt attention. In a typical bacterial corneal ulcer, there is a milky white stromal infiltrate. The surrounding cornea is hazy (edematous). (*From* Baum J, Barza M: Infections of the eye and adjacent sinuses. *In* Gorbach S, Bartlett J, Blacklow NR (eds.): *Infectious Diseases*. Philadelphia: W.B. Saunders; 1992:1140; with permission.)

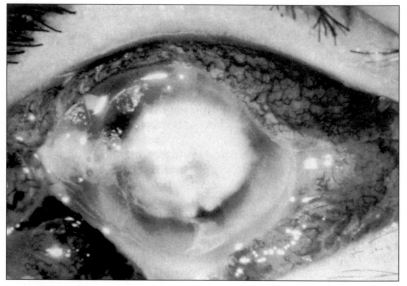

FIGURE 1-36 Fungal keratitis. It may be clinically impossible to distinguish fungal keratitis from bacterial keratitis. Fungal infection presents as a corneal fungal infiltrate that typically enlarges over a few weeks and has characteristic fine feathery margins, heaped-up edges, and adjacent satellite lesions. (*From* Baum J, Barza M: Infections of the eye and adjacent sinuses. *In* Gorbach S, Bartlett J, Blacklow NR (eds.): *Infectious Diseases*. Philadelphia: W.B. Saunders; 1992:1140; with permission.)

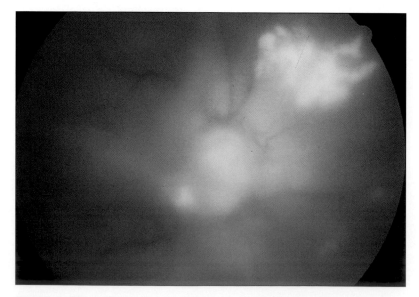

FIGURE 1-37 Endogenous (candida) endophthalmitis. Endophthalmitis may be endogenous or exogenous. Endogenous endophthalmitis

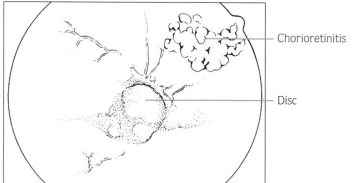

is a complication of blood-borne infection, either bacterial or fungal, that seeds the globe. Usually, a site of infection exists elsewhere that is either the source or a consequence of the blood-borne infection. This case is an example of endophthalmitis caused by *Candida albicans*. Vitritis has made the vitreous hazy; accordingly, the view of the optic disc and retinal vasculature is not clear. An area of chorioretinitis and exudate is seen to the right and superior to the optic disc. (*Courtesy of* R. Olsen, MD.)

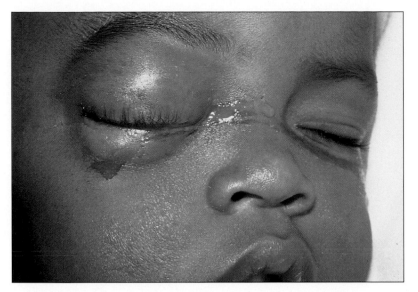

FIGURE 1-38 Exogenous endophthalmitis. Exogenous endoph-thalmitis is most often a postsurgical complication. It can also result from foreign-body penetration. *Staphylococcus epidermidis* and *Bacillus cereus* are the most common bacterial agents involved. This child presented with a high fever and eye swelling, which was initially treated as conjunctivitis. When his eyelids were everted, the right globe was proptotic and the cornea was a cloudy white. An ophthalmologist diagnosed this as a panoph-thalmitis; enucleation was necessary.

Microbiology of endophthalmitis

Organism	Postoperative infections	Traumatic infections
Staphylococcus epidermidis	38%	20%
Staphylococcus aureus	21%	0%
Streptococcus spp.	11%	13%
Bacillus spp.	0%	27%
Haemophilus influenzae	3%	0%
Other gram-negative species	13%	20%
Fungi	8%	17%
Other	6%	3%
Mixed flora	2%	11%

FIGURE 1-39 Microbiology of endophthalmitis. (Forster RK: Endophthalmitis. *In* Duane TD, Jaeger AE (eds.): *Clinical Ophthalmology*, vol. 4. Philadelphia: J.B. Lippincott; 1988.)

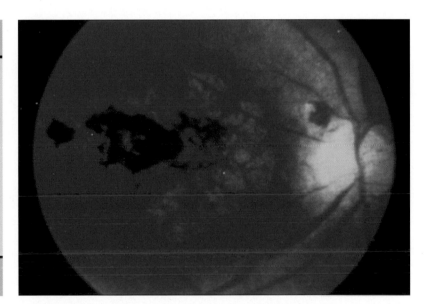

FIGURE 1-40 Chorioretinitis. Chorioretinitis may be seen in cases of congenital toxoplasmosis, cytomegalovirus infection, or acquired histoplasmosis; the lesions caused by these various agents are indistinguishable from one another. The black areas represent scarring.

SELECTED BIBLIOGRAPHY

Lusk RP, Tychsen L, Park TS: Complications of sinusitis. *In* Lusk RP (ed.): *Pediatric Sinusitis*. New York: Raven Press; 1992.

Van Dyke RB, Desky AB, Daum RS: Infections of the eye and periorbital structures. *Adv Pediatr Infect* 1988, 3:125–180.

Weiss A, Brinser JH, Nazar-Stewart V: Acute conjunctivitis in childhood. *J Pediatr* 1993, 122:10–14.

CHAPTER 2

Otitis Media and Infections of the Inner Ear

Ayal Willner
Kenneth M. Grundfast
Rande H. Lazar

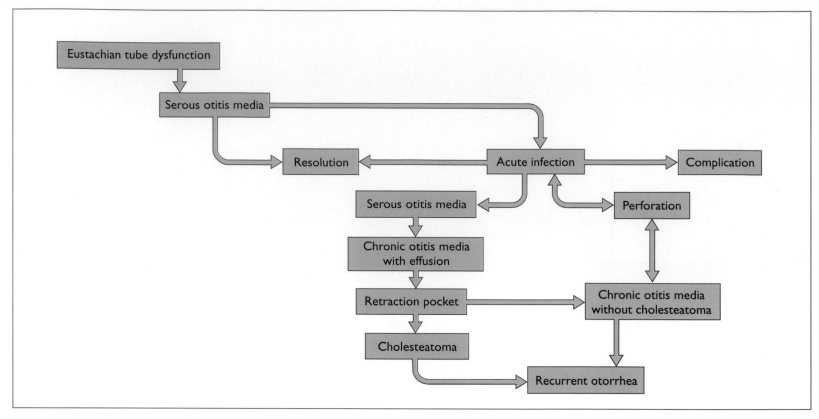

FIGURE 2-1   Natural history of otitis media. Otitis media develops after a disturbance of eustachian tube function. Acute otitis media occurs when fluid, which is initially serous, accumulates behind the tympanic membrane and may become infected. With treatment, and sometimes without, the acutely infected ear usually returns to the serous state. With return of eustachian tube function, the fluid drains. In some cases, the acute infection can lead to a perforation of the drum or a complication. If eustachian tube function does not return, persistent otitis media with effusion may result, as may chronic changes in the tympanic membrane. Over time, recurrent infection and persistent effusion may result in chronic inflammation and may lead to mastoiditis, with or without cholesteatoma, chronic otorrhea, and late complications.

NORMAL ANATOMY

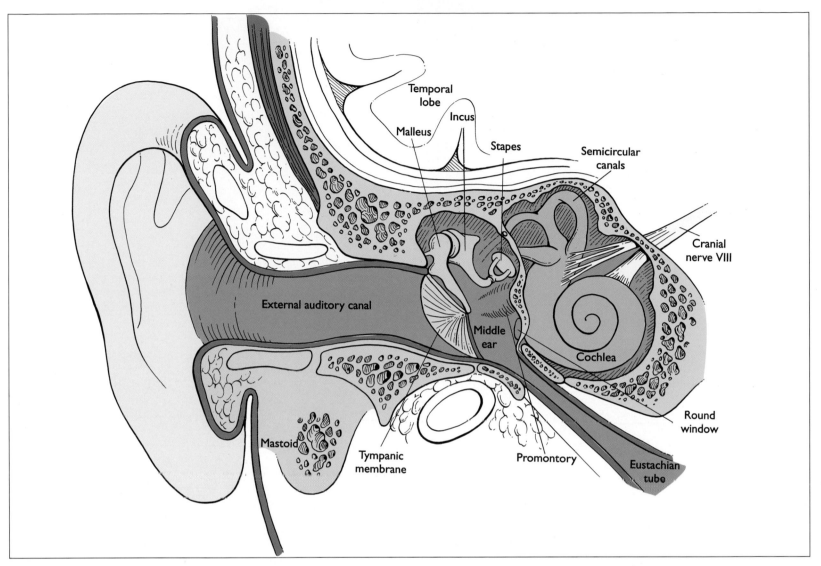

FIGURE 2-2 Normal cross-sectional anatomy of the ear. The external, middle, and inner ear comprise a compact group of components situated in the temporal bone. Sound is funneled by the pinna into the external auditory canal, where it causes vibration of the tympanic membrane. Attached to the tympanic membrane is the malleus, which, with the incus, increases sound pressure by 30%. The stapes articulates with the long process of the incus, and the stapes footplate acts as a piston to transfer the sound vibrations to the cochlea, where the vibratory stimuli are transformed to nerve impulses. The inner ear also houses the semicircular canals, which, via a portion of the eighth cranial nerve, give dynamic and static information on the motion and position of the head.

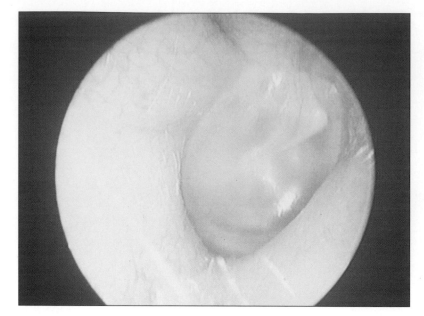

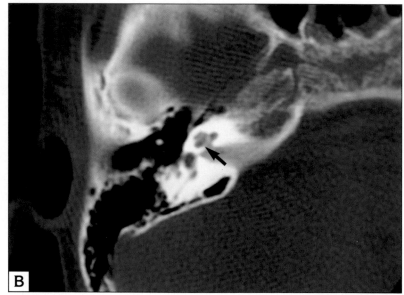

Pars flaccida
Incus long process
Lateral process
Stapedial tendon
Manubrium
Umbo
Pars tensa
Promontory
Round window niche

FIGURE 2-3 Normal eardrum (tympanic membrane). The normal eardrum, as viewed with an otoscope, is a translucent gray structure. During physical examination, two parts of the drum normally can be seen: the pars tensa, which encompasses the area of the drum inferior to the lateral process, and the pars flaccida, above the level of the lateral process. Several bony landmarks can be identified: the lateral process, manubrium of the malleus, umbo, incus, stapedial tendon, promontory, and round window niche.

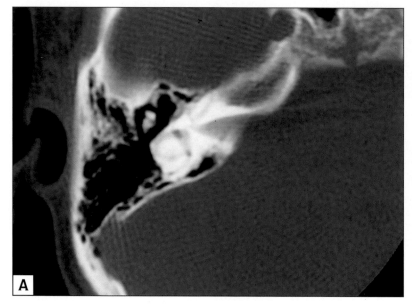

A

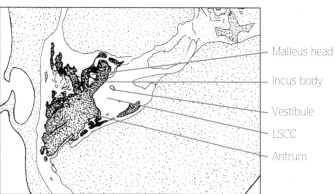

Malleus head
Incus body
Vestibule
LSCC
Antrum

B

FIGURE 2-4 Axial computed tomographic (CT) scan of the normal ear. In an axial CT scan, several anatomic landmarks can be identified. These structures are important because their obliteration or alteration provides important clues in the diagnosis of otitic infections. **A,** A superior CT section shows the head of the malleus and body of the incus, as well as the lateral semicircular canal (LSCC) and vestibule. The mastoid air cell system is well developed, with abundant pneumatization that emanates from the antrum. **B,** A CT section taken from a slightly more inferior position shows the turns of the cochlea (*arrow*). Acute infection of the inner ear structures can lead to permanent loss of vestibular function and profound deafness in the affected ear. Acute otitis media does not usually cause ossicular destruction. However, acute necrotizing otitis media, caused by β-hemolytic streptococci, can lead to destruction of the blood supply to the ossicles and subsequent bony loss.

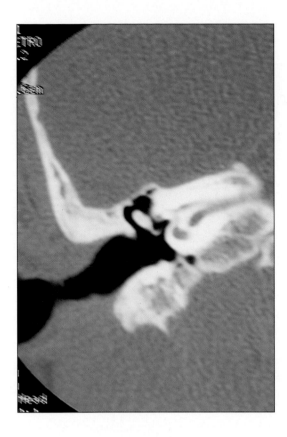

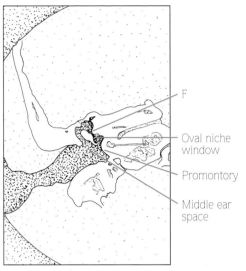

FIGURE 2-5 Coronal CT scan of the normal ear canal. A coronal CT scan shows the pathway into the inner ear. The middle ear space is well aerated. The long process of the incus articulates with the stapes. The stapes footplate and oval window are seen as an area of very thin bone above the promontory. The superior margin of the oval window niche is formed by the tympanic segment and second genu of the seventh cranial nerve (*F*). Acute or chronic infection can lead to suppurative labyrinthitis or facial nerve dysfunction.

F
Oval niche window
Promontory
Middle ear space

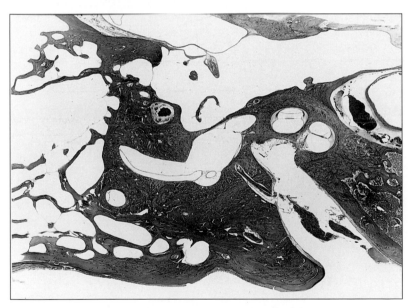

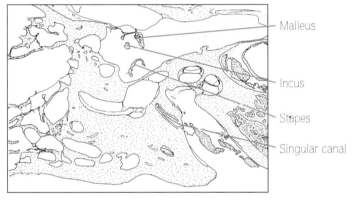

Malleus
Incus
Stapes
Singular canal

FIGURE 2-6 Histologic section of normal tympanic membrane and inner ear. The tympanic membrane is normally thin and firmly bound to the malleus. Behind the manubrium of the malleus is the long process of the incus, which turns medially to articulate with the stapes. A turn of the cochlea is seen, as is the vestibule and a portion of the lateral semicircular canal. (Periodic acid–Schiff stain.) (*From* Paparella MM, Shumrick DA, Gluckman JL, Meyerhoff WL (eds.): *Otolaryngology*, vol. I, 3rd ed. Philadelphia: W.B. Saunders; 1991:429; with permission.)

ACUTE OTITIS MEDIA

Epidemiology and Pathophysiology

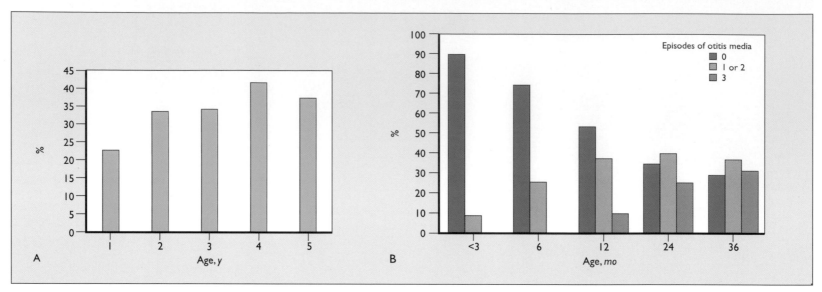

FIGURE 2-7 Epidemiology of otitis media. Otitis media is a common health problem. In 1986, there were 31 million visits to physicians for otitis media, and the direct and indirect cost has been estimated at $3.5 billion annually. **A,** Proportion of office visits for otitis media. Otitis media is one of the complaints most frequently addressed by pediatricians. In children under 5 years of age, otitis media makes up 22% to 42% of office visits. **B,** Incidence of otitis media by age. By 36 months of age, less than 30% of children will *not* have had at least one episode of otitis media, whereas more than 30% will have had three episodes. Numerous studies have shown that, in general, the incidence and prevalence of otitis media peak in children in the preschool years and decrease as age increases.

Possible factors predisposing to otitis media	
Male sex	Winter season
American Indian or Alaskan Eskimo ethnic group	Altered host defenses (acquired and/or congenital)
Poor social conditions	Genetic predisposition
Daycare attendance	

FIGURE 2-8 Predisposing factors to otitis media. Studies examining the effects of various factors that may predispose children to otitis media have identified several to be associated with an increased incidence of otitis media. Some other factors, such as breast-feeding, may have a protective effect, but this association has not been shown conclusively.

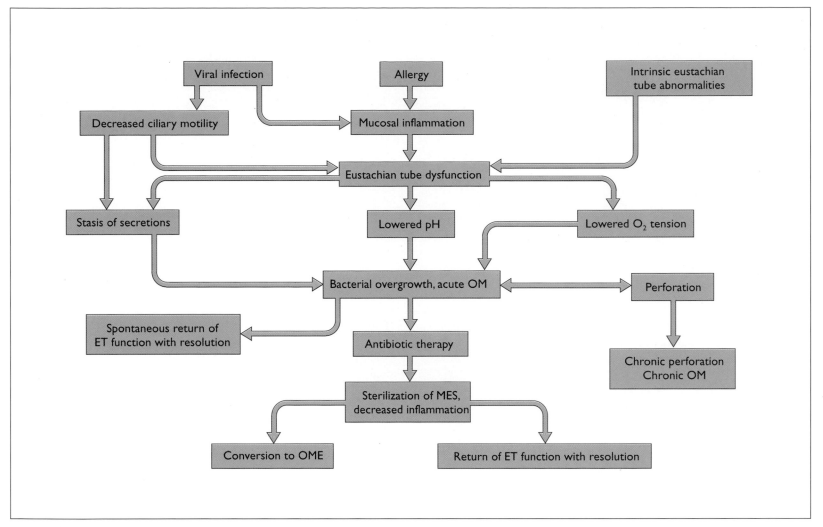

FIGURE 2-9 Pathophysiology of otitis media (OM). Otitis media occurs after interaction of a multitude of genetic and environmental factors. The cornerstone is disruption of eustachian tube (ET) function by either viral, bacterial, or, possibly, allergic causes. The closure of the ET may be due to direct mucosal swelling within the lumen of the tube or due to blockage by obstructive adenoids. In addition, structural factors specific to the individual patient (*ie*, strength, angle, and length of ET) effect the likelihood of ET dysfunction. With ET dysfunction, and worsened by mucosal swelling and decreased ciliary motility, comes stasis of secretions, lowered oxygen tension, and lowered pH. These changes in the microenvironment may lead to bacterial overgrowth and acute otitis media. Resolution occurs by spontaneous return of ET function, by creation of an alternate drainage and aeration pathway by rupture of the tympanic membrane, or by antimicrobial treatment that sterilizes the effusion. With resolution of swelling and return of ET function, the effusion should drain. If the fluid does not drain, persistent serous otitis media results. (MES—middle ear space.)

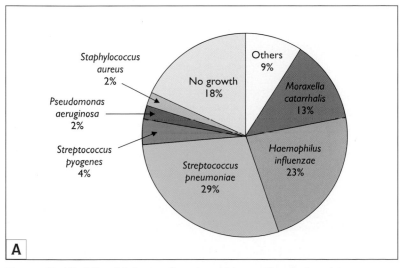

A

FIGURE 2-10 Microbiology of acute otitis media. **A**, Aerobic organisms causing acute otitis media. Sixty-five percent of cases of acute otitis media are caused by *Streptococcus pneumoniae*, *Haemophilus influenzae*, and *Moraxella catarrhalis*. Significantly, 20% of effusions in acute otitis media fail to grow an organism in culture.

B. Predominant organisms isolated in acute otitis media	
Aerobic bacteria	**Anaerobic bacteria**
Haemophilus influenzae	*Peptostreptococcus* spp.
Streptococcus pneumoniae	*Peptococcus* spp.
Moraxella catarrhalis	

Anaerobic organisms increasingly are being cultured in cases of acute otitis media. This increase probably reflects improvements in the ability to culture these organisms rather than an actual increase in anaerobes as pathogens. Also, viruses have been cultured from approximately 15% of patients with otitis media. Viruses may play a synergistic role by causing swelling or decreasing ciliary motility. **B**, Predominant organisms causing acute otitis media. (Panel 10A *adapted from* Bluestone CD: The ear and mastoid infections. *In* Gorbach S, *et al.* (eds.): *Textbook of Infectious Diseases*. Philadelphia: W.B. Saunders; 1992:442; with permission.)

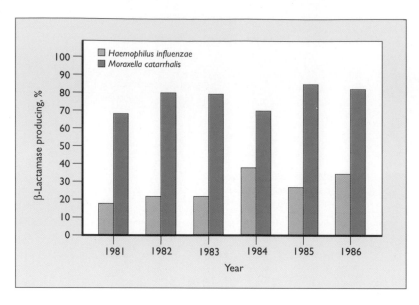

FIGURE 2-11 Antibiotic resistance in acute otitis media. An increasing rate of β-lactamase production is being seen in *Haemophilus influenzae* and *Moraxella catarrhalis*, approaching 50% and 90%, respectively. (*Adapted from* Bluestone CD: The ear and mastoid infections. *In* Gorbach S, *et al.* (eds.): *Textbook of Infectious Diseases*. Philadelphia: W.B. Saunders; 1992:443; with permission.)

Diagnosis and Treatment

Signs and symptoms of acute otitis media	
Fever	Lethargy
Otalgia	Headache
Hearing loss	Anorexia
Otorrhea	Vomiting
Vertigo/unsteadiness	Diarrhea
Irritability	

FIGURE 2-12 Signs and symptoms of acute otitis media. Young patients with otitis media often exhibit few localized symptoms. With older patients, otalgia, complaints of hearing loss, and headache are more commonly seen.

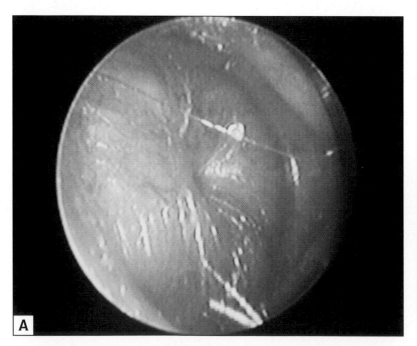

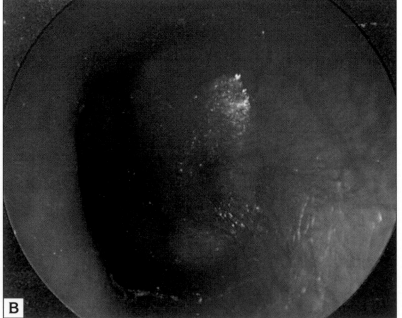

FIGURE 2-13 Acute otitis media with bulging drum. **A**, An operative photograph of acute otitis media shows the drum to be inflamed with thickening and erythema, and the landmarks have been obliterated by the bulging drum. This acute process usually, though not invariably, is accompanied by fever and otalgia. Of note, bulging of the tympanic membrane may be seen in any acute inflammatory process of the ear, including acute mastoiditis, coalescent mastoiditis, and complicated mastoiditis. **B**, Acute otitis media with bulging and hyperemia of the posterosuperior quadrant of the tympanic membrane. (*From* Bull TR: *A Color Atlas of E.N.T. Diagnosis*, 2nd ed. London: Wolfe Medical Publications; 1987:96; with permission.)

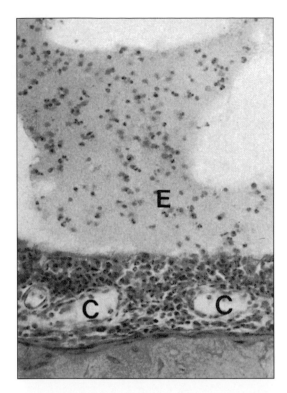

FIGURE 2-14 Histologic section of middle ear in acute otitis media. In this specimen from a feline middle ear that has had the eustachian tube blocked, the effusion (E) of the resultant acute otitis media is markedly purulent. Also, there is cellular infiltration and capillary dilatation (C) in the subepithelial space. (*From* Paparella MM, Shumrick DA, Gluckman JL, Meyerhoff WL (eds.): *Otolaryngology*, 3rd ed. Philadelphia: W.B. Saunders; 1991:1522; with permission.)

A. Oral antibiotic therapy for acute otitis media

Initial infection	Recurrent infection or failed initial therapy
Amoxicillin	Amoxicillin-clavulanate
Trimethoprim-sulfamethoxazole (penicillin allergic)	Cefaclor
	Cefuroxime-axetil
	Cefixime
Erythromycin-sulfisoxazole (penicillin allergic)	Cefprozil
	Cefpodoxime proxetil
	Loracarbef
	Trimethoprim-sulfamethoxazole
	Erythromycin-sulfisoxazole

FIGURE 2-15 Antibiotic therapy for acute otitis media. The management of acute otitis media is with antimicrobial agents for 10 to 14 days. Usually, an antibiotic such as amoxicillin is sufficient and cost-effective initial therapy. If the initial course of therapy is unsuccessful in relieving the symptoms and converting acute otitis media to serous otitis media, treatment with a different antibiotic that has β-lactamase resistance is indicated. **A,** Oral antibiotic therapy for acute otitis media. **B,** Efficacy of antimicrobial agents against common pathogens in acute otitis media. (Panel 15B *from* Bluestone CD: The ear and mastoid infections. *In* Gorbach S, *et al.* (eds.): *Textbook of Infectious Diseases*. Philadelphia: W.B. Saunders; 1992:443; with permission.)

B. Efficacy of antimicrobial agents against common pathogens in acute otitis media

Antimicrobial agent	*Streptococcus pneumoniae* (30%)*	*Haemophilus influenzae* (20%)	*Moraxella catarrhalis* (< 20%)	*Streptococcus pyogenes* (< 10%)	*Staphylococcus aureus* (< 5%)
Ampicillin or amoxicillin	+	±	±	+	±
Amoxicillin-clavulanate	+	+	+	+	+
Penicillin	+	-	±	+	±
Clindamycin	+	-	±	+	+
Erythromycin	+	-	±	+	+
Sulfonamides	-	+	+	-	-
Erythromycin-sulfisoxazole	+	+	+	+	±
Trimethoprim-sulfamethoxazole	±	+	+	-	+
Cefaclor	+	±	±	+	+
Cefuroxime axetil	+	+	+	+	+
Cefixime	±	+	+	±	-

*Numbers in parentheses denote approximate percentages of the cases of acute otitis media caused by each pathogen.
+—effective; ±—effective for strains not producing β-lactamase; -—not effective.

<table>
<tr><td>

Indications for myringotomy or tympanocentesis

Patients who are seriously ill, have severe otalgia, or appear toxic
Unsatisfactory response to antimicrobial therapy
Onset in a child on appropriate and adequate antimicrobial
  therapy
Confirmed or suspected suppurative complication
Otitis media in a newborn, immunocompromised patient, or
  patient in whom an unusual organism is suspected

</td></tr>
</table>

FIGURE 2-16 Indications for myringotomy or tympanocentesis. Myringotomy or tympanocentesis is reserved for those patients who meet the criteria.

Uncommon Pathogenic Organisms

<table>
<tr><td>

Uncommon organisms in acute otitis media

Corynebacterium diphtheriae
Mycobacterium tuberculosis
Clostridium tetani
Ascaris lumbricoides
Pneumocystis carinii

</td></tr>
</table>

FIGURE 2-17 Uncommon pathogenic organisms in acute otitis media. Occasionally, acute otitis media can be caused by unusual pathogens. These cases often do not present with the typical bulging drum but instead may present with a polyp in the external auditory canal.

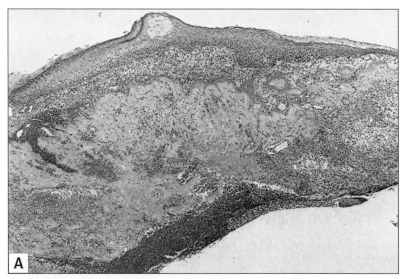

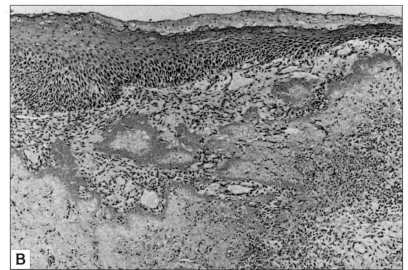

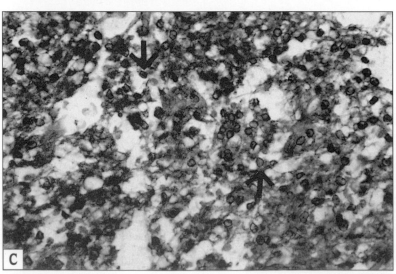

FIGURE 2-18 *Pneumocystis carinii* otitis media. In recent years, the incidence of otitis media caused by *P. carinii* has increased along with the increasing numbers of patients with AIDS. Otitis media due to *P. carinii* infection often presents with a fleshy friable mass with small areas of ulceration. Purulent discharge may drain through an accompanying perforation. **A,** Histologic examination of a specimen reveals an irregularly shaped, nodular mass lined with squamous epithelium. **B,** On medium-power examination, lymphocytes and neutrophils are prominent, and lakes of foamy eosinophilic material are noted in the upper dermis. **C,** On high-power view, Grocott-Gomori methenamine-silver nitrate stain reveals spherical organisms characteristic of *P. carinii* cysts (*arrows*) in the foamy areas. Treatment includes local debridement of the infected tissue and treatment with antibiotics. (*From* Sandler ED, Sandler JM, LeBoit PE, *et al.*: *Pneumocystis carinii* otitis media in AIDS: A case report and review of the literature regarding extrapulmonary pneumocystosis. *Otolaryngol Head Neck Surg* 1990, 103:817–821; with permission.)

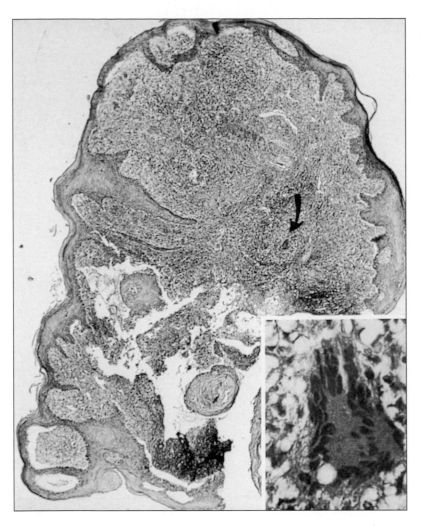

FIGURE 2-19 Tuberculous otitis media. An inflammatory aural polyp was removed from a patient with tuberculous otitis media. The inset shows the typical granulomatous inflammatory reaction with giant cell formation (*arrow*). (Hematoxylin-eosin stain; × 650.) (*From* Paparella MM, Shumrick DA, Gluckman JL, Meyerhoff WL (eds.): *Otolaryngology*, 3rd ed. Philadelphia: W.B. Saunders; 1991:1533; with permission.)

Acute Mastoiditis

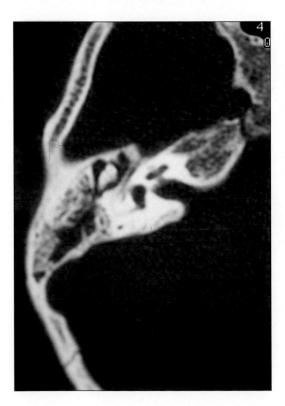

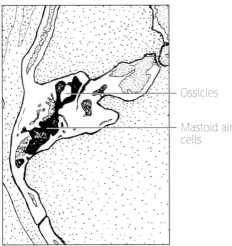

Ossicles

Mastoid air cells

FIGURE 2-20 Axial CT scan showing acute mastoiditis. Acute mastoiditis accompanies almost any acute middle ear inflammation. The middle ear and mastoid air cell system are opacified, but there is no destruction of bony septa. It is likely that the soft tissue density seen is both fluid and thickened mucosal surfaces throughout the mastoid air cell system and middle ear space. This process is an entirely reversible one, and with antibiotic therapy and resolution of the inflammatory process, the findings on CT scan will revert to normal.

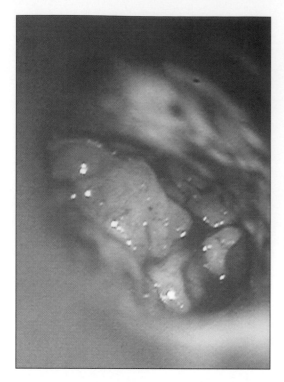

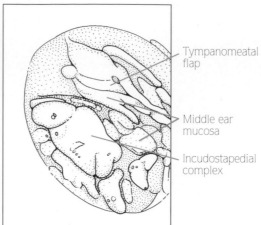

FIGURE 2-21 Operative photograph of acute mastoiditis showing granulations in the middle ear. In general, management of acute mastoiditis is with antibiotics alone. In cases of complication, however, this approach may be insufficient, and mastoidectomy is required to remove the infected tissue or drain the abscess that has led to the complication. In this photograph, the tympanic membrane has been lifted to expose the middle ear space. The incus and incudostapedial joint are encased in glistening edematous mucosa that must be removed to open the passage to the antrum. The mucosa of the middle ear space also is inflamed.

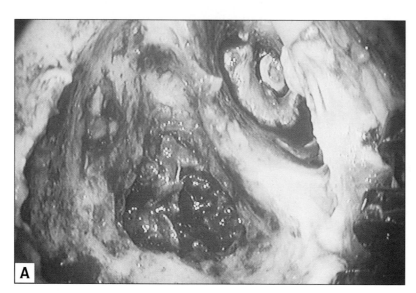

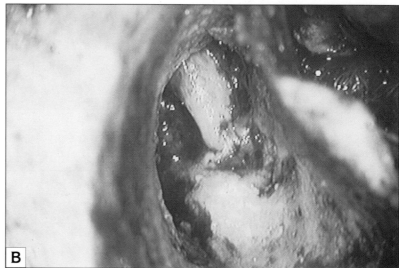

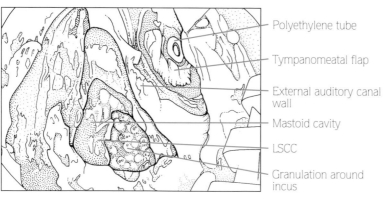

FIGURE 2-22 Operative photograph of acute mastoiditis with granulations covering the incus. **A,** In this photograph, the mastoid air cells and mastoid cortex have been drilled away to form a common mastoid cavity. The incudal fossa, which houses the body of the incus, is filled with granulation tissue, and the incus cannot be seen. When enveloped in this tissue, the ossicles block adequate drainage of the mastoid air cell system. (LSCC—lateral semicircular canal.) **B,** The incus has been denuded of the surrounding granulation tissue. By thorough removal of this edematous mucosa from the superior and lateral surfaces of the incus, aeration of the mastoid via the middle ear can be reestablished.

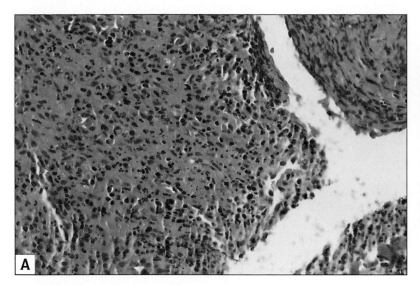

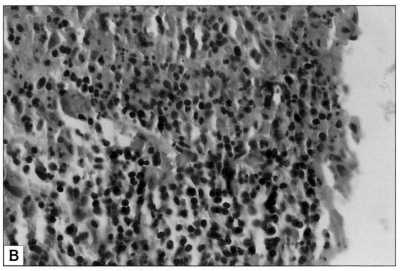

FIGURE 2-23 Histologic section of granulation tissue in acute mastoiditis. **A**, Low-power view of granulation tissue removed during mastoidectomy. This sample is representative of the entire mastoid contents, which was extremely inflamed, and shows a highly cellular infiltrate. **B**, High-power magnification shows abundant lymphocytes and many polymorphonuclear cells. Although the amount of tissue injury is substantial, this area is supplied by a rich vascular network, and prompt institution of antibiotic therapy will usually resolve the infection. (Hematoxylin-eosin stain. Magnification: panel 23A, × 22.5; panel 23B, × 300.)

OTITIS MEDIA WITH EFFUSION

Etiology and Pathogenesis

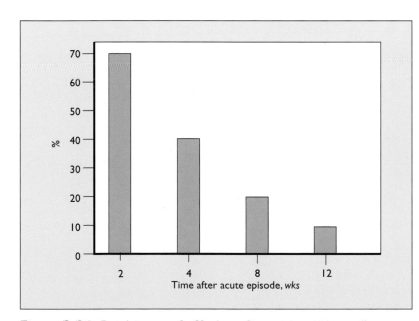

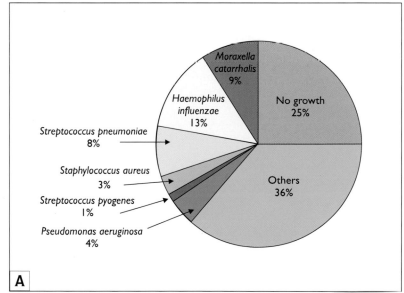

FIGURE 2-24 Persistence of effusion after acute otitis media. Otitis media with effusion results from eustachian tube dysfunction. The effusion may occur on its own, as a prelude to acute otitis media, or during the resolution of acute otitis media. In approximately 90% of cases of acute otitis media, the effusion will resolve by 12 weeks.

FIGURE 2-25 Microbiology of chronic otitis media with effusion. Of the bacteria cultured from cases of chronic otitis media with effusion (lasting > 3 months), *Haemophilus influenzae*, *Streptococcus pneumoniae*, and *Moraxella catarrhalis* are the most frequent isolates. However, anaerobes are also frequently isolated, and in many cases, no organism can be recovered. **A**, Frequency of isolates in chronic otitis media with effusion. (*continued*)

B. Predominant organisms isolated in chronic otitis media with purulent effusion

Aerobic bacteria	Anaerobic bacteria
Staphylococcus aureus	Pigmented *Prevotella* and *Porphyromonas* spp.
Escherichia coli	*Fusobacterium* spp.
Klebsiella pneumoniae	*Peptostreptococcus* spp.
Pseudomonas aeruginosa	

Figure 2-25 (*continued*) **B,** Predominant organisms isolated in chronic otitis media with purulent effusion. (Panel 25A *adapted from* Bluestone CD: The ear and mastoid infections. *In* Gorbach S, *et al.* (eds.): *Textbook of Infectious Diseases.* Philadelphia: W.B. Saunders; 1992:442; with permission.)

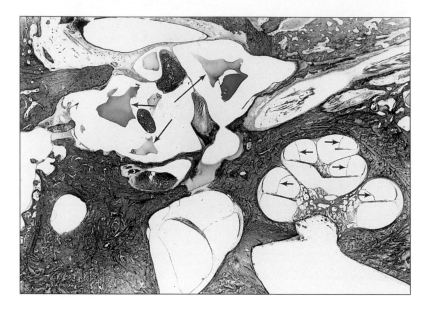

Figure 2-26 Histologic section showing otitis media with effusion. In this axial histologic section, serous fluid (*arrows*) is seen in the middle ear cleft. The tympanic membrane is thickened behind the malleus, but anteriorly it remains thin. In this case, the lining of the mesotympanum is not thickened, but as the otitis becomes chronic, thickening of this lining epithelium and granulation tissue may develop. (Hematoxylin-eosin stain.) (*From* Paparella MM, Shumrick DA, Gluckman JL, Meyerhoff WL (eds.): *Otolaryngology*, 3rd ed. Philadelphia: W.B. Saunders; 1991:431; with permission.)

Signs and symptoms of otitis media with effusion

No symptoms	Imbalance
Decreased hearing	Irritability
Pulling at ear	Lethargy
Head banging	Anorexia

Figure 2-27 Symptoms and signs of otitis media with effusion. In many cases, there are no early symptoms of otitis media effusion. In addition, the symptoms that do exist may be nonlocalizing or difficult to interpret. Unfortunately, although otitis media effusion may be symptomatically silent, deleterious changes in the structure and function of the tympanic membrane may occur over time.

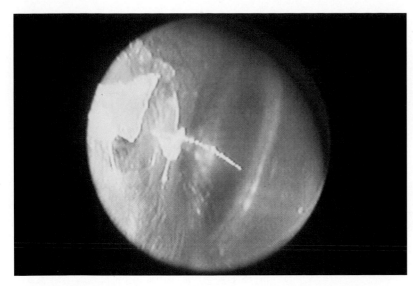

FIGURE 2-28 Otoscopic view of otitis media with effusion, showing retracted drum and serous fluid. When otitis media effusion occurs without an antecedent acute otitis media, air trapped within the middle ear space is absorbed, resulting in negative pressure and retraction of the tympanic membrane.

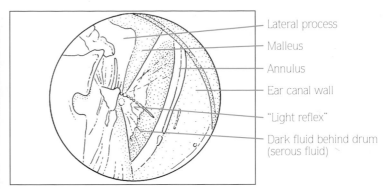

In addition, the negative pressure leads to transudation of fluid into the mesotympanum. As the photograph illustrates, the tympanic membrane is retracted, leading to a relative prominence of the lateral process. The drum is still thin and translucent. Serous fluid can be seen as a dullness of the anterior inferior drum below the umbo. Retraction is an early tympanic membrane change but can lead to further flaccidity and retraction pocket formation. This process is reversible with either return of eustachian tube function, myringotomy and evacuation of the fluid, or evacuation of the fluid and placement of pressure-equalizing tubes.

FIGURE 2-29 Otoscopic view of otitis media with effusion showing trapped air. Another common otoscopic finding in a patient with otitis media effusion is a dark immobile drum with air bubbles and an air-fluid level behind it. Trapped air provides an obvious diagnosis of otitis media effusion. (*From* Bull TR: *A Color Atlas of E.N.T. Diagnosis*, 2nd ed. London: Wolfe Medical Publications; 1987:89; with permission.)

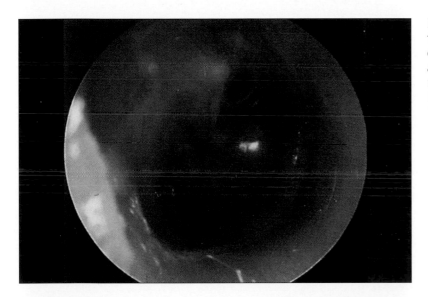

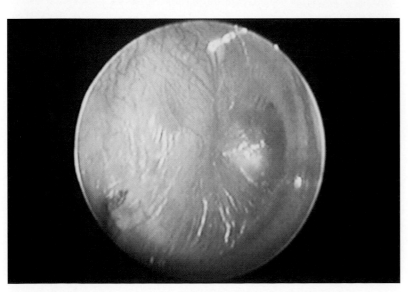

FIGURE 2-30 Otoscopic view of otitis media with effusion, showing bulging drum. As early inflammation progresses, there is an increase in the amount of fluid produced by the cells lining the

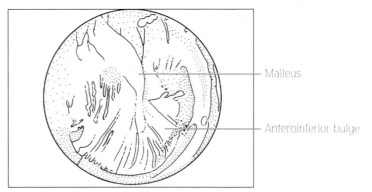

middle ear cleft and mastoid air cell system. In such cases, the drum may be seen to bulge. Generally, otitis media effusion is painless. However, as the amount of fluid increases and the drum bulges, pain may develop. In this photograph, the bulging of the drum is most prominent at the anteroinferior quadrant. This area may have been the site of a previous perforation or ventilation tube. The fluid seen at this stage of otitis media with effusion is usually clear or may give a bluish hue to the drum, because purulent material has not yet developed.

Pneumatic otoscopy						Middle ear	
		Eardrum movement					
		Positive pressure		Negative pressure			
Eardrum position		Low	High	Low	High	Contents	Pressure
Neutral	External canal / Middle ear	1+	2+	1+	2+	Air	Ambient
Neutral		2+	3+	2+	3+	Air	Ambient
Neutral		0	1+	0	1+	Air or air and effusion	Ambient
Retracted		0	0	1+	2+	Air or air and effusion	Low negative
Retracted		0	0	0	1+	Air or air and effusion	High negative
Retracted		0	0	0	0	Air or effusion or both	Very high negative or intermediate
Full		0	1+	0	0	Air and effusion	Positive or indeterminate
Bulging		0	0	0	0	Effusion	Positive or indeterminate

FIGURE 2-31 Pneumatic otoscopy. Movement of the drum on pneumatic otoscopy can be used to determine the pressure difference between the middle ear space and the external auditory canal and to detect fluid within the middle ear space. On the illustration, the position of the eardrum is shown at rest (*solid line*), with positive pressure applied (bulb compressed; *dashed line*), and with negative pressure applied (bulb released; *dotted lines*). The degree of tympanic membrane movement as visualized through the otoscope is noted as none (0), slight (1+), moderate (2+), or excessive (3+). (*Adapted from* Bluestone CD, Klein JO: *Otitis Media in Infants and Children*, 2nd ed. Philadelphia: W.B. Saunders; 1995:76; with permission.)

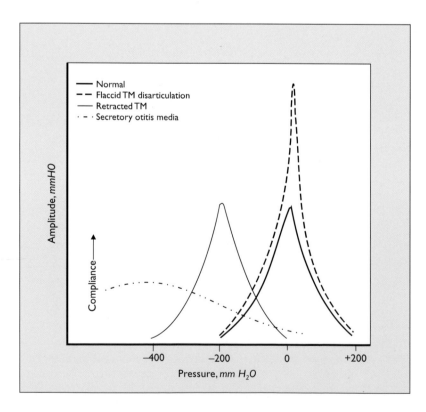

Legend:
— Normal
-- Flaccid TM disarticulation
— Retracted TM
· - · Secretory otitis media

Amplitude, *mmHO*
Compliance →
Pressure, mm H₂O
−400   −200   0   +200

FIGURE 2-32 Tympanometry. The tympanogram measures the amount of sound that is reflected off the drum from a source in the external auditory canal. By varying the pressure within the external auditory canal, the tympanic membrane (TM) can be brought to the position that will transmit rather than reflect the sound. (*From* Feigin RD, Kline MW, Hyatt SR, Ford KL III: Otitis media. *In* Feigin RD, Cherry JD (eds.): *Textbook of Pediatric Infectious Diseases*, 3rd ed. Philadelphia: W.B. Saunders: 1992:178; with permission.)

Treatment

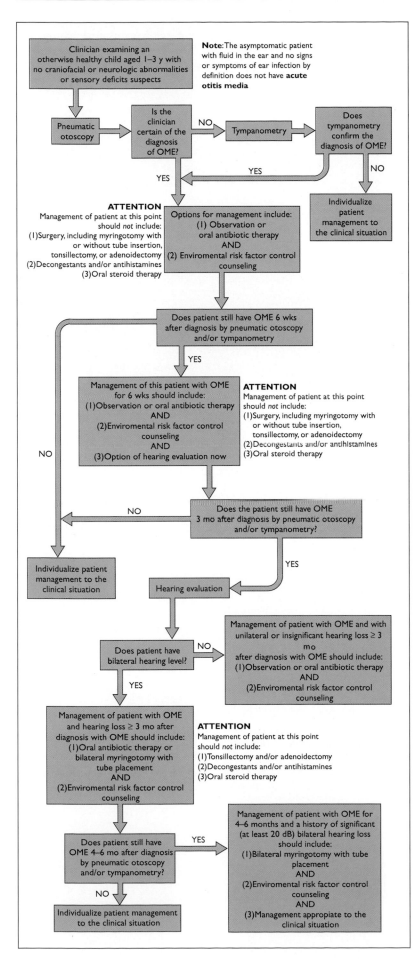

FIGURE 2-33 Management of chronic otitis media with effusion. In an otherwise healthy child aged 1 to 3 years, the treatment of chronic otitis media with effusion (OME) combines initial antibiotic therapy with reassessment by physical examination pneumatic otoscopy, and tympanometry. Patients in whom the effusion does not resolve within 3 months require hearing evaluation. Patients who show a significant hearing loss should undergo myringotomy and tube placement, whereas those who have normal hearing may be either reassessed after another 3 months or undergo surgery. No beneficial role of steroids or decongestants has been shown. Of importance, this algorithm applies only to patients aged 1 to 3 years with chronic otitis media effusion. (*Adapted from* Agency for Health Care Policy and Research: *Otitis Media With Effusion in Young Children* [*Clinical Practice Guideline No. 12*]. Rockville, MD: U.S. Department of Health and Human Services; 1994. AHCPR publ. no. 94-0622; with permission.)

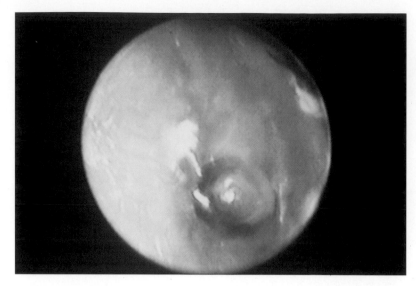

FIGURE 2-34 Evacuation of fluid in otitis media with effusion. For recurrent acute otitis media that has failed to resolve with medical therapy, or for chronic serous otitis media with either hearing loss or changes in the tympanic membrane, treatment is myringotomy and placement of ventilation tubes. In cases of otitis media with complications, including subperiosteal abscess, petrositis, extra- or intracranial abscess, and cranial nerve dysfunction, myringotomy is used in conjunction with external drainage procedures. After incision of the anteroinferior tympanic membrane, a drop of fluid may form, as seen here. In this case, the fluid was viscous and required vigorous suctioning to evacuate it from the mesotympanum. This type of fluid decreases the conductive abilities of the tympanic membrane and ossicular chain, resulting in conductive hearing loss.

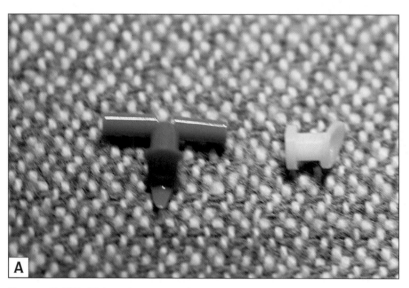

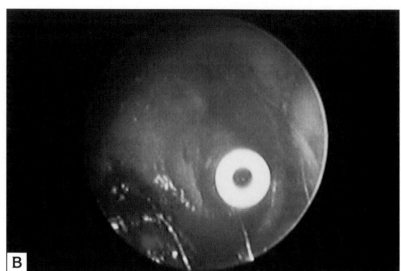

FIGURE 2-35 Tube placement for treatment of otitis media. **A**, In general, tubes can be classified as long- or short-acting. On the right in the illustration is the short-acting (6–18 months)

Armstrong tube. On the left is a long-acting (> 2 years) butterfly tube. **B**, Armstrong tube in place.

COMPLICATIONS OF OTITIS MEDIA

Complications of otitis media	
Intratemporal	**Extratemporal**
Tympanic membrane perforation	Meningitis
Cholesteotoma	Extradural abscess
Adhesive otitis media	Subdural empyema
Ossicular discontinuity	Otitis hydrocephalus
Mastoiditis	Focal otitic encephalitis
Petrositis	Brain abscess
Cholesterol granuloma	Neck abscess
Labyrinthitis	Lateral sinus thrombosis

FIGURE 2-36 Complications of otitis media. The complications of otitis media occur as a result of infection with a particularly virulent organism, repeated infection, or prolonged effusion or eustachian tube dysfunction leading to tympanic membrane changes. The ratio of complicated infections resulting from a fulminant course of an acute infection versus complications that are sequelae of long-standing ear disease is approximately 1:2.

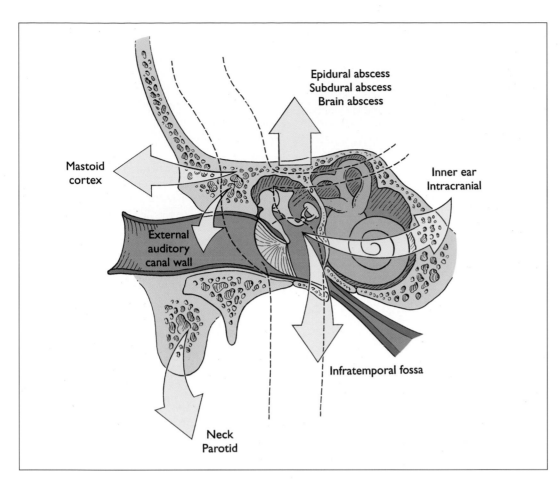

FIGURE 2-37 Directions of spread in complicated otitis media. Complicated otitis media occurs when the infection spreads beyond the confines of the temporal bone. This spread occurs via three mechanisms: 1) direct extension with loss of bone leading to direct inflammation and infection of the surrounding tissues; 2) extension via preformed pathways in which natural dehiscences in the temporal bone allow spread of infectious material; and 3) extension via thrombophlebitic veins that traverse the bone to join the dural sinuses or the internal jugular vein.

Bacteriology of complicated acute otitis media	
Microorganism	**%**
Streptococcus pyogenes	20
Streptococcus pneumoniae	16
Staphylococcus aureus	11
Haemophilus influenzae	4

FIGURE 2-38 Bacteriology of complicated acute otitis media. Among bacterial isolates from the middle ear, subperiosteal abscess, or mastoid, *Streptococcus pneumoniae* and *Haemophilus influenzae* are still commonly isolated organisms in cases of complications. However, *Streptococcus pyogenes* and *Staphylococcus aureus* assume a more important role in these cases.

Extracranial Complications

Coalescent Mastoiditis

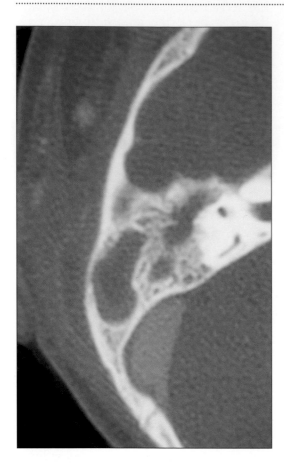

FIGURE 2-39 CT scan showing coalescent mastoiditis. In this axial CT scan, the mastoid cavity is opacified, and there is loss of definition of the bony septa between individual air cells. In coalescent mastoiditis, osteoclastic resorption of the septa results in an abscess cavity. As the abscess enlarges, the center becomes increasingly removed from any blood supply, which decreases the likelihood that conservative management with antibiotics alone will resolve the infection. However, as in other abscesses of the head and neck, intravenous antibiotic therapy may sterilize the abscess, and myringotomy may be the only surgical intervention necessary. In this case, myringotomy serves to provide drainage of the abscess through the middle ear and to obtain material for culture. With resorption of the abscess or drainage through the eustachian tube or ventilation tube, reaeration of the mastoid will proceed.

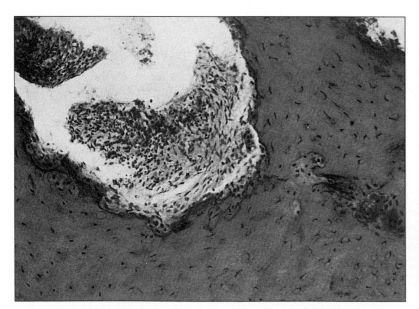

FIGURE 2-40 Histologic examination of coalescent mastoiditis during osteoclastic phase. A histologic section shows a focus of bony erosion. In coalescent mastoiditis, destruction of bony tissue is not through direct infection or dissolution by bacteria or their mediators. Rather, it occurs by an active process of osteoclastic resorption. Multinucleated osteoclasts and the typical scalloped appearance of osteoclastic resorption can be seen. Through this process, the fine septa separating the individual air cells are destroyed, leading to an abscess within the mastoid bone. (*From* Glassock ME III, Shambaugh GE Jr (eds.): *Surgery of the Ear*, 4th ed. Philadelphia: W.B. Saunders; 1990:174; with permission.)

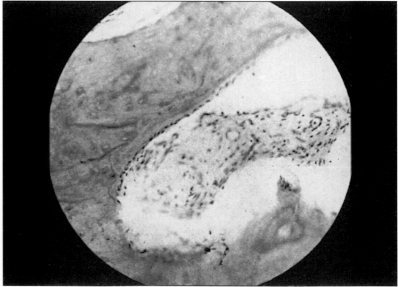

FIGURE 2-41 Histologic examination of coalescent mastoiditis during osteoblastic phase. A photomicrograph of resolving coalescent mastoiditis shows that the multinucleated osteoclasts have been replaced by a single layer of uninuclear osteoblasts. These osteoblasts will deposit bone and return the architecture to normal. The exact bony makeup of the septa of the mastoid air cell system, however, will not be fully reconstituted. (*From* Glassock ME III, Shambaugh GE Jr (eds.): *Surgery of the Ear*, 4th ed. Philadelphia: W.B. Saunders; 1990:175; with permission.)

Subperiosteal Abscess

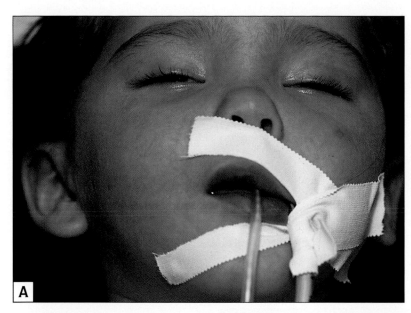

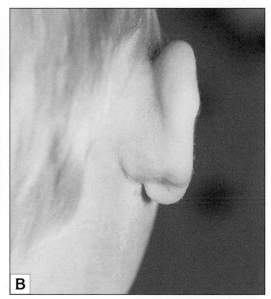

FIGURE 2-42 Lopped ear of subperiosteal abscess. Subperiosteal abscess arises when a focus of infection erodes through the lateral cortex of the mastoid bone or through the posterosuperior wall of the external auditory canal. This is an example of direct extension of infection. **A**, Anterior view. The patient has acute mastoiditis with the formation of a subperiosteal abscess, which has produced the classic "lop ear" on the right. This ear protrudes away from the head when compared with the normal left ear. **B**, Posterior view. Pus has broken through the mastoid cortex to form a pocket on the lateral aspect of the mastoid, causing postauricular swelling and inflammation and pushing the pinna forward. Although a subperiosteal abscess almost always creates this deformity, lopping of the ear may be caused by any postauricular inflammatory process. Interestingly, these patients often do not have a history of recurrent otitis media and may not complain of pain or fever. The postauricular area is, however, almost always tender to touch.

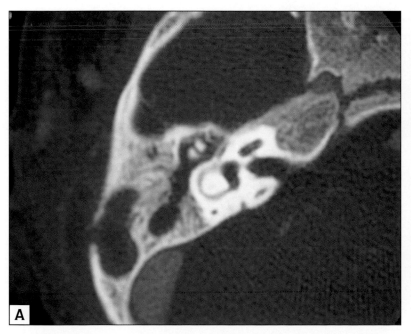

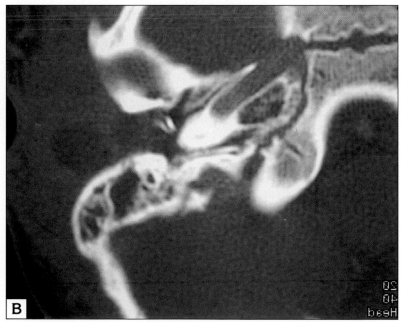

FIGURE 2-43 CT scan of subperiosteal abscess. **A**, An axial CT scan with intravenous contrast enhancement shows the typical radiographic appearance of a subperiosteal abscess. There is a defect in the lateral mastoid cortex and an area of hypodensity just lateral to the bone of the mastoid. Around this is a rim of enhancing tissue, which is the periosteum of the mastoid cortex. **B**, A more inferior CT section in a different patient shows an area of rarefied bone in the posterior wall of the external auditory canal. Around this thinned bone is another hypodense subperiosteal abscess. On physical examination, this abscess may appear as sagging of the posterior canal wall. Of note, a tube is in place in the tympanic membrane, and in fact, pus was draining from the ear. This case illustrates how, even with a ventilation tube in place, acute inflammation may lead to severe swelling of the mucosal lining of the ossicles and blockage of the drainage pathways.

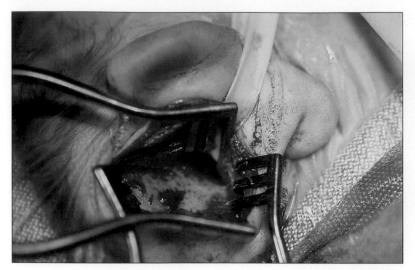

FIGURE 2-44 Operative view of subperiosteal abscess. The ear has been pulled forward with a drain, and the postauricular incision has been made. On dissection of the postauricular wound, pus was encountered. With further exploration, a large defect in the mastoid cortex was uncovered. In most cases in which frank pus is encountered on division of the mastoid periosteum, an area of erosion of the underlying mastoid cortex or eternal auditory canal can be found. There is disagreement as to whether complete removal of the mastoid cortex and air cells is necessary for effective treatment of this complication, or if a limited drainage procedure can be used to allow resolution of the acute problem with later reassessment. With either method, once drainage is established, resolution of the infectious process usually occurs after a few days of intravenous antibiotic therapy.

Neck Abscess

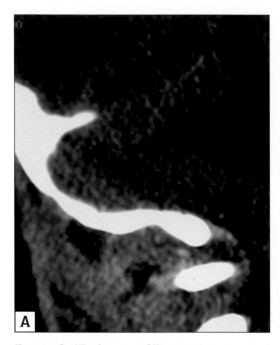

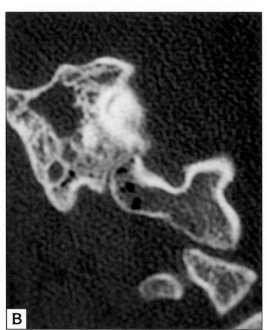

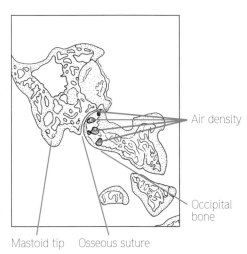

Air density

Occipital bone

Mastoid tip   Osseous suture

FIGURE 2-45 Coronal CT scan showing neck abscess. Neck abscesses can occur through two mechanisms. In the first, direct extension of infection with bony erosion through the mastoid tip may lead to spread into the neck. The second route of spread is through naturally occurring dehiscences in the hypotympanum, which may allow bacteria access to the infratemporal fossae. **A,** In this coronal CT scan using the soft tissue algorithm, a lucent area can be seen abutting the occipital bone, but it does not have the typical lenticular appearance of a subperiosteal abscess. This area represents an abscess cavity related to an episode of acute otitis media, but whether it arose from an infected cervical lymph node, as a direct extension from the overlying occipital bone, or from extension through a preformed pathway is not certain. **B,** A coronal CT scan, taken slightly anterior to the previous scan, uses an algorithm that highlights bony detail. The mastoid is opacified except for the tip, which has a few "bubbles" of gas density. Similarly, there are bubbles of gas density in the occipital bone. In this patient, no direct connection was found between these two areas at operation. As well, it is unlikely that the infection would have traveled via direct extension through the suture line between the temporal and occipital bones. Seeding of the occipital bone with bacteria probably occurred through a thrombophlebitic process.

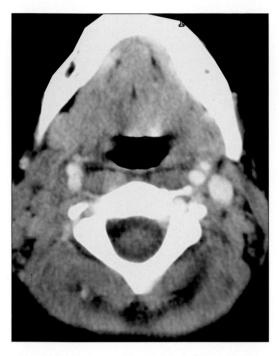

FIGURE 2-46 CT scan showing neck cellulitis. Diffuse swelling of the deep neck structures on the right can be seen on this CT scan, but no ring-enhancing low-density areas indicative of abscess are present. The internal jugular vein cannot be visualized on the right side. The internal jugular vein was thrombosed as a result of a complicated acute otitis media that lead to sigmoid sinus thrombosis and neck cellulitis. The patient presented with a chief complaint of neck pain, swelling, and stiffness. In such cases, the practitioner must also be concerned about a Bezold's abscess, which occurs when coalescent mastoiditis breaks through the mastoid tip and spreads into the neck. Symptoms are indistinguishable from the current presentation, and careful diagnostic imaging must be used to ensure that there is no frank abscess in the neck, and that the bone of the mastoid tip is intact.

Suppurative Labyrinthitis

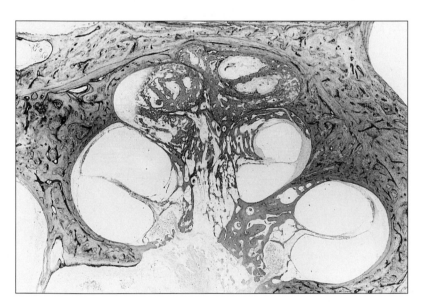

FIGURE 2-47 Suppurative labyrinthitis. Acute otitis media can infrequently enter the inner ear from the mesotympanum. Infection is believed to spread to the inner ear in most cases via the round or, less frequently, the oval window. In suppurative labyrinthitis, destruction of the inner ear structures leads to profound deafness. Histologically, there is an initial influx of young fibroblasts, followed by an ingrowth of capillaries and pathologic bone formation. In this photograph, the bony trabeculae have obliterated the area of the apical turn. (Hematoxylin-eosin stain.) (*From* Paparella MM, Shumrick DA, Gluckman JL, Meyerhoff WL (eds.): *Otolaryngology*, 3rd ed. Philadelphia: W.B. Saunders; 1991: 434; with permission.)

Intracranial Complications

Signs and symptoms of intracranial complications	
Fever	Nausea and vomiting
Headache	Localizing sign
Diminished consciousness	Postauricular swelling
Otalgia	Papilledema

FIGURE 2-48 Signs and symptoms of intracranial complications. The signs and symptoms of an intracranial process secondary to otitis media are not significantly different from those of other etiologies. However, otalgia and postauricular swelling in a patient with otorrhea or a history of acute otitis media can help identify the otitic nature of the complication.

Bacteriology of intracranial complications of otitis media	
Anaerobes	**Aerobes**
Microaerophilic streptococci	Group A streptococcus
Peptostreptococcus spp.	*Staphylococcus* spp.
Fusobacterium spp.	*Haemophilus* spp.
Pigmented *Prevotella* and	*Enterobacteriaceae* spp.
Porphyromonas spp.	*Pseudomonas aeruginosa*

FIGURE 2-49 Bacteriology of intracranial complications of otitis media. In a study of 102 Thai patients with complications from acute and chronic otitis media, organisms were isolated from 13 of 43 intracranial complications. Similar organisms were isolated from ears of these patients. Interestingly, these organisms differ from those isolated in cases of extracranial complication. This difference may relate to the differing pathogenesis of the two types of complications or to differences in the sample populations. (Brook I: Aerobic and anaerobic bacteriology of intracranial abscesses. *Pediatr Neurol* 1992, 8:210–214.)

Venous Sinus Thrombosis

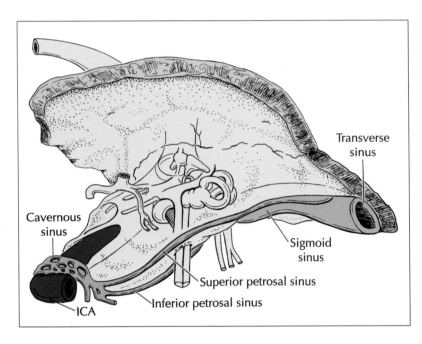

FIGURE 2-50 The dural sinuses. A three-quarter view of the skull base shows the dural sinuses: the transverse sinus, sigmoid sinus, superior petrosal sinus, inferior petrosal sinus, and cavernous sinus. In addition, the internal carotid artery (ICA) is shown. Thrombophlebitis occurs as bacteria spreads from the mastoid through small communicating veins to infect the dural sinuses. Progressive inflammation can lead to thrombosis of the affected sinus. This clot can propagate to neighboring sinuses and eventually may compromise effective venous outflow. (*From* Glassock ME III, Shambaugh GE Jr (eds.): *Surgery of the Ear*, 4th ed. Philadelphia: W.B. Saunders; 1990:48; with permission.)

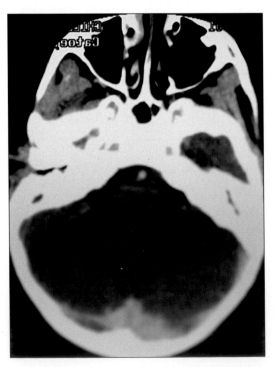

FIGURE 2-51 Axial CT scan showing venous sinus thrombosis. On the patient's left side, contrast is seen passing through the transverse sinus and the superior portion of the sigmoid sinus. On the right, however, only a thin ribbon of contrast is able to pass by the portion of thrombosed transverse and sigmoid sinuses.

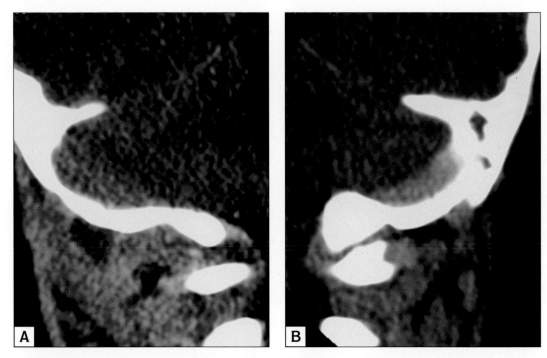

FIGURE 2-52 Coronal CT scan showing venous sinus thrombosis. **A,** On the patient's right side, there is no corresponding blush. This finding is characteristic of sigmoid sinus thrombosis. **B,** On the patient's left side, however, a crescent of contrast flows unimpeded through the left sigmoid sinus.

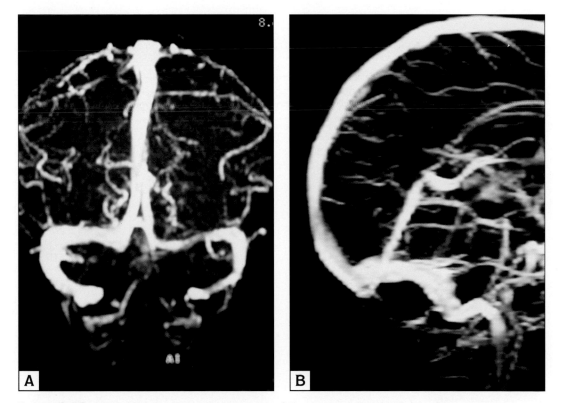

FIGURE 2-53 Magnetic resonance venogram of the normal dural sinuses. The superior sagittal sinus drains into two transverse sinuses. Each transverse sinus, in turn, leads to the sigmoid sinus, which traverses the mastoid, turns up briefly at the jugular bulb, and exits the skull as the internal jugular vein. Thrombosis of a single transverse or sigmoid sinus is usually well tolerated by the patient. However, if propagation of the clot leads to sagittal sinus thrombosis, decreased venous outflow and precipitous elevation of intracranial pressure may develop. In addition, the clot can release septic emboli and lead to infection or thrombosis within the pulmonary vasculature. **A,** Axial view. **B,** Sagittal view.

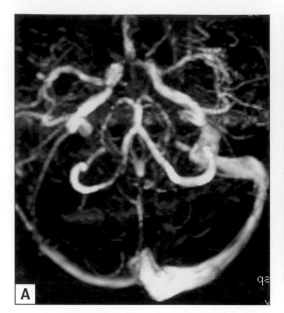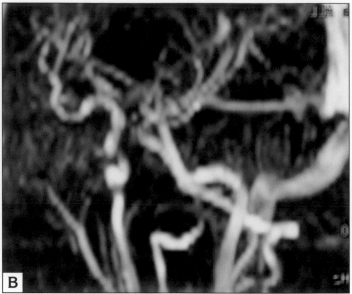

FIGURE 2-54 Magnetic resonance venogram showing venous sinus thrombosis. Magnetic resonance venography can readily demonstrate the venous drainage of the brain. **A**, On the axial projection, the transverse and sigmoid sinuses are easily identified on the left but conspicuously absent on the right. **B**, In the coronal projection, the lack of venous drainage is equally evident. In this case, thrombosis followed thrombophlebitis during an episode of acute otitis media. Treatment with long-term intravenous antibiotic therapy stabilized the clot. The role of anticoagulants in such cases is not yet fully determined. Although they appear to decrease the rate of clot propagation and emboli, concerns exist about the risks of intracranial hemorrhage.

Intracranial Abscess

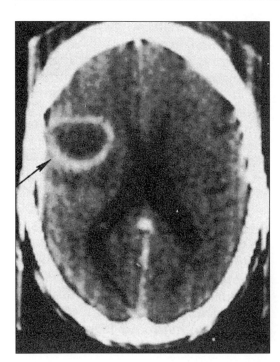

FIGURE 2-55 Intracranial abscess. Via direct extension or as a further complication of sinus thrombosis, an abscess may occur in the epidural space, the subdural space, or within the brain parenchyma. A large right-sided brain abscess, resulting from an episode of otitis media is pictured in this axial CT scan. Such abscesses can result from either an episode of acute otitis media or from chronic otomastoiditis. (*From* Feigin RD, Kline MW, Hyatt SR, Ford KL III: Otitis media. *In* Feigin RD, Cherry JD (eds.): *Textbook of Pediatric Infectious Diseases*, 3rd ed. Philadelphia: W.B. Saunders; 1992:180; with permission.)

CHRONIC OTOMASTOIDITIS

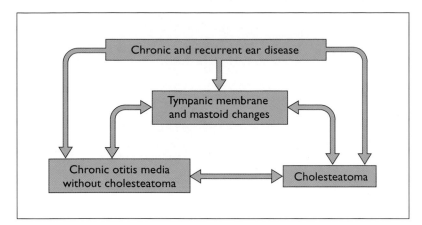

FIGURE 2-56 Chronic ear disease. Recurrent and chronic infections of the ear lead to three broad categories of chronic ear disease: tympanic membrane and mastoid changes, chronic otitis media without cholesteatoma, and cholesteatoma. Although each can occur independently, it is common to find two or all three processes active in one patient.

Tympanic Membrane Changes

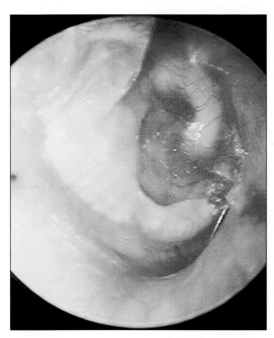

FIGURE 2-57 Tympanosclerosis. Tympanosclerosis is the deposition of hyaline material within the middle layer of the tympanic membrane. This condition results from recurrent infection and sometimes as a consequence of ventilation tube placement. Usually, this phenomenon is of no importance, but when severe, it can progress to involve the entire drum and ossicular chain, resulting in a conductive hearing loss.

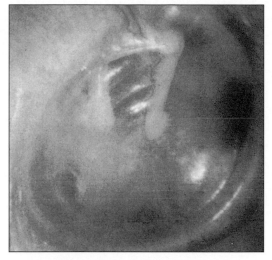

FIGURE 2-58 Myringo-incudo-pexy (shrink-wrap ear). In cases of chronic otitis media with effusion or recurrent acute otitis media, changes in the tympanic membrane develop. In this photograph, the drum has retracted and become adherent to the incus and incudostapedial joint. This condition develops after a long period of retraction that has led to flaccidity of the tympanic membrane. In addition, recurrent infection can lead to scar bands that bind the drum to the ossicles and medial wall of the mesotympanum. At this stage of chronic ear disease, ventilation tubes do not, in general, return the drum to its normal position. Fortunately, hearing in these ears is usually normal. Such ears must be carefully monitored for progression to more severe chronic ear disease. (*From* Tos M, Stangerup S-E, Larsen P: Incidence and progression of myringo-incudo-pexy after secretory otitis. *Acta Otolaryngol (Stockh)* 1992, 112:512–517; with permission.)

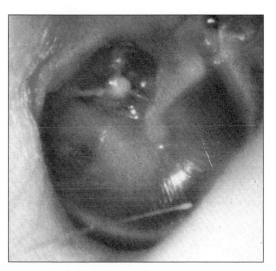

FIGURE 2-59 Myringo-stapedio-pexy (retraction pocket). Continued negative pressures within the mesotympanum, in an ear that already has a myringo-incudo-pexy, may lead to necrosis of the long process of the incus. The drum then lies directly on the head of the stapes. Hearing in these patients, and in those with myringo-incudo-pexy, is usually at or near normal. However, such progression may continue and lead to dissolution of the stapes superstructure of development of a cholesteatoma. (*From* Tos M, Stangerup S-E, Larsen P: Incidence and progression of myringo-incudo-pexy after secretory otitis. *Acta Otolaryngol (Stockh)* 1992, 112:512–517; with permission.)

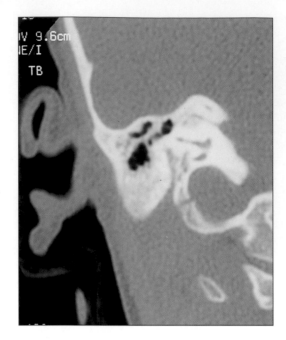
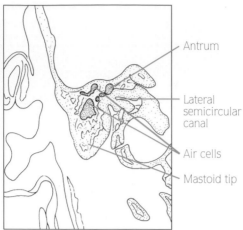

Antrum

Lateral
semicircular
canal

Air cells

Mastoid tip

FIGURE 2-60 Poorly pneumatized mastoid. This child, born with Pierre Robin syndrome, has had persistent problems with otitis media with effusion due to the cleft palate that is part of this congenital abnormality. Several studies have demonstrated that chronic middle ear fluid leads to poor development of the mastoid air cell system. This effect also is seen in patients who do not have branchial apparatus deformities. Ventilation tubes appear to mitigate this retardation of mastoid development. The antrum and some air cells are present, but the inferior half of the mastoid tip has failed to be pneumatized. This is the most benign long-term effect of chronic otitis media.

Tympanic Membrane Perforation

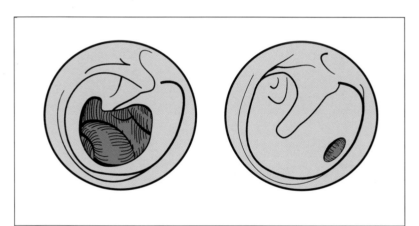

FIGURE 2-61 Tympanic membrane perforations. Perforations are generally described as being central (*left*) or marginal (*right*).

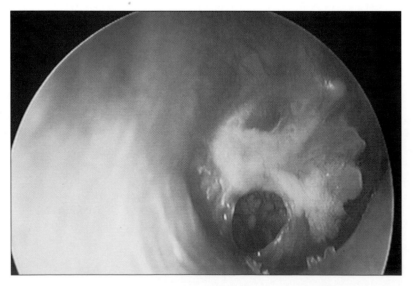

FIGURE 2-62 Central perforation of the tympanic membrane. The most common perforation occurs within the pars tensa and has a rim of surrounding tympanic membrane. Recurrent infection with repeated rupture of the drum may lead to a persistent perforation. Prolonged drainage may prevent closure of an acute rupture, and when the epithelial surfaces from the lateral and medial layers of the drum merge, the perforation will persist even after resolution of infection. Often, as illustrated here, the drum also shows other evidence of chronic infection. Fibrosis of the middle fibrous layer of the drum, due to chronic inflammation, leads to the white tympanosclerotic plaques.

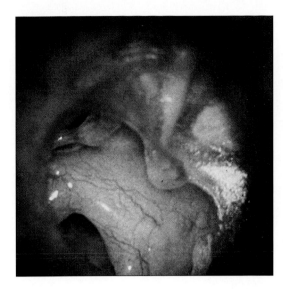

FIGURE 2-63 Marginal perforation of the tympanic membrane. Marginal perforations are less common but require a more complex repair. This perforation extends to the edge of the drum. In general, grafts used to repair tympanic membrane perforations are placed under the edge of the remaining drum to prevent blunting of the angle between the external auditory canal wall and the new drum to avoid lateralization of the graft and distraction of the new drum from the malleus, situations that lead to a poor conduction of sound to the inner ear. In the marginal perforation shown here, there is no rim of intact tympanic membrane inferiorly. Other strategies must therefore be employed to ensure effective closure of this drum and recovery of the conductive hearing loss. (*From* Bull TR: *A Color Atlas of E.N.T. Diagnosis*, 2nd ed. London: Wolfe Medical Publications; 1987:81; with permission.)

Chronic Otitis Media Without Cholesteatoma

Signs and symptoms of chronic otomastoiditis vs acute otitis media

Acute otitis media	Chronic otomastoiditis
Pain	Painless
Fever	No fever
Episodic otorrhea	Chronic/recurrent otorrhea
Good response to oral antibiotics	Poor response to oral antibiotics

FIGURE 2-64 Signs and symptoms of chronic otomastoiditis versus acute otitis media. Chronic otomastoiditis is the culmination of recurrent episodes of acute otitis media and chronic otitis media with effusion. These infections have led to changes in the tympanic membrane and mastoid that may range from mild to severe. Chronic infection leads to mucosal changes around the ossicles and disruption of normal airflow in and out of the mastoid air cell system and results in recurrent inflammation, formation of granulation tissue, and chronic otorrhea. Although usually painless, chronic otomastoiditis is poorly responsive to most antibiotics.

Bacteriology of chronic otomastoiditis without cholesteatoma

Common	Rare
Pseudomonas aeruginosa	*Streptococcus pneumoniae*
Escherchia coli	*Staphylococcus epidermidis*
Staphylococcus aureus	α-Hemolytic streptococci
Peptostreptococcus spp.	*Fusobacterium* spp.
Pigmented *Prevotella* and	*Actinomyces* spp.
Porphyromonas spp.	*Bacteroides* spp.

FIGURE 2-65 Bacteriology of chronic otomastoiditis without cholesteatoma. The bacteriology of chronic otitis media without cholesteatoma is different than that of acute otitis media or chronic otitis media with effusion. (Brook I: Aerobic and anaerobic bacteriology of chronic mastoiditis in children. *Am J Dis Child* 1981, 135:47.)

A. Antimicrobial therapy for chronic otitis media without cholesteatoma

Systemic	Topical
Oral ciprofloxacin (adults)	Gentamicin drops
An aminoglycoside	Tobramycin drops
Ceftazidime	Tobramycin/dexamethasone drops
Ticarcillin-clavulanate	
Clindamycin	

FIGURE 2-66 Antimicrobial therapy for chronic otitis media without cholesteatoma. **A,** Treatment reflects the different microflora from that seen in acute and chronic otitis media and is generally directed at eradicating *Pseudomonas aeruginosa* and also anaerobic bacteria whenever present. In general, systemic and topical agents are used. (*continued*)

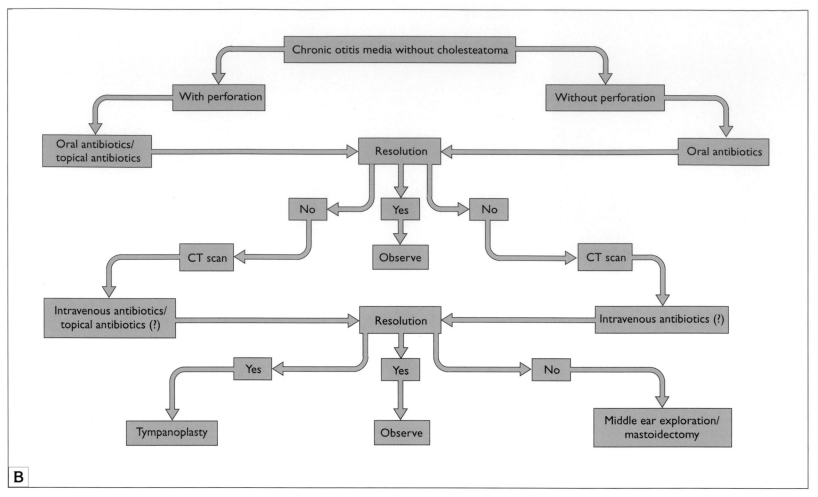

B

FIGURE 2-66 (*continued*) **B,** Depending on whether the drum is currently intact or not, different oral and topical antibiotic regimens may be employed. If oral therapy fails to render the ear quiescent, intravenous and topical therapy may be necessary. Often, however, surgery is required to eradicate the diseased mucosa and reestablish aeration pathways.

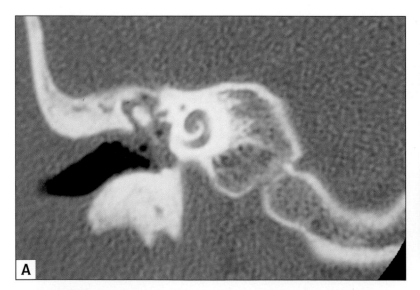

A

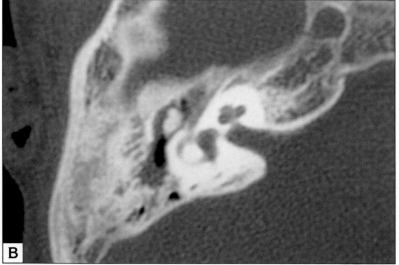

B

FIGURE 2-67 CT scan of chronic inflammation of the middle ear. **A,** A coronal CT scan illustrates the epitympanic soft tissue density seen in cases of chronic otitis media without (and with) cholesteatoma. The lateral aspect of the tympanic membrane is poorly defined due to infected debris and otorrhea. Behind the drum and around the malleus is soft tissue density consisting of fluid, inflamed mucosa, or cholesteatoma. A few small pockets of air may indicate that the tympanic membrane is not intact. **B,** An axial CT section through the mastoid shows diffuse soft tissue density with scattered pockets of air density. No obvious destruction of septa is noted, making the diagnosis of chronic otitis media without cholesteatoma more likely than a diagnosis of cholesteatoma. The patient underwent middle ear exploration because of his clinical and radiographic findings. On elevation of a tympanomeatal flap, mucoid material as well as chronically inflamed mucosa were noted. Because of the chronic nature of the inflammation, the obvious block of effective mastoid aeration, and the CT findings, mastoidectomy was performed. In addition to the inflammation, ossicular discontinuity with erosion of the long process of the incus was discovered.

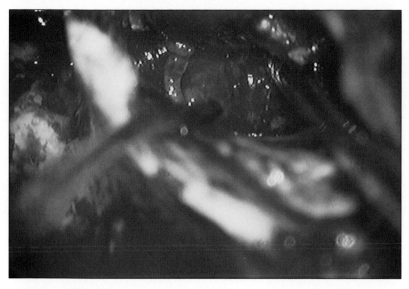

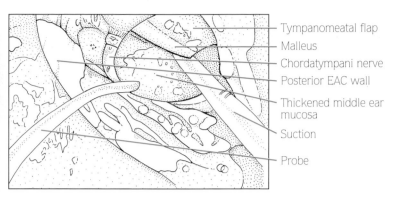

Tympanomeatal flap
Malleus
Chordatympani nerve
Posterior EAC wall
Thickened middle ear mucosa
Suction
Probe

FIGURE 2-68 Operative photograph of chronic otomastoiditis without cholesteatoma. The tympanic membrane has been lifted to reveal chronically inflamed middle ear mucosa. Unlike the case with acute mastoiditis, the mucosa is not pale and edematous, but rather it is firm and adherent to the underlying ossicles. Like acute mastoiditis, this thickened mucosa leads to poor aeration and drainage of the mastoid secretions. The secretions pool and become recurrently infected. This infection will often lead to a chronic perforation of the drum with recurrent drainage or to a granulation polyp that constantly weeps. As shown, the incus and incudostapedial joint are encased in edematous mucosa that must be removed to open the passage to the antrum. The mucosa of the middle ear space, as well, is inflamed. The probe holds the tympanomeatal flap up, exposing the medial surface of the malleus. The suction catheter evacuates fluid from the area medial to the long process of the incus and the stapes head. (EAC—external auditory canal.)

Chronic Otitis Media With Cholesteatoma

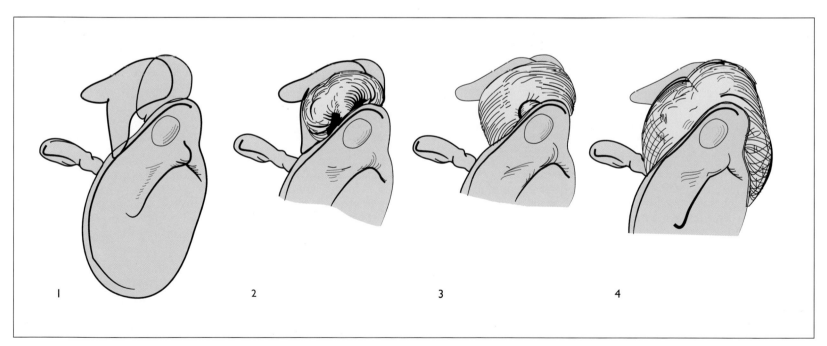

1   2   3   4

FIGURE 2-69 Pathogenesis of chronic otitis media with cholesteatoma. When invagination of the tympanic membrane into the middle ear space (from the pars tensa) or into the epitympanum (from the pars flaccida) occurs, cholesteatoma may form. This squamous-lined sac exfoliates cells internally, resulting in expansion of the sac. Dissolution of bone by the sac lining disrupts the ossicular chain and allows progression into the epitympanum and mastoid. (*Adapted from* Bluestone CD, Klein JO: *Otitis Media in Infants and Children*, 2nd ed. Philadelphia: W.B. Saunders; 1995:225; with permission.)

Bacteriology of cholesteatoma

Aerobes	Anaerobes
Pseudomonas aeruginosa	*Bacteroides* spp.
Proteus spp.	Pigmented *Prevotella* and
Escherichia coli	*Porphyromonas* spp.
Streptococcus spp.	*Peptostreptococcus* spp.
Staphylococcus epidermidis	*Propionibacterium acnes*
Staphylococcus aureus	*Fusobacterium* spp.
	Clostridium spp.

Management of cholesteatoma: Surgical options

Removal of disease	Prevention of recurrence
Atticotomy	Ventilation tube placement
Simple mastoidectomy	Silastic sheet placement
Modified radical mastoidec-tomy	Ossicular chain recon-struction
Radical mastoidectomy	

FIGURE 2-70 Bacteriology of cholesteatoma. The process of cholesteatoma formation is usually the result of chronic infection and may follow chronic otitis media without cholesteatoma. It is not surprising, therefore, that the bacteriology of this entity is similar to that of chronic otomastoiditis without cholesteatoma. (Brook I: Aerobic and anaerobic bacteriology of cholesteatoma. *Laryngoscope* 1981, 9:251.)

FIGURE 2-71 Management of cholesteatoma: surgical options. Cholesteatoma is a surgical disease. Antibiotics may be helpful in controlling an associated infection, but otologic surgery is necessary to remove all disease, create a safe middle ear space, and preserve or restore hearing.

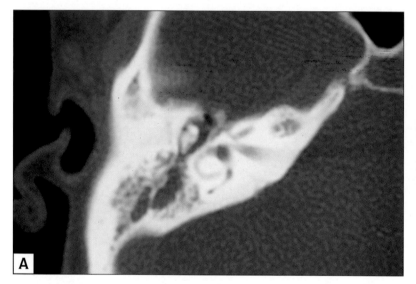

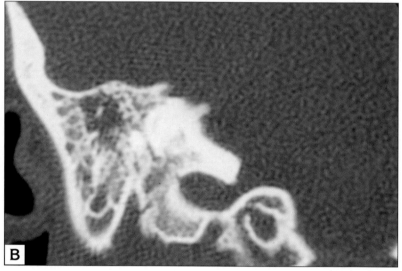

FIGURE 2-72 CT scan of cholesteatoma showing soft tissue density. **A,** An axial CT section at the level of the incus body and the malleus head shows the typical soft tissue density of cholesteatoma. Unlike chronic otitis media without cholesteatoma, no air is seen in the mastoid. In addition, the septa of the air cells are being eroded by the advancing sac. A small linear bone density may represent a ridge of bone that has not yet been eroded by the cholesteatoma. **B,** On a coronal CT view, the destruction of the septa is more pronounced. Such lesions usually arise from retraction pockets in chronically infected ears. They present with a long history of recurrent otorrhea. Pain is not usually a symptom, and these patients rarely have fever. High fever or severe pain that accompanies otorrhea must raise the concern of malignancy or necrotizing (malignant) otitis externa.

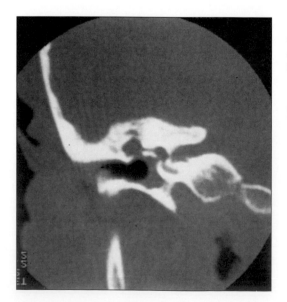

FIGURE 2-73 CT scan of advanced cholesteatoma. Untreated cholesteatoma can have dire consequences, including deafness, loss of ipsilateral vestibular function on the affected side, intracranial infection, and paralysis of the facial nerve. This CT scan shows a cholesteatoma that has eroded onto the lateral semicircular canal. This patient had vertigo and was at risk for suppurative labyrinthitis or an intracranial complication. (*From* Glassock ME III, Shambaugh GE Jr (eds.): *Surgery of the Ear*, 4th ed. Philadelphia: W.B. Saunders; 1990:123; with permission.)

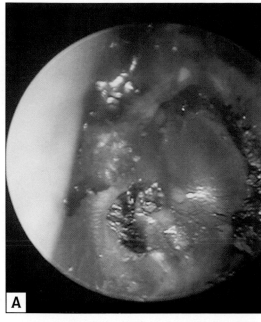

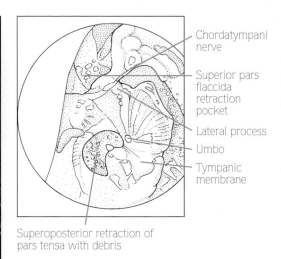

Chordatympani nerve

Superior pars flaccida retraction pocket

Lateral process

Umbo

Tympanic membrane

Superoposterior retraction of pars tensa with debris

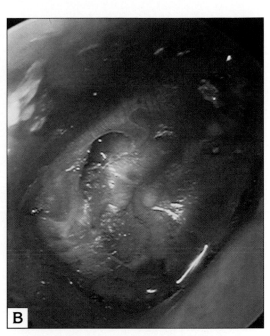

FIGURE 2-74 Tympanic membrane changes associated with cholesteatoma. **A,** A view of the tympanic membrane shows debris in the posterosuperior quadrant of the pars tensa. Often, in a patient with recurrent or chronic otorrhea, this debris hides a retraction pocket underneath. **B,** After cleaning, a slitlike opening can be seen. Over a long period of time, negative pressure within the middle ear, along with recurrent and chronic infection, can lead to flaccidity of the drum and creation of a retraction pocket. As keratinaceous debris and desquamated cells build up within this pocket, it enlarges to form a sac. With further buildup of debris, the advancing surface of this sac will fill the interstices of the epitympanum and erode the middle and inner ear structures. In addition, chronic otorrhea results from infection arising from both the underlying chronic ear disease and the inspissated debris within the sac itself.

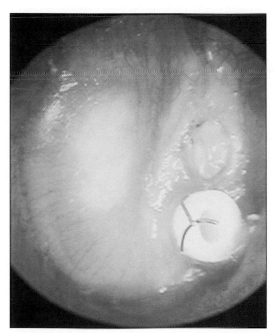

FIGURE 2-75 Cholesteatoma behind the tympanic membrane. An otoscopic view shows a white sac behind an anterosuperior perforation. A ventilation tube is seen in the anteroinferior quadrant. In this case, insertion of a tube did not prevent the formation of cholesteatoma. It may be that the process of cholesteatoma development had started before insertion of the tube or that this case represents a congenital cholesteatoma that developed in the mesotympanum but which has eroded through the tympanic membrane.

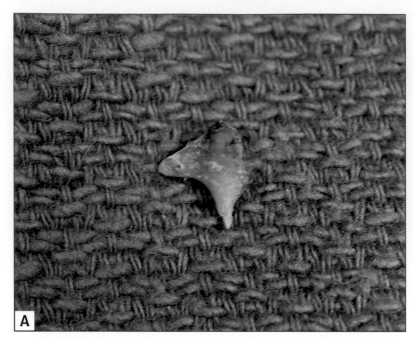
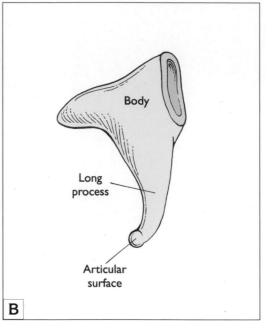

FIGURE 2-76 Gross specimen of an eroded incus. The long process of the incus is most frequently eroded because it is in the direct line of the advancing cholesteatoma sac and, because of the ossicular structures, it has the poorest blood supply. During mastoidectomy for cholesteatoma, this eroded incus was removed to allow complete exploration of the epitympanum and to facilitate complete removal of disease. Unlike mastoidectomy for chronic otitis media without cholesteatoma, mastoidectomy for cholesteatoma requires that all disease be removed to prevent recurrence. **A,** The incus pictured here is missing the long process. **B,** A drawing of the normal incus shows the long process intact.

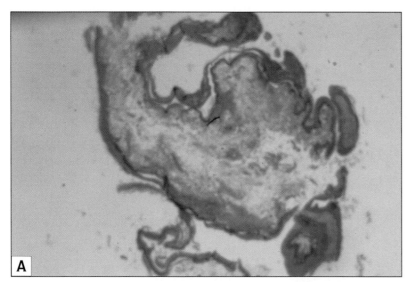
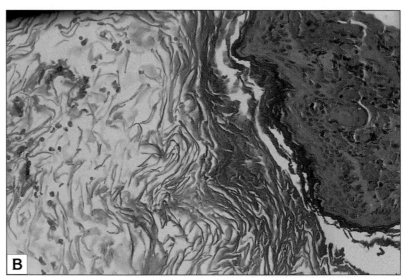

FIGURE 2-77 Histologic section of cholesteatoma. **A,** A low-power photomicrograph of a removed cholesteatoma shows a lobule of eosinophilic material surrounded by a layer of cellular material with increased staining. This lobule consists of keratinaceous debris within a portion of the cholesteatoma sac. The material within the sac easily supports the growth of microorganisms and leads to the recurrent otorrhea seen in these patients. **B,** On higher magnification, the desquamated keratin layer is seen. The sac is lined by keratinizing stratified squamous epithelium and is surrounded by chronically inflamed tissue with many lymphocytes. (Hematoxylin-eosin stain. Magnification: panel 77A, × 22.5; panel 77B, × 300.)

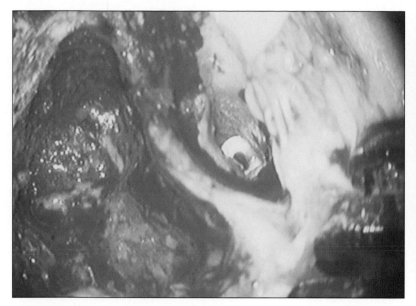

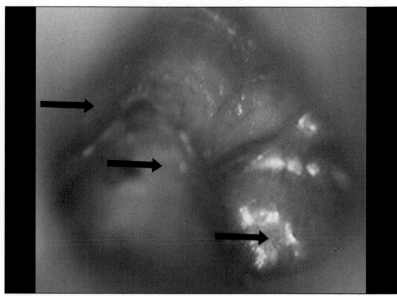

FIGURE 2-78 Mastoidectomy cavity with intact canal wall. With newer equipment, techniques, and possibilities of reconstruction of the conductive mechanism, many surgeons choose to leave the posterior wall of the external auditory canal intact. The mastoid cortex is removed, and the mastoid air cell walls and mucosa are then removed until the antrum and epitympanum are reached. The posterior wall of the external auditory canal is left intact to leave a more natural middle ear space. In cases of intact canal wall mastoidectomy for cholesteatoma, the patient undergoes a "second-look" procedure 6 to 12 months after the initial mastoidectomy. During this procedure, small spheres (pearls) of residual choles-teatoma, if present, can be removed, and the ossicular chain may be reconstructed with grafts, if needed. If a large recurrence of cholesteatoma is found, this cavity can be converted to a modified radical cavity that can be better monitored for recurrent or persis-tent disease.

FIGURE 2-79 Modified radical mastoidectomy. Radical or modified-radical mastoidectomy is frequently the preferred treatment for chronic otitis media with cholesteatoma. During this procedure, the posterior wall of the external auditory canal is removed to form a common cavity with the mastoid, creating a large mastoid bowl (*top arrow*). The posterior wall of the external auditory canal is removed medially to the level of the descending, or mastoid, portion of the facial nerve (*middle arrow*). The tympanic membrane (*bottom arrow*) is then draped over this ridge to create a small middle ear space. Also, the external auditory meatus is enlarged. The result of this procedure is a cavity that is easily monitored for recurrence of disease and one that can be regularly and effectively cleaned. (*From* Bull TR: *A Color Atlas of E.N.T. Diagnosis*, 2nd ed. London: Wolfe Medical Publications; 1987:87; with permission.)

SELECTED BIBLIOGRAPHY

Bluestone CD, Klein JO: *Otitis Media in Infants and Children*, 2nd ed. Philadel-phia: W.B. Saunders; 1995.

Brook I: Otitis media: Microbiology and management. *J Otolaryngol* 1994, 23:269–275.

Bull TR: *A Color Atlas of E.N.T. Diagnosis*, 2nd ed. London: Wolfe Medical Publi-cations; 1987.

Feigin RD, Kline MW, Hyatt SR, Ford KL III: Otitis media. *In* Feigin RD, Cherry JD (eds.): *Textbook of Pediatric Infectious Diseases*. Philadelphia: W.B. Saun-ders; 1992:174–189.

Glassock ME III, Shambaugh GE Jr (eds.): *Surgery of the Ear*, 4th ed. Philadel-phia: W.B. Saunders; 1990.

Paparella MM, Shumrick DA, Gluckman JL, Meyerhoff WL (eds.): *Otolaryngology*, 3rd ed. Philadelphia: W.B. Saunders; 1991.

CHAPTER 3

Infections of the External Ear

Theodore W. Fetter

NORMAL ANATOMY

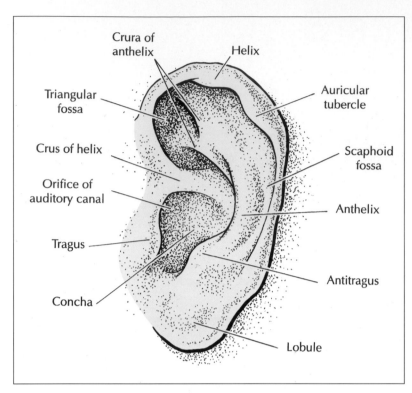

FIGURE 3-1 Lateral surface of the auricle. The external ear is composed of a flexible, potentially mobile auricle (pinna) and the external auditory canal, formed of fibrous tissue, elastic cartilage, and bone. The skin is tight over these structures, leaving little room for soft tissue swelling. When infection occurs, pain develops very quickly. (*Adapted from* Anson B, Donaldson J: *Surgical Anatomy of the Temporal Bone and Ear.* Philadelphia: W.B. Saunders; 1967; with permission.)

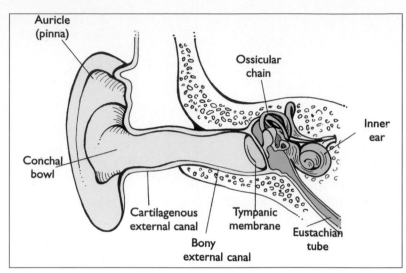

FIGURE 3-2 Cross-sectional anatomy of the external ear. The external auditory canal is approximately 2.5 cm in length and extends in a curving course from the conchal bowl to the tympanic membrane. The outer one third of the canal is surrounded by cartilage and runs backward and upward. The inner two thirds has bony walls and runs slightly backward and then turns forward and downward. The narrowest portion of the canal, the isthmus, is just lateral to the junction of the outer cartilaginous and inner bony portions.

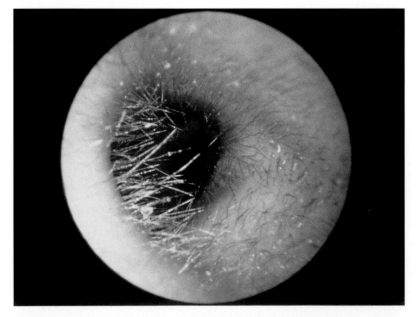

FIGURE 3-3 Otoscopic view of the cartilaginous external auditory canal. The cartilaginous portion of the external auditory canal contains numerous tiny villous hairs. The skin lining the outer canal is relatively thick, with a well-developed dermis and subcutaneous layer containing many sebaceous and modified (ceruminous) apocrine glands. The cerumen from these glands produces an acid pH that inhibits the growth of bacteria. The lateral portion of the canal is relatively mobile within the surrounding connective tissue and cartilaginous framework. (*From* Hawke M, Keene M, Alberti PW: *Clinical Otoscopy: An Introduction to Ear Diseases*, 2nd ed. Edinburgh: Churchill Livingstone; 1990:21; with permission.)

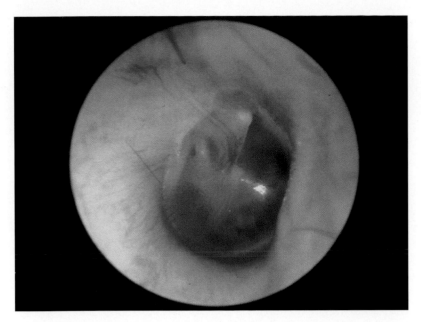

FIGURE 3-4 Otoscopic view of the bony external auditory canal. The inner two thirds of the external auditory canal is surrounded by a bony framework. The skin lining the bony portion is thin and lacks the adnexal structures (hairs and glands) seen in the outer portion. The skin is firmly attached to the underlying bone and is both immobile and easily traumatized. (*From* Hawke M, Keene M, Alberti PW: *Clinical Otoscopy: An Introduction to Ear Diseases*, 2nd ed. Edinburgh: Churchill Livingstone; 1990:21; with permission.)

PATHOGENESIS AND ETIOLOGY

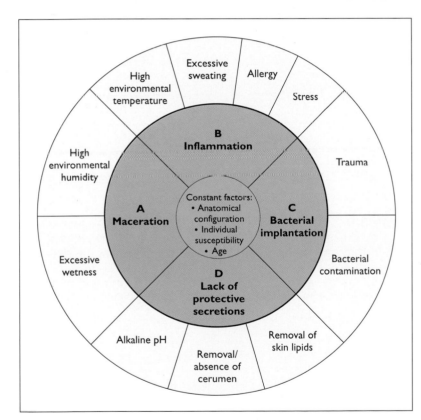

FIGURE 3-5 Factors involved in the etiology of external otitis. Anatomic and physiologic characteristics of the external ear canal provide protective factors against infection. The self-debriding mechanism of desquamation by centrifugal migration provides a cleansing of the external ear canal skin. The acidic pH of the ear canal inhibits growth of pathogenic organisms. The firmly adherent skin of the ear canal is water resistant. The ample blood and lymphatic supply of the ear canal skin and subcutaneous tissues are protective. Cerumen is antibacterial and water repellent. Factors that disrupt the natural protective mechanisms of the ear canal produce conditions that are favorable to the development of otitis externa. Prolonged exposure to water and excessive ear cleaning are major factors believed to be associated with infection. *A)* Excessive wetness, such as that caused by swimming, bathing, or increased environmental humidity, can lead to maceration of the skin in the ear canal, allowing penetration by bacteria. *B)* Obstruction of the gland ducts that produce cerumen may result from inflammation, keratin, or secretion. *C)* Foreign bodies lodged in the ear canal, repeated ear cleansing, or insertion of fingernails, cotton swabs, or other objects may result in mechanical trauma, allowing implantation of exogenous organisms onto or through the damaged skin. *D)* Cerumen creates a protective acid pH in the ear canal, and its removal by excessive ear cleansing, bathing, or swimming can lead to an alkaline pH that is favorable to bacterial growth. Various systemic illnesses also have been associated with otitis externa and include anemia, diabetes, allergy, dermatitis, and anxiety (neurodermatosis). (*Adapted from* Senturia BH, Marcus MD, Lucente FE: *Diseases of the External Ear: An Otologic-Dermatologic Manual.* New York: Grune & Stratton; 1980:32; with permission.)

Normal flora of the external auditory canal

Staphylococcus epidermidis
Corynebacterium spp. (diphtheroids)
Micrococcus spp.
Staphylococcus aureus
Viridans streptococci
Pseudomonas aeruginosa
Propionibacterium acnes

FIGURE 3-6 Normal flora of the external auditory canal. The microbial flora of the external canal is similar to the flora of skin elsewhere. There is a predominance of *Staphylococcus epidermidis, Staphylococcus aureus, Corynebacterium*, and, to a lesser extent, aerobic bacteria such as *Propionibacterium acnes.* Fungal organisms are found in approximately 25% of individuals. In approximately 30% of individuals, the ear canal is sterile.

Microbiology of otitis externa

Common (isolated in > 75% of cases)
  Pseudomonas aeruginosa
  Staphylococcus aureus
Less common
  Enterobacteriaceae
    Proteus spp.
    Klebsiella spp.
    Escherichia coli
  Peptostreptococcus spp.
  Propionibacterium acnes
  Aspergillus spp.
Rare
  Candida albicans
  α-Streptococci

FIGURE 3-7 Microbiology of otitis externa. *Pseudomonas aeruginosa* and *Staphylococcus aureus* are the predominant isolates recovered from cases of otitis externa. In a retrospective study of 46 cases, Brook and colleagues recovered a total of 42 aerobic bacteria, 22 anaerobic bacteria, and 3 *Candida albicans* organisms. Thirty-five percent of cases had multiple organisms isolated, illustrating the polymicrobial nature of much otitis externa. (*From* Brook I, Frazier EH, Thompson DH: Aerobic and anaerobic microbiology of external otitis. *Clin Infect Dis* 1992, 15:955–958; with permission.)

Types of external ear infections

Bacterial infections
  Acute diffuse bacterial otitis (swimmer's ear)
  Acute localized otitis externa (furunculosis)
  Impetigo
  Erysipelas
  Perichondritis and chondritis
Fungal infections
  Otomycoses
Viral infections
  Herpes zoster
  Herpes simplex
Mixed etiology infections
  Chronic otitis externa
  Necrotizing (malignant) otitis externa
  Bullous myringitis
  Granular myringitis

FIGURE 3-8 Types of external ear infections. Many patients with otitis externa present with aural pain, which can be significant, as part of their many presenting symptoms. Other symptoms that may predominate include itching, hearing loss, aural fullness, or aural discharge. Additional symptoms may include tragal or auricular tenderness on movement and occasionally cellulitis and fever.

BACTERIAL OTITIS EXTERNA

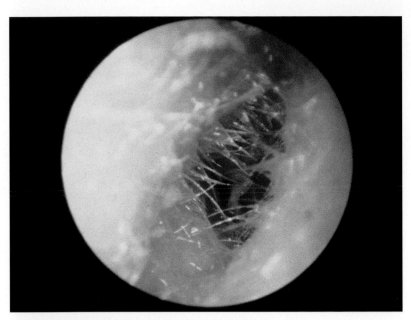

FIGURE 3-9 Otoscopic view of early acute diffuse otitis externa. Acute diffuse otitis externa (swimmer's ear) is a nonlocalized inflammation of the external auditory canal and is the most commonly seen type of otitis externa. It is commonly associated with swimming and hot, humid climates. The patient presents with complaints of itching, pain (which may be severe), a blocked feeling or sense of pressure in the ear, and possible aural discharge. On otoscopy, the skin of the cartilaginous external canal is edematous and tender and has a shiny, red appearance. The lumen is narrowed, and a yellow mucopurulent exudate may be seen. Gram-negative bacteria, particularly *Pseudomonas aeruginosa*, are the usual pathogens, but *Staphylococcus aureus* also is isolated frequently. (*From* Hawke M, Keene M, Alberti PW: *Clinical Otoscopy: A Text and Color Atlas.* Edinburgh: Churchill Livingstone; 1990:59; with permission.)

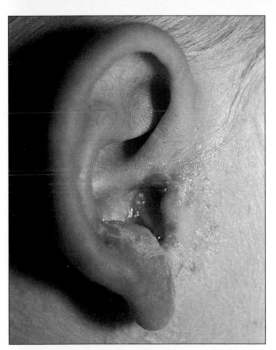

FIGURE 3-10 Lateral view of the ear in acute diffuse otitis externa. External examination shows swelling of the ear canal and lymphadenopathy anterior to the tragus. A yellow, mucopurulent discharge may ooze from the ear opening, especially as the condition progresses. Movement of the tragus or auricle is extremely painful, which may limit or prevent otoscopic examination. (*Courtesy of* A. Willner, MD.)

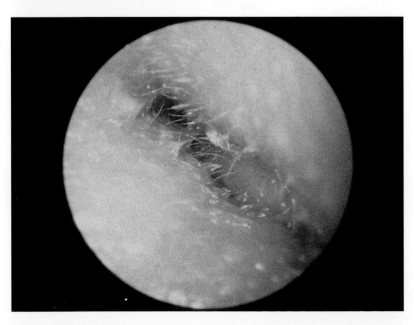

FIGURE 3-11 Otoscopic view of severe acute diffuse otitis externa. As the acute otitis external progresses, the swelling of the canal wall may increase, occluding the lumen and causing hearing loss. Severe pain is usually present. (*From* Benjamin B, Bingham B, Hawke M, Stammberger H: *A Color Atlas of Otorhinolaryngology.* Philadelphia: J.B. Lippincott; 1995:37; with permission.)

A. Basic treatment concepts for external ear canal infections

Selection of otic drops: antiseptic vs. antibiotic
Ensure adequate application of otic drops to infected ear canal skin
  Cleanse ear canal
  Use ear canal wick
Option: use of otic drops with a corticosteroid
Oral (systemic) antibiotics—usually not necessary
Adequate analgesics to relieve pain

FIGURE 3-12 A and **B**, Basic treatment concepts for external ear canal infections and treatment of acute diffuse externa. Either antiseptic or antibiotic otic drops are the mainstay of the treatment of most routine external ear infections, including acute diffuse otitis externa. Antibiotic drops usually contain contain a combination of antibiotics effective against staphylococci and gram-negative organisms. Antiseptic drops can be antibacterial and antifungal and do not risk development of cutaneous sensitivity, particularly to neomycin. The acid pH of optic drops is antimicrobial and helps to restore the normal protective acid pH of the canal wall. Topical corticosteroids in otic drops are anti-inflammatory and help decrease swelling of the canal skin. Topical drops are ineffective unless they are in contact with the canal skin. Thorough initial and periodic cleaning of the canal wall is essential to obtain the desired response from the otic drops. In marked swelling of the ear canal skin, a wick is necessary to ensure wicking of the otic drops along the entire length

of the ear canal skin. Placement of sterile cotton in the external ear canal meatus after application of otic drops maintains contact of the drops with the canal skin. Oral antibiotics are usually not required unless there are associated regional or systemic indications such as cellulitis, cervical lymphadenopathy, or fever. Otitis externa is often very painful. Adequate oral analgesics, including oral narcotics, should be provided.

B. Treatment of acute diffuse otitis externa

Likely pathogens	Treatment

Pseudomonas aeruginosa *Staphylococcus aureus*	Topical
	  Burow's solution—2 tablets in pint of water, irrigate 3–4 times daily
	  Acetic acid (VoSol), with hydrocortisone (VoSol HC)—5 drops, 4 times daily
	  Polymyxin, neomycin, hydrocortisone (Cortisporin)
	Systemic
	  Ciprofloxacin (Cipro)—500 mg orally, twice daily
	  Cefuroxime axetil (Ceftin)—250–500 mg orally, twice daily
	  Cefixime (Suprax)—400 mg once daily
	  Amoxicillin/clavulante (Augmentin)—500 mg, 3 times daily

FIGURE 3-13 Acute localized otitis externa (furunculosis). Localized otitis externa may occur as a pustule or furuncle associated with infected hair follicles. *Staphylococcus aureus* is the most common pathogen, although group A streptococci are also recovered. Furuncles occur only in the outer cartilaginous, hair-bearing portion of the external canal. They appear as an extremely painful, red, localized swelling. (*From* Hawke M, Keene M, Alberti PW: *Clinical Otoscopy: A Text and Color Atlas.* Edinburgh: Churchill Livingstone; 1990:58; with permission.)

Treatment of acute localized otitis externa (furunculosis)

Likely pathogens	Treatment

Staphylococcus aureus Group A streptococcus	Topical
	  Acetic acid (VoSol) with hydrocortisone (VoSolHC)—5 drops, 4 times daily
	  Burow's solution soak
	  Polymyxin, neomycin, hydrocortisone (Cortisporin)—4 drops, 4 times daily
	Systemic
	  Dicloxacillin (Cloxacin)—500 mg orally, 4 times daily
	  Amoxicillin/clavulanate (Augmentin)—500 mg orally, 3 times daily
	  Cefuroxime axetil (Ceftin)—250–500 mg orally, twice daily
	  Ciprofloxacin (Cipro)—500 mg orally, twice daily
	Incision and drainage may be necessary

FIGURE 3-14 Treatment of acute localized otitis externa (furunculosis). Treatment with topical otic drops and systemic (oral) antibiotics, analgesics, and local heat may be curative. Incision and drainage of a pointing furuncle or small abscess is necessary to relieve severe pain and achieve resolution when these conditions are present. (*Adapted from* Cheever LW, Johnson MP: Otitis externa. *In* Rakel RE (ed.): *Conn's Current Therapy, 1995.* Philadelphia: W.B. Saunders; 1995:106; with permission.)

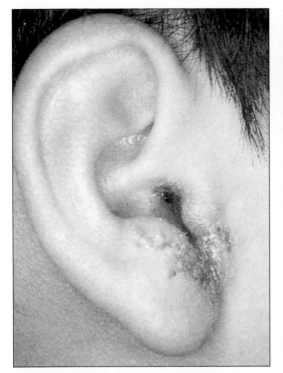

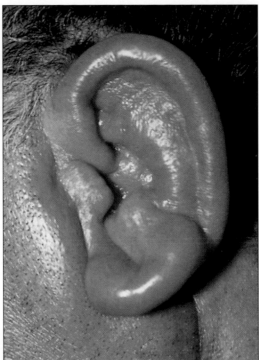

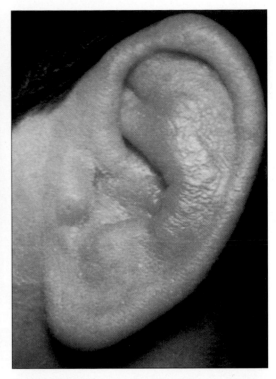

FIGURE 3-15 Impetigo of the auricle. The superficial layers of epidermis may become infected with *Staphylococcus aureus* or *Streptococcus pyogenes*, the usual causes of impetigo. These lesions appear initially as a vesicle or infected scratch and may develop into a chronic weeping and crusted lesion. In this patient, *Staphylococcus aureus*–laden discharge from an infected middle ear resulted in impetigo over the upper portion of the lobule. (*From* Hawke M, Keene M, Alberti PW: *Clinical Otoscopy: A Text and Color Atlas.* Edinburgh: Churchill Livingstone; 1984:43; with permission.)

FIGURE 3-16 Auricular erysipelas. Erysipelas is an acute, localized but spreading form of superficial cellulitis. It usually involves only the pinna in the ear and can spread to adjacent facial areas. It is caused mainly by group A β-hemolytic streptococci. The lesions are characteristically bright red, well demarcated, and tender, with an elevated and distinct advancing peripheral margin. Penicillin therapy brings a rapid response. (*Courtesy of* B. Benjamin, MD.)

FIGURE 3-17 Perichondritis of the auricle. Perichondritis is an infection or inflammation of the cartilage of the pinna, usually arising after trauma, external otitis, or surgery and leading to necrosis of the underlying cartilage. Clinically, the skin of the ear is diffusely swollen, red, and tender. The lobule is spared infection because it contains no cartilage. Gram-negative organisms are the most common organism isolated in this infection, especially *Pseudomonas aeruginosa* and *Proteus*. Treatment is with systemic antibiotics and, often, surgical debridement. (*From* Hawke M, Keene M, Alberti PW: *Clinical Otoscopy: An Introduction to Ear Diseases*, 2nd ed. Edinburgh: Churchill Livingstone; 1990:56; with permission.)

FUNGAL OTITIS EXTERNA (OTOMYCOSIS)

Pathogenic fungi in otomycosis

Common yeast and fungi	Uncommon yeast and fungi
Aspergillus niger	*Trichophyton*
Aspergillus flavus	*Geotrichum*
Aspergillus fumigatus	*Torulopsis*
Candida albicans	*Candida krusei*
Candida parapsilosis	*Candida tropicalis*
Penicillium	*Cryptococcus*
Alternaria	*Chaetomium*
Actinomyces	*Beauveria*
	Rhizopus
	Nocardia caviae
	Mucor

FIGURE 3-18 Pathogenic fungi in otomycosis. Many species of fungi have been identified in cases of otomycosis. The most common organisms are *Aspergillus* and *Candida* species. Often these cases are mixed bacterial and fungal infections, with the most common bacterial co-isolates being *Staphylococcus aureus*, *Pseudomonas*, and *Proteus* species. Otomycosis occurs frequently in hot, humid climates and in persons with diabetes or a history of instrumentation of the ear canal. Fungal mycelia and hyphae are often visible on microotoscopic examination of the ear canals or low-power microscopic examination of lesion scrapings, enabling a quick diagnosis without the need for culture. (*Adapted from* Lucente FE: Fungal infections of the external ear. *Otolaryngol Clin North Am* 1993, 26(6):995–1007; with permission.)

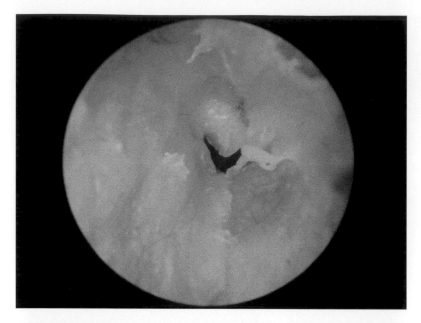

FIGURE 3-19 *Candida albicans* otomycosis. Most patients with otomycosis present with intense itching of the involved canal, persistent otorrhea, and pain. In advanced cases, as seen in this photograph, a creamy white exudate is seen within the deep canal. Infection with *C. albicans* does not show any morphologic evidence of fungi, and diagnosis can only be made by culture. (*From* Benjamin B, Bingham B, Hawke M, Stammberger H: *A Color Atlas of Otorhinolaryngology.* Philadelphia: J.B. Lippincott; 1995:39; with permission.)

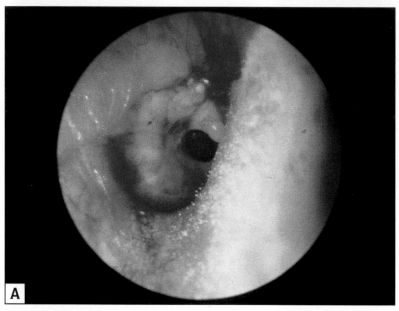

A

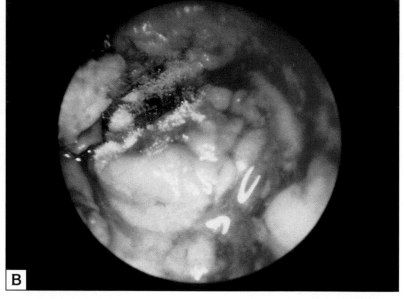

B

FIGURE 3-20 *Aspergillus niger* otomycosis. *Aspergillus* is responsible for up to 90% of cases of otomycosis. **A,** Otomycosis due to *A. niger* can usually be diagnosed by the presence of white, fluffy, cottonlike material, which represents the fungal hyphae. A creamy white mucopurulent exudate may fill the ear canal. **B,** Numerous mycelia with grayish-black or brown fruiting heads (conidio-phores) can be seen in *Aspergillus* infection. A brownish-yellow mucopurulent exudate is present behind, and often the underlying canal skin is inflamed and granular due to invasion by the fungal mycelia. (*From* Hawke M, Keene M, Alberti PW: *Clinical Otoscopy: An Introduction to Ear Diseases,* 2nd ed. Edinburgh: Churchill Livingstone; 1990:79–80; with permission.)

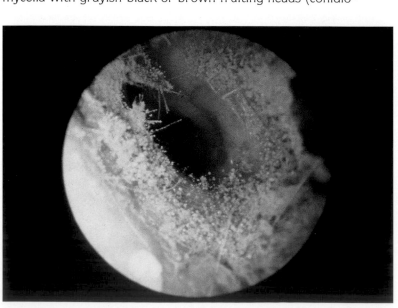

FIGURE 3-21 *Aspergillus flavus* otomycosis. Multiple golden yellow dots are visible, representing the conidiophores of *A. flavus.* (*From* Benjamin B, Bingham B, Hawke M, Stammberger H: *A Color Atlas of Otorhinolaryngology.* Philadelphia: J.B. Lippincott; 1995:40; with permission.)

Topical agents used in the treatment of otomycosis

m-Cresyl acetate	Miconazole
Thimerosal (merthiolate)	Natamycin
Gentian violet	Flucytosine
Nystatin	Merthiolate
Clotrimazole	Iodochlorhydroxyquin
Amphotericin B	
Tolnaftate	

FIGURE 3-22 Agents used in the treatment of otomycosis. Management of otomycosis consists of careful and repeated cleaning of the ear to remove all fungal debris, followed by application of topical antifungal drops, ointment, or powder. Nystatin is usually effective against *Candida* infections, and clotrimazole is most effective against *Aspergillus*. Systemic therapy with oral ketoconazole, fluconazole, or mycostatin can be used in refractory cases. Treatment of invasive otomycosis with intravenous amphotericin B has been reported in patients with AIDS. (*Adapted from* Lucente FE: Fungal infections of the external ear. *Otolaryngol Clin North Am* 1993, 26(6):995–1007; with permission.)

VIRAL OTITIS EXTERNA

Clinical characteristics of herpes zoster oticus

Preceded by hot feeling in ear, developing into severe pain

Clumps of blisters appear along specific dermatomes

Blisters begin as raised reddish papules, then vesiculate and crust over

Blisters may involve concha and superficial ear canal, extending to the lower auricle, lobule, and adjacent upper neck

Generalized or extensive dissemination may occur in immunocompromised patients

Associated findings may include malaise, hearing loss, vertigo, and facial paralysis

FIGURE 3-23 Clinical characteristics of herpes zoster oticus. Ramsey Hunt syndrome (geniculate or cephalic herpes zoster) results from reactivation of a dormant varicella infection of the facial nerve roots. It is characterized by a cutaneous herpetic eruption of the external ear and pinna. It may or may not occur with an associated facial paralysis, vertigo, and hearing loss. The reason for the reactivation is often unknown but may be associated with a decrease in immune function (*eg*, as with malignancy) or stress. Clinically, the initial hot feeling in the ear develops into pain, which is often severe, and is followed by the eruption of the skin lesions.

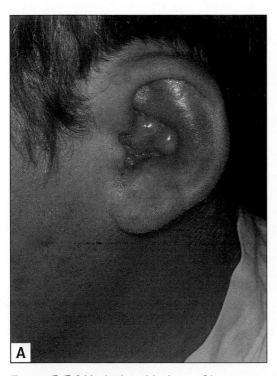

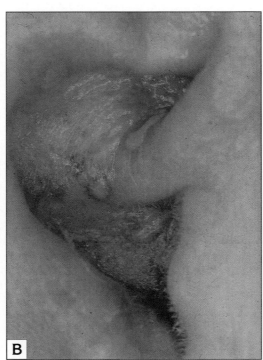

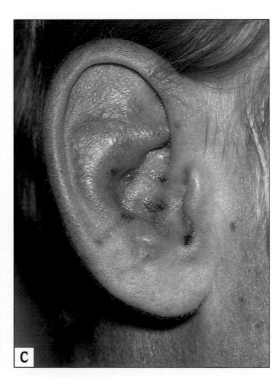

FIGURE 3-24 Vesiculated lesions of herpes zoster oticus. The lesions appear as clusters of raised, reddish papules that vesiculate and then crust over. **A** and **B**, In the early stages, clusters of papules and vesicles are visible in the conchal bowl. **C**, Over days, the blisters rupture and dry out and then become crusted. (Panel 24A *courtesy of* R. Crane, MD; panel 24B *from* Hawke M, Keene M, Alberti PW: *Clinical Otoscopy: An Introduction to Ear Diseases*, 2nd ed. Edinburgh: Churchill Livingstone; 1990:86; with permission.)

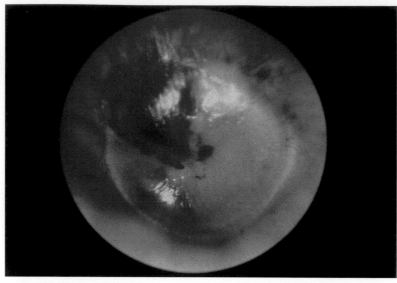

FIGURE 3-25 Herpes zoster of tympanic membrane. A hemorrhagic bleb due to herpes zoster is seen on the anteriosuperior surface of the tympanic membrane. Herpes zoster infrequently affects the tympanic membrane. (*From* Hawke M, Keene M, Alberti PW: *Clinical Otoscopy: An Introduction to Ear Diseases*, 2nd ed. Edinburgh: Churchill Livingstone; 1990:86; with permission.)

Treatment of herpes zoster oticus

Topical cleansing/debridement of ear blisters
Topical acyclovir ointment applied to skin lesions
Oral antiviral agents (*eg*, acyclovir, famciclovir) are started early
  to decrease sequella
Oral prednisone to reduce postherpetic neuralgia
Appropriate analgesics

FIGURE 3-26 Treatment of herpes zoster oticus. When the diagnosis of herpes zoster oticus is suspected, the patient should be started on a course of oral acyclovir or famciclovir. Vesicles should be cleaned to avoid a subsequent secondary bacterial infection. Oral prednisone can be used to minimize the postherpetic neuralgia.

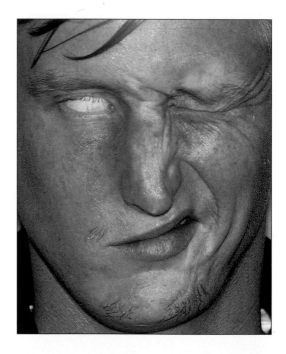

FIGURE 3-27 Facial palsy in Ramsay Hunt syndrome. Herpes zoster oticus may involve the VIIth and VIIIth cranial nerves, resulting in ipsilateral facial paralysis, usually transitory, hearing loss, and vertigo. Herpetic vesicles on the external ear or tympanic membrane may be an early and transient finding that is easily overlooked. The syndrome is frequently characterized by severe aural pain. This patient (*see also* Fig. 3-24C) shows a maximal facial grimace with a complete right facial paralysis and the associated doll's-eye phenomenon.

Treatment of Ramsay Hunt syndrome with facial paralysis

Oral antiviral agents
Intravenous acyclovir therapy for complete facial paralysis
Oral prednisone therapy
Appropriate eye care for facial paralysis

FIGURE 3-28 Treatment of Ramsay Hunt syndrome with facial paralysis. The facial paralysis associated with herpes zoster oticus is frequently more severe than that of idiopathic (Bell's) facial palsy. Thus, aggressive medical therapy is indicated to minimize the sequella of facial paralysis. Oral prednisone is considered to decrease facial nerve swelling. Intravenous antiviral therapy is especially important if electrodiagnostic testing reveals severe facial denervation.

INFECTIONS OF MIXED ETIOLOGY

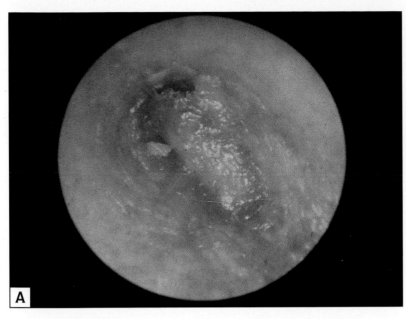

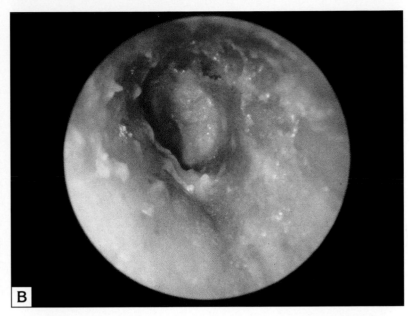

FIGURE 3-29 Otologic view of chronic otitis externa. Chronic forms of otitis externa may result from recurrent or incompletely treated acute disease, untreated underlying dermatologic conditions, or chronic drainage from suppurative otitis media. Bacterial, fungal, or mixed infections may be responsible, and culture is required to help select the appropriate antimicrobial therapy. Treatment of the underlying cause is crucial. Unusual etiologies including tuberculosis, syphilis, leprosy, sarcoidosis, and malignancy should be considered. **A,** On otoscopy, the skin of the external bony canal is thickened and the lumen is blocked with a yellowish-brown plug of infected cerumen. A purulent exudate sometimes is seen in the meatus. **B,** After debridement, the lumen is seen to be narrowed due to chronic thickening and fibrosis within the lining skin. A small hematoma that occurred during cleaning is seen on the anterior canal wall. (*From* Hawke M, Keene M, Alberti PW: *Clinical Otoscopy: An Introduction to Ear Diseases,* 2nd ed. Edinburgh: Churchill Livingstone; 1990:81; with permission.)

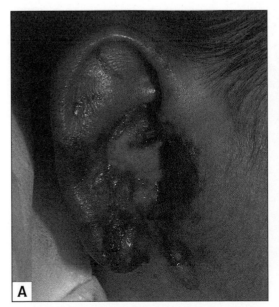

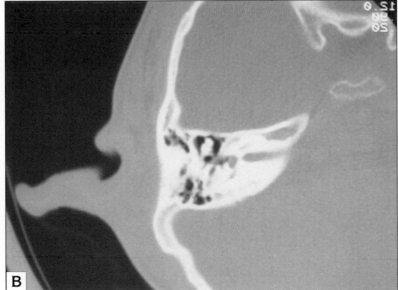

FIGURE 3-30 Chronic otitis externa with pinna involvement. Severe chronic otitis externa can result if prompt intervention is not undertaken for an acute infection. **A,** In this child, a delay of 3 weeks resulted in severe swelling and erythema of the pinna, with areas of necrotic skin and denuded cartilage. There was also a loss of skin connecting the lobule to the side of the head. **B,** An axial computed tomography scan shows extensive auricular and periauricular swelling. Swelling has turned the pinna perpendicular to the mastoid cortex, which remains free of disease. Treatment was with topical sulfadiazine cream and parenteral antibiotics. (*Courtesy of* A. Willner, MD.)

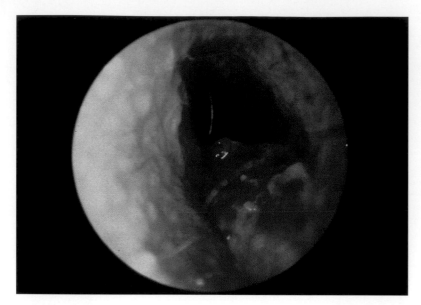

FIGURE 3-31 Otoscopic view of necrotizing (malignant) otitis externa. Necrotizing otitis externa is a severe, invasive, locally aggressive infection that occurs primarily in elderly diabetics and immunocompromised patients. The condition almost always is caused by *Pseudomonas aeruginosa* infection. Classically, necrotizing otitis externa presents as severe otalgia associated with the presence of exuberant granulation tissue arising from the floor of the external auditory canal at the junction of the bony and cartilaginous portions with persistent purulent otorrhea. Despite the misleading nomenclature, this is a bacterial infection, not a neoplastic condition. (*From* Hawke M, Keene M, Alberti PW: *Clinical Otoscopy: A Text and Color Atlas*. Edinburgh: Churchill Livingstone; 1984:65; with permission.)

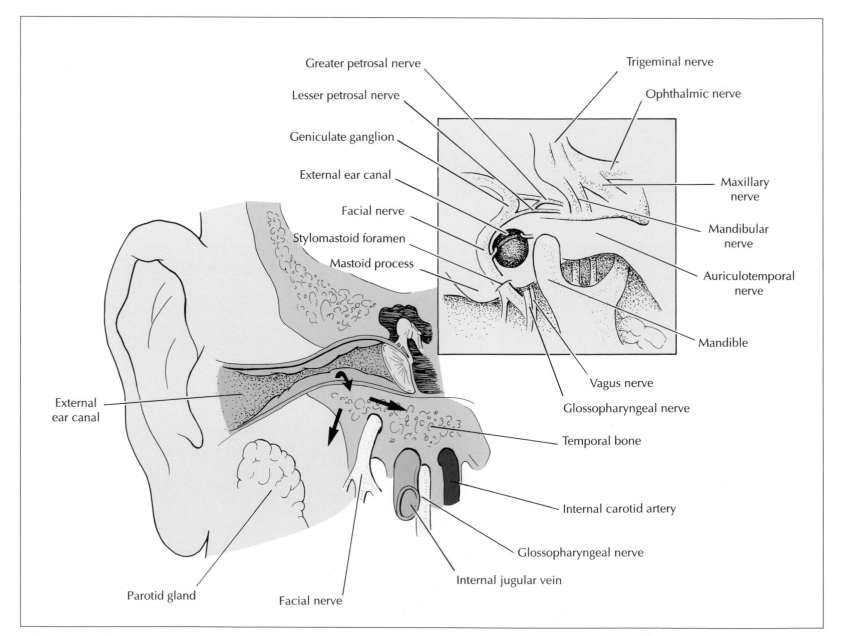

FIGURE 3-32 Anatomic spread of necrotizing (malignant) otitis externa. The spread of necrotizing otitis externa follows a characteristic route that results in a pattern of cranial neuropathies. The infection begins at the junction of the cartilaginous and bony portions of the external canal. It spreads into the temporal bone and the mastoid, where the facial nerve is involved as it exits the stylo- mastoid foramen, resulting in facial palsy. Osteomyelitis of the skull base follows as well as progressive cranial nerve palsies; complications may include venous thrombosis, meningitis, and brain abscess, leading to death. The spread can be rapid. (*Adapted from* Evans P, Hofmann L: Malignant external otitis: A case report and review. *Am Fam Physician* 1994, 49:427–431; with permission.)

Clinical features of necrotizing (malignant) otitis externa

Usually affects elderly diabetics and immunocompromised patients

Presents as refractive, progressive form of diffuse otitis externa

Severe, persistent otalgia (worse at night) and purulent otorrhea

Absence of fever

Progressive cranial nerve palsies (usually VIIth cranial nerve)

Granulation tissue present in external auditory canal

Pseudomonas aeruginosa isolated on culture

Bony erosion noted on imaging studies

FIGURE 3-33 Clinical features of necrotizing (malignant) otitis externa. Necrotizing otitis externa often must be differentiated from chronic otitis externa. Patients present with a refractory, persistent otitis externa and generally report persistent and severe ear pain, which is worse at night and wakes them from sleep. Granulation tissue at the junction of the cartilaginous and osseous canals is an invariable finding. Facial nerve palsies occur in 20% to 30% of patients and are an ominous finding. (Rubin J, Yu VL: Malignant external otitis. *Am J Med* 1988, 85:391.)

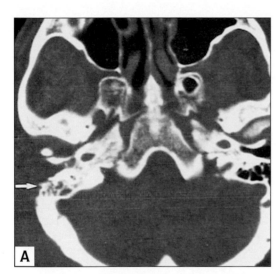
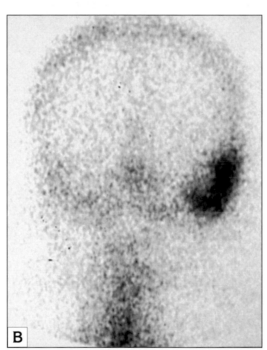
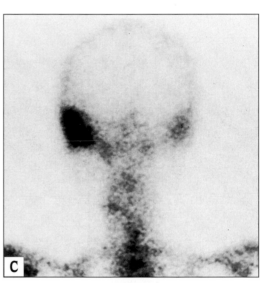

FIGURE 3-34 Radiographic studies in necrotizing otitis externa. The patient with suspected necrotizing (malignant) otitis externa should be studied with computed tomography (CT) to rule out bony involvement. Radionuclide imaging is very sensitive but lacks specificity and is often used to confirm the diagnosis and follow clinical resolution. The role of magnetic resonance imaging remains to be determined. **A,** An axial CT scan shows erosion of the mastoid cortex (*arrow*) with clouding of the mastoid air cells on the right. CT is useful in delineating soft tissue involvement, but significant bone loss must occur to be detected by CT. **B,** Technetium-99m bone scintigraphy shows increased uptake (infection) in the right mastoid region. These scans can detect early bone loss, making them useful in confirming the diagnosis, but are unable to differen-

tiate among various inflammatory conditions. In addition, the radionuclide is incorporated into bone, and scans remain positive even following clinical resolution. **C,** Gallium-67 scintigraphy shows an area of intense uptake in the right temporal lobe. The technique requires 48 to 72 hours to complete, but because gallium is not taken up by osteoclasts, it can be used to follow the course of infection. (Panels 34A and 34B *from* Guy RL, Wylie E, Hickey SA, Tonge KA: Computed tomography in malignant otitis externa. *Clin Radiol* 1991, 43:166–170; with permission; panel 34C *from* Caruso VG, Meyerhoff WL: Trauma and infection of the external ear. *In* Paparella MM, Shumrick DA, Gluckman JL, Meyerhoff WL (eds.): *Otolaryngology,* 3rd ed. Philadelphia: W.B. Saunders; 1991:1231; with permission.)

Treatment of necrotizing (malignant) otitis externa

Systemic
   Ceftazidime (Fortaz)—2 g intravenously, every 8–12 hours
   Ciprofloxacin (Cipro)—750 mg orally, twice daily
   Tobramycin—1–1.5 mg/kg intravenously, every 8 hours
   Plus ticarcillin (Ticar)—3 g intravenously, every 4 hours
Surgical
   Local debridement of ear canal
   Rarely, extensive surgical debridement

Figure 3-35 Treatment of necrotizing otitis externa. Before the advent of effective antipseudomonal antibiotics, treatment of the condition was primarily surgical debridement and the mortality rate was 30%. Today, most patients receive prolonged courses of systemic antibiotics and local debridement of the involved area, with cure rates of approximately 90%. Patients should be followed for at least 1 year after discontinuing antibiotics. (*Adapted from* Cheever LW, Johnson MP: Otitis externa. *In* Rakel RE (ed.): *Conn's Current Therapy, 1995.* Philadelphia: W.B. Saunders; 1995:106; with permission.)

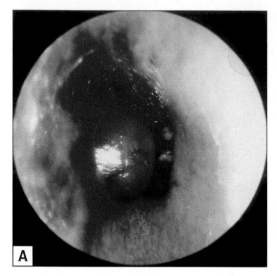 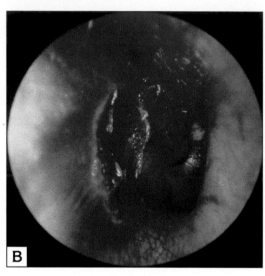 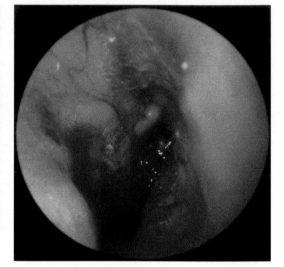

Figure 3-36 Otoscopic view of bullous myringitis. Bullous myringitis is an acute inflammation of the tympanic membrane and surrounding meatal skin that is characterized by severe pain and the presence of hemorrhagic blebs. The condition is thought to be due to an influenza-like virus, but in some cases, *Mycoplasma pneumoniae* has been cultured. **A,** A large hemorrhagic bleb is present on the posterior bony canal wall and adjacent tympanic membrane. The bleb contains a serous effusion with a collection of blood in the inferior portion. **B,** After rupture and aspiration of the bleb, extensive subcutaneous and intracutaneous hemorrhage can be seen. There is extensive hemorrhage along the handle of the malleus. (*From* Hawke M, Keene M, Alberti PW: *Clinical Otoscopy: A Text and Color Atlas.* Edinburgh: Churchill Livingstone; 1984:76; with permission.)

Figure 3-37 Otoscopic view of granular myringitis. Granular myringitis is a chronic infection of the tympanic membrane associated with the development of painless, bright red granulation tissue. The condition appears to be the result of chronic superficial infection, by bacteria or fungi, of the epithelium covering the lateral surface of the tympanic membrane. Granulation tissue may be diffuse or localized, as it is in this photograph. (*From* Hawke M, Keene M, Alberti PW: *Clinical Otoscopy: A Text and Color Atlas.* Edinburgh: Churchill Livingstone; 1984:77; with permission.)

SELECTED BIBLIOGRAPHY

Caruso VG, Meyerhoff WL: Trauma and infection of the external ear. *In* Paparella MM, Shumrick DA, Gluckman JL, Meyerhoff WL (eds.): *Otolaryngology,* 3rd ed. Philadelphia: W.B. Saunders; 1991:12

Hawke M, Keene M, Alberti PW: *Clinical Otoscopy: An Introduction to Ear Diseases,* 2nd ed. Edinburgh: Churchill Livingstone; 1990.

Jahn AF, Hawke M: Infections of the external ear. *In* Cummings CW, Krause CJ, Schuller DE, *et al.* (eds.): *Otolaryngology—Head and Neck Surgery,* 2nd ed. St. Louis: Mosby Year-Book; 1993:154.

Rubin J, Yu VL: Malignant external otitis. *Am J Med* 1988, 85:391.

Senturia BH, Marcus MD, Lucente FE: *Diseases of the External Ear: An Otologic-Dermatologic Manual.* New York: Grune & Stratton; 1980.

CHAPTER 4

Sinusitis

Ellen R. Wald

ANATOMY OF THE PARANASAL SINUSES

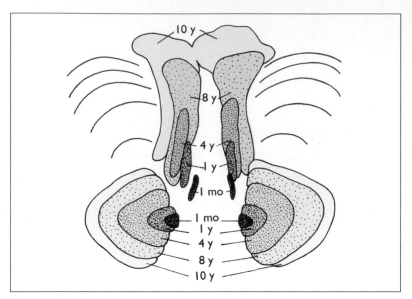

FIGURE 4-1 Developmental anatomy of the maxillary and frontal sinuses. The maxillary and ethmoid sinuses form during the third to fourth gestational month. At birth, the maxillary sinus is a slit-like cavity running in an anteroposterior direction parallel to the middle third of the nose. Gradually, the maxillary sinus increases in width and height until in the adult it holds a volume of 15 mL. The frontal sinuses develop embryologically from an anterior ethmoid and move from an infraorbital to supraorbital position sometime between 6 and 10 years of age. The frontal sinuses evaginate the frontal bone and may not be completely formed until late adolescence. This composite drawing shows changes in the size and shape of the maxillary and frontal sinuses during infancy and childhood.

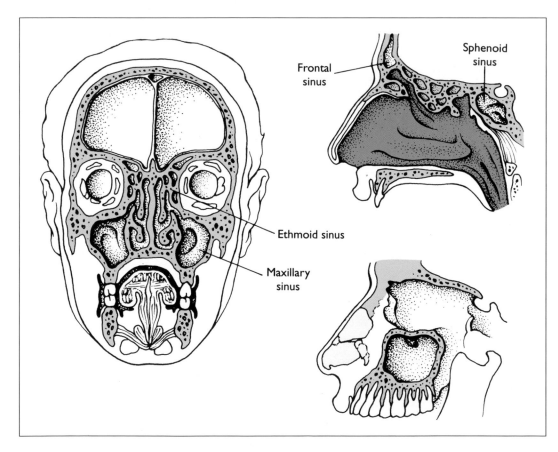

FIGURE 4-2 Anatomy of the paranasal sinuses. The relationship between the nose and the paranasal sinuses is shown. It is important to note the outflow tract of the maxillary sinus high on the medial wall of that sinus. This awkward positioning of the outflow tract predisposes to maxillary sinusitis as a complication of a viral upper respiratory tract infection. The numerous ethmoid sinuses each drain by a tiny independent ostium into the middle meatus. The very narrow caliber of these draining ostia sets the stage for obstruction to occur easily and often during a viral upper respiratory tract infection. (*From* Wald ER: Acute sinusitis in children. *Pediatr Infect Dis J* 1983, 2:61–68; with permission.)

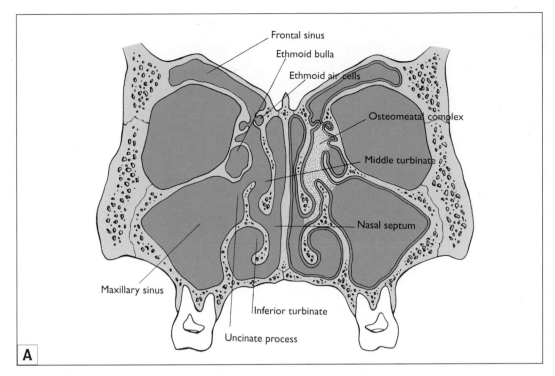

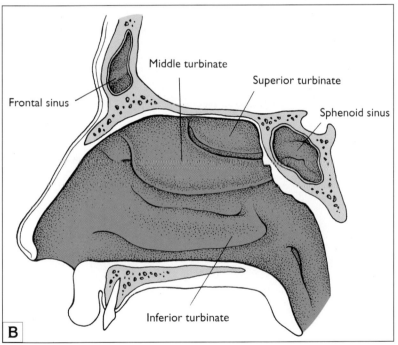

FIGURE 4-3 Anatomy of the turbinates. **A,** The inferior and middle turbinates in the coronal plane. The ethmoid bulla is the most inferior of the ethmoid air cells. If enlarged, it can impinge on the outflow tract of the maxillary sinus. The osteomeatal complex is the area between the inferior and middle turbinates; it represents the confluence of the drainage from the frontal, ethmoid, and maxillary sinuses. Within the osteomeatal complex, there are several areas in which mucosa abuts mucosa. When this occurs, ciliary function may be impaired even without actual physical obstruction. **B,** Sagittal view of the nose and paranasal sinuses, depicting the relationship of the inferior, middle, and superior turbinates, which originate from the lateral wall of the nose. Beneath the middle and superior turbinates, there is a meatus that drains two or more of the paranasal sinuses. The maxillary, anterior ethmoids, and frontal sinuses drain to the middle meatus, whereas the posterior ethmoids and sphenoid sinus drain to the superior meatus. Only the lacrimal duct drains to the inferior meatus. (*From* Wald ER: Sinusitis in children. *N Engl J Med* 1992, 326:319–323; with permission.)

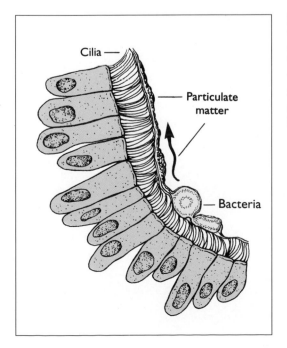

FIGURE 4-4 Nasal mucosa and cilia. In the posterior two thirds of the nasal cavity and within the sinuses, the epithelium is composed of pseudostratified columnar cells, of which most are ciliated. There are also interspersed goblet cells that contribute to the mucus secretions. There appears to be a double layer of mucus in the airways: the gel layer (superficial viscid fluid) and the sol layer (underlying serous fluid). The gel layer entraps particles such as bacteria and other debris; the thinner sol layer allows the cilia to beat rhythmically. The tips of the cilia touch the gel layer during forward movement and thereby move the particulate matter into the nasopharynx to be expectorated or swallowed.

Factors predisposing to sinus ostial obstruction	
Mucosal swelling	**Mechanical obstruction**
Systemic disorder	Choanal atresia
Viral URI	Deviated septum
Allergic inflammation	Nasal polyps
Cystic fibrosis	Foreign body
Immune disorders	Tumor
Immotile cilia	
Local insult	
Facial trauma	
Swimming or diving	
Rhinitis medicamentosa	

URI—upper respiratory tract infection.

FIGURE 4-5 Factors predisposing to sinus ostial obstruction. (*From* Wald ER: Sinusitis in infants and children. *Ann Otol Rhinol Laryngol* 1992, 101(suppl 55):37–41; with permission.)

CLINICAL PRESENTATIONS AND MANAGEMENT OF SINUSITIS

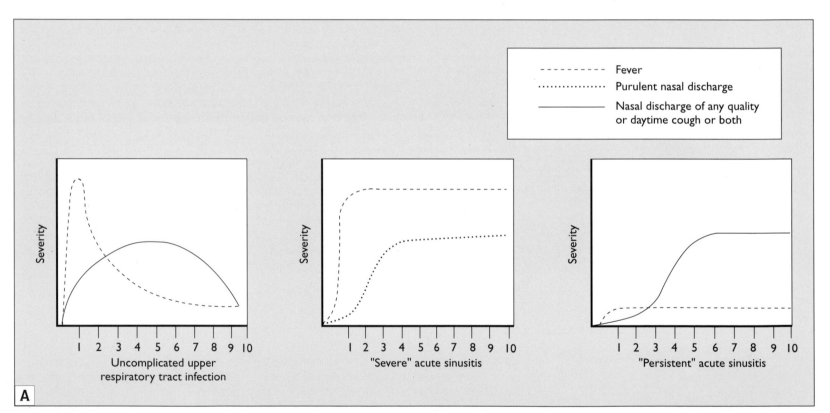

A

FIGURE 4-6 Clinical course and presentations of sinusitis. **A**, There are two common clinical presentations for patients with acute sinusitis that must be differentiated from that of a simple uncomplicated viral upper respiratory tract infection. In the child with a viral upper respiratory tract infection, fever, if present, occurs early in the illness, usually in concert with other constitutional symptoms such as myalgia and headache. The fever resolves in a day or two, and then the respiratory symptoms become prominent. Respiratory symptoms such as nasal discharge (of any quality—serous, mucoid, or purulent), nasal congestion, and cough peak in 5–7 days. Although the patient may not be symptom-free at 10 days, the symptoms have usually diminished, and improvement is apparent. (*continued*)

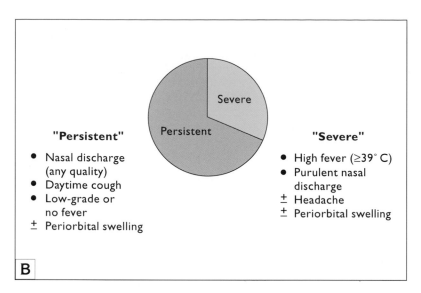

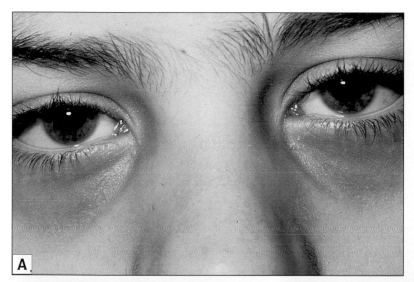

B

"Persistent"

- Nasal discharge (any quality)
- Daytime cough
- Low-grade or no fever
- ± Periorbital swelling

"Severe"

- High fever (≥39° C)
- Purulent nasal discharge
- ± Headache
- ± Periorbital swelling

FIGURE 4-6 (*continued*) **B**, In patients with "severe" acute sinusitis, the fever persists and the nasal discharge is purulent (thick, colored, and opaque). In patients with "persistent" acute sinusitis, fever is low-grade or absent, but respiratory symptoms (nasal discharge of any quality or daytime cough, or both) persist beyond 10 days without evidence of improvement.

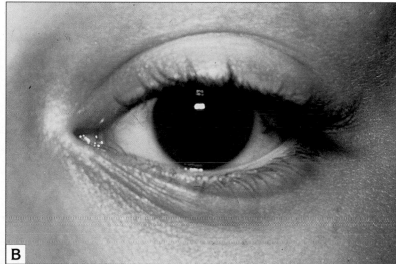

A

B

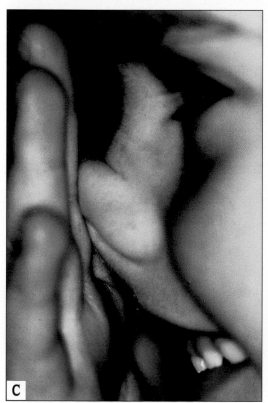

C

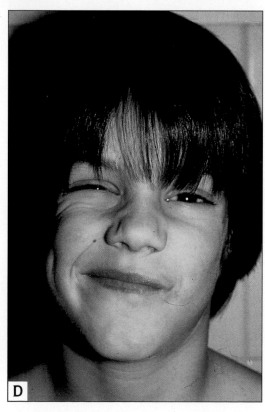

D

FIGURE 4-7 Allergy as a risk factor for sinusitis. Allergy is second to viral upper respiratory tract infections as a risk factor for sinusitis. Allergy should be suspected in patients with any of the following findings: **A**, Allergic "shiners," or discoloration of the area below the eyes. **B**, Dennies' lines, which are additional transverse creases in the infraorbital area. **C**, Allergic salute, which is an upward movement of the nose in response to pruritus. **D**, Excessive facial grimacing in response to pruritus.

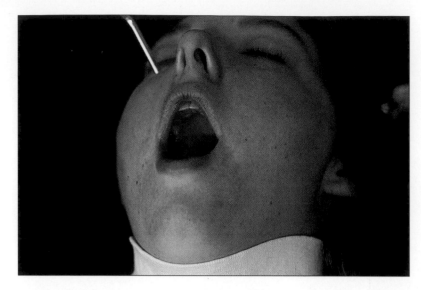

FIGURE 4-8 Transillumination technique. Three evaluations can be helpful in confirming a diagnosis of sinus infection: transillumination, imaging, and sinus aspiration. Transillumination is a procedure that is used to assess the maxillary and frontal sinuses in older children, adolescents, and adults. In a darkened room, the transilluminator, connected to an otoscope handle, is placed at the midpoint of the inferior orbital rim to see if light comes through the hard palate (excluding the alveolar ridge). When the transmission of light is normal, as shown in this example, the maxillary sinus is air-filled. If the light is absent, the maxillary sinus is fluid-filled. The results correlate well with the findings of sinus aspiration, provided the interpretation is limited to the extremes of normal or absent. This technique can also be used to evaluate the frontal sinuses. (*From* Wald ER: Rhinitis and acute and chronic sinusitis. *In* Bluestone CB, Stool SE (eds.): *Pediatric Otolaryngology*, 2nd ed. Philadelphia: W.B. Saunders; 1990:735; with permission.)

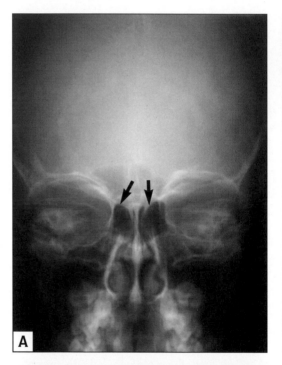

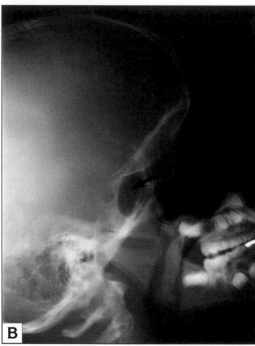

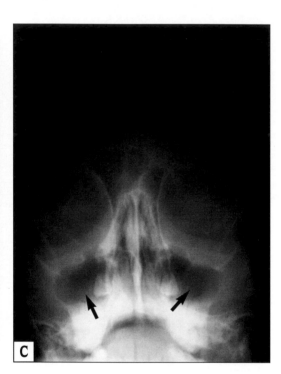

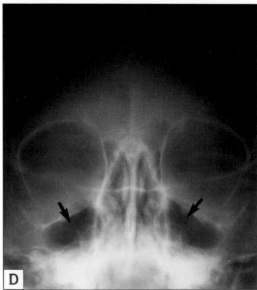

FIGURE 4-9 Radiographic evaluation. Radiographs can be used to confirm the clinical suspicion of acute sinusitis. Three radiographic views should be obtained as follows: **A**, Anteroposterior, to visualize the ethmoid air cells (*arrows*); **B**, Lateral, to visualize the frontal and sphenoid sinuses (*arrow*); **C**, Occipitomental, to visualize the maxillary sinuses (*arrows*). These radiographs show normal findings. **D**, This is another example of an occipitomental view demonstrating normal aeration of the maxillary sinuses bilaterally (*arrows*).

Radiographic criteria for sinusitis
Complete opacification
Mucosal thickening of at least 4 mm
Presence of an air-fluid level

FIGURE 4-10 The radiographic findings indicative of a diagnosis of acute sinusitis are complete opacification, mucosal thickening of at least 4 mm, or the presence of an air-fluid level. The most common radiologic finding in sinus-aspiration–proven bacterial sinusitis is complete opacification. Air-fluid levels are observed in 30% of adults and < 10% of children with bacterial sinusitis.

FIGURE 4-11 Diagnostic radiographic findings. **A**, An occipitomental view shows complete opacification of the left maxillary sinus (*arrow*). The right maxillary sinus is well aerated. **B**, An occipitomental view demonstrates significant mucosal thickening in the right maxillary sinus. There is an air-fluid level in the left maxillary sinus, an unusual finding in children with acute sinusitis. The left frontal sinus, although rudimentary, is opacified. **C**, An occipitomental view demonstrates mucosal thickening in the right maxillary sinus and > 75% opacification of the left maxillary sinus. **D**, This occipitomental radiograph shows dramatic mucosal thickening of the right maxillary sinus and a normal left maxillary sinus. (*continued*)

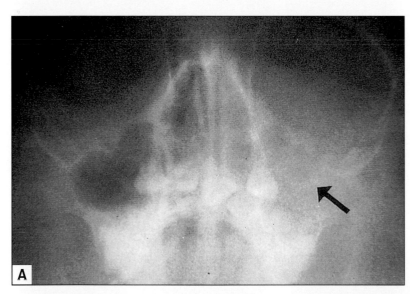

A

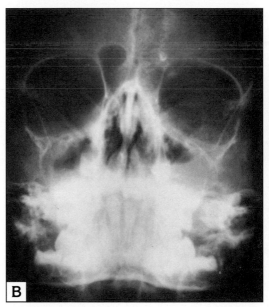

B

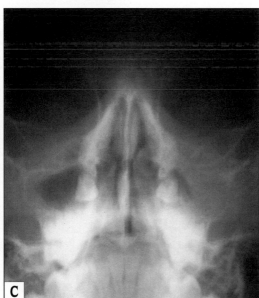

C

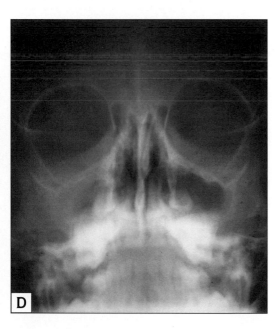

D

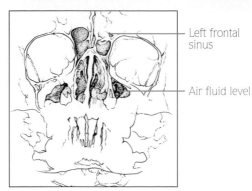

Left frontal sinus

Air fluid level

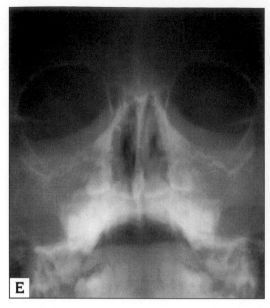

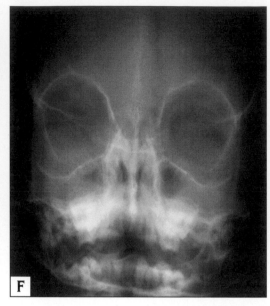

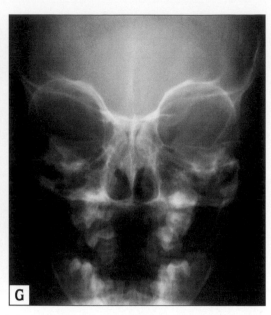

FIGURE 4-11 (*continued*) **E**, An occipitomental view demonstrates complete opacification of both maxillary sinuses. **F**, An occipitomental view shows dramatic bilateral mucosal thickening with better aeration of the left maxillary sinus. **G**, An anteroposterior view shows opacification of the ethmoid sinuses bilaterally.

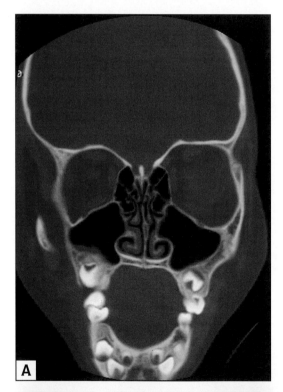

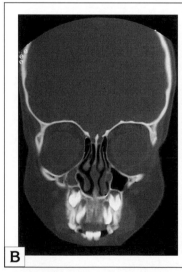

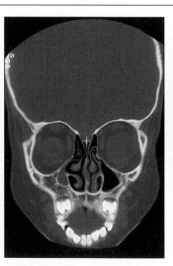

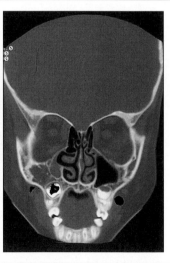

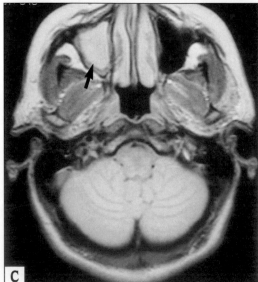

FIGURE 4-12 Computed tomographic (CT) and magnetic resonance (MR) evaluations. Other imaging modalities used to confirm a diagnosis of sinusitis include CT and MR imaging. These studies are usually reserved for patients with very protracted symptoms or patients in whom complications of sinusitis have developed. **A**, A coronal CT scan demonstrates completely aerated maxillary and ethmoid sinuses bilaterally. **B**, This CT scan was done because of recurrent episodes of right-sided maxillary sinusitis. The coronal CT demonstrates that the right maxillary sinus is actually hypoplastic. **C**, This axial MR image shows complete opacification of the left maxillary sinus (*arrow*). MR imaging is a particularly good modality to demonstrate neoplasms or vascular abnormalities. (*continued*)

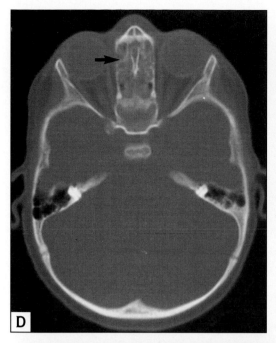

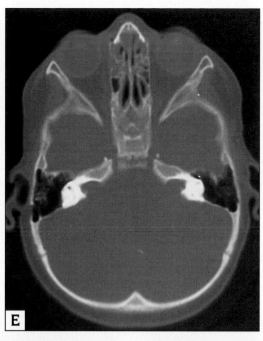

FIGURE 4-12 (*continued*) **D** and **E**, An axial CT scan was performed to evaluate a child with recurrent eye swelling associated with recurrent upper respiratory tract infection. These views show the bony dehiscence in the left lateral ethmoid bone (*panel 12D, arrow*). These dehiscences may occur naturally as the bones of the orbit and skull form. **F**, A coronal CT shows a completely opacified right maxillary sinus (*arrow*), significant mucosal thickening in the left maxillary sinus (*arrowhead*), and opacification of the ethmoids bilaterally (*open arrows*). **G**, This coronal CT scan shows complete opacification of the left sphenoid sinus (*arrow*) in a posterior cut. (Panels 9F and 9G *courtesy of* M. Casselbrant, MD.)

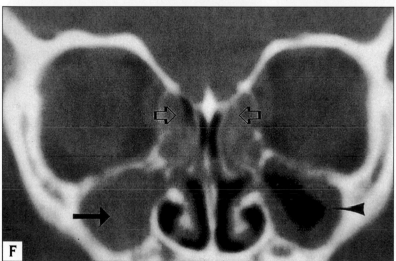

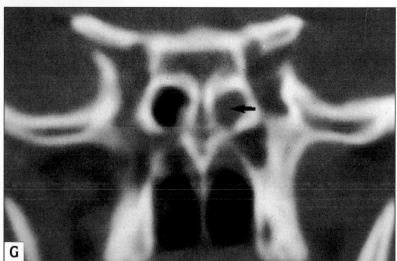

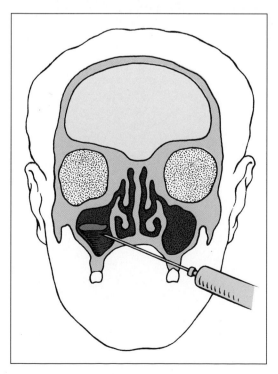

FIGURE 4-13 Sinus aspiration. Sinus aspiration is the best measure (gold standard) for diagnosis of acute sinusitis. The trocar is passed beneath the inferior turbinate and across the lateral nasal wall. Secretions are aspirated into the syringe and sent to the laboratory for Gram stain and culture. The area beneath the inferior turbinate must be sterilized so that the culture is not contaminated by normal nasal flora. An infection is defined as the recovery of bacteria in very high colony counts of at least 10^4 cfu/mL. (*From* Wald ER: Rhinitis and acute and chronic sinusitis. *In* Bluestone CB, Stool SE (eds.): *Pediatric Otolaryngology*, 2nd ed. Philadelphia: W.B. Saunders; 1990:738; with permission.)

Indications for sinus aspiration in children

Suppurative complications of acute sinusitis
  Orbital
  Central nervous system
Failure to improve on appropriate antimicrobial therapy
Severe symptoms or toxicity
Immunocompromised host

FIGURE 4-14 Indications for sinus aspiration in children. Aspiration is performed on selected patients who are either seriously ill or likely to harbor unusual microbiologic agents in their sinus cavities. Aspiration is indicated in patients who fail to respond to antimicrobial therapy, those who present with serious intracranial complications, or immunosuppressed persons in whom a broad range of pathogens may be causative.

Microbiology of acute maxillary sinusitis in 50 children

Bacterial species	%
Streptococcus pneumoniae	28
Haemophilus influenzae	19
(20% of isolates β-lactamase positive)	
Moraxella catarrhalis	19
(27% of isolates β-lactamase positive)	
Other	6
Sterile	30

FIGURE 4-15 Microbiology of acute sinusitis in children. The data are derived from maxillary sinus aspirations performed on 50 symptomatic patients. *Streptococcus pneumoniae* is the most common cause of acute sinusitis in all age groups, both children and adults, with *Haemophilus influenzae* (nontypeable) being the next most common cause in both groups. *Moraxella catarrhalis* (previously known as *Neisseria catarrhalis* and *Branhamella catarrhalis*) is also a frequent maxillary sinus isolate in children. Currently, nearly 100% of *M. catarrhalis* are β-lactamase positive. Neither staphylococci nor anaerobes are frequently recovered from patients with acute sinusitis. Viral agents, recovered from maxillary sinus aspirates in approximately 10% of patients, include adenovirus, parainfluenza, and influenza virus. (Wald ER, Milmoe GJ, Bowen AD, *et al.*: Acute maxillary sinusitis in children. *N Engl J Med* 1981, 304:749.)

Microbiology of acute sinusitis in adults

Bacterial species	%
Streptococcus pneumoniae	31
Haemophilus influenzae (unencapsulated)	21
Rhinovirus	15
Gram-negative bacteria	9
Anaerobic bacteria	6
Combined *S. pneumoniae* and *H. influenzae*	5
Influenza virus	5
Moraxella catarrhalis	2

FIGURE 4-16 Microbiology of acute sinusitis in adults. *Streptococcus pneumoniae* and *Haemophilus influenzae* account for about one half of all cases in adults as well as children. Less-frequent causes include *Staphylococcus aureus*, *Streptococcus pyogenes*, and the parainfluenza and adenoviruses. (Gwaltney JM Jr: Sinusitis. *In* Mandell GL, Douglas RG Jr, Bennett JE (eds): *Principles and Practice of Infectious Diseases*, 3rd ed. New York: Churchill Livingstone; 1990:510–514.)

Symptoms of subacute sinusitis in children

Nasal discharge
Daytime cough
Intermittent low-grade fever
Malodorous breath
Headache

FIGURE 4-17 Symptoms of subacute sinusitis in children. Subacute sinusitis in children is characterized by respiratory symptoms that persist for > 30 but < 120 days. Fever is a frequent complaint but is rarely documented. Headache may be present but is mild.

Bacteria cultured from 40 children with subacute sinusitis

Bacterial species	n
Streptococcus pneumoniae	12
Haemophilus influenzae	11
Moraxella catarrhalis	8
Streptococcus pyogenes	2
Other	2

FIGURE 4-18 Microbiology of subacute sinusitis in children. Bacteria cultured from 40 children with subacute sinusitis are recorded. (Wald ER, Byers C, Guerra N, *et al.*: Subacute sinusitis in children. *J Pediatr* 1989, 115:28–32.)

Comparison of microbiology of acute, subacute, and chronic sinusitis in children

Bacterial species	Acute	Subacute	Chronic
Streptococcus pneumoniae	+	+	+
Haemophilus influenzae	+	+	+
Moraxella catarrhalis	+	+	+
Staphylococci			+
Respiratory anaerobes			+

FIGURE 4-19 Comparison of microbiology of acute, subacute, and chronic sinusitis in children. The respiratory anaerobes include anaerobic cocci, *Bacteroides* spp., and *Veillonella* spp.

Antimicrobials and dosages for sinusitis in children

Antimicrobial	Daily dosage
Amoxicillin	40 mg/kg/d ÷ 3
Amoxicillin/potassium clavulanate	40/10 mg/kg/d ÷ 3
Erythromycin/sulfisoxazole	50/150 mg/kg/d ÷ 4
Sulfamethoxazole/trimethoprim	40/8 mg/kg/d ÷ 2
Cefaclor	40 mg/kg/d ÷ 3
Cefuroxime axetil	30 mg/kg ÷ 2
Cefprozil	30 mg/kg/d ÷ 2
Cefixime	8 mg/kg/d ÷ 1 or 2
Cefpodoxime proxetil	10 mg/kg/d ÷ 2
Loracarbef	30 mg/kg/d ÷ 2

FIGURE 4-20 Antimicrobials and dosages for the treatment of sinusitis in children. Amoxicillin is the drug of choice for uncomplicated sinusitis. Amoxicillin/potassium clavulanate, erythromycin/sulfisoxazole, cefuroxime axetil, and cefpodoxime proxetil have the most comprehensive antimicrobial spectrum. The dosages provided are total daily amounts and should be administered in divided doses as indicated. Therapy should be continued until the patient is symptom-free for at least 7 days.

Fungi causing sinusitis

Phycomycetes (esp. *Mucor* spp.; also *Absidia, Rhizopus*)
Aspergillus (esp. fumigatus; *also* niger, flavus, oryzae, nidulans*)*
Histoplasma
Candida
Coccidioides
Alternaria

FIGURE 4-21 Fungi causing sinusitis. The most common fungal pathogens are of the class Phycomycetes and *Aspergillus* spp. All these fungi are saprophytic and ubiquitous in soil and can be found in the oral cavity. They may become pathogenic in individuals with altered immune functions (*eg*, prolonged steroid or other immunosuppressive therapy, organ transplant recipients, malignancy, diabetes mellitus, AIDS). (White JA: Paranasal sinus infections. *In* Ballenger JJ (ed.): *Diseases of the Nose, Throat, Ear, Head, and Neck*, 14th ed. Philadelphia: Lea & Febiger; 1991:184–202.) (*Courtesy of* H-W Pfister, MD.)

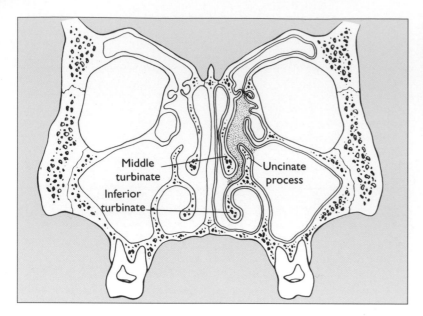

FIGURE 4-22 Endoscopic sinus surgery. In patients who fail to respond to antimicrobial and adjunctive therapy, functional endoscopic surgery may be performed. The focus of endoscopic sinus surgery is the osteomeatal complex, which is located between the inferior and middle turbinates. It represents the confluence of the outflow tracts of the ethmoid, frontal, and maxillary sinuses. The natural ostium is widened by excising the uncinate process and ethmoid bullae, and an anterior ethmoidectomy is performed.

COMPLICATIONS

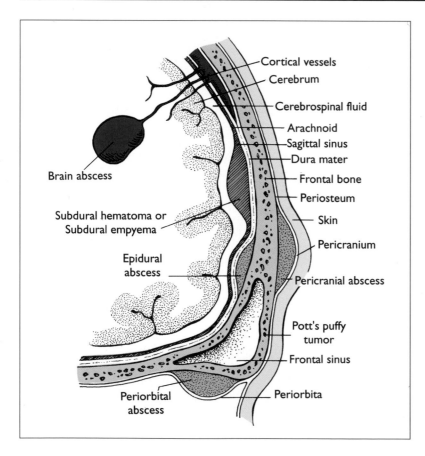

FIGURE 4-23 Suppurative complications of frontal sinusitis involving the central nervous system, bone, and eye. The central nervous system problems include brain abscess, subdural empyema, and epidural abscess. Infections involving the orbit usually result from an intact or ruptured periorbital or subperiosteal abscess. These subperiosteal abscesses may also point toward the skin and give rise to subperiosteal abscess of the frontal bone or Pott's puffy tumor.

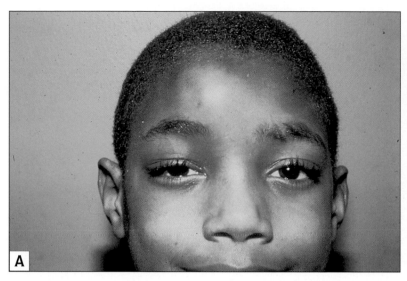
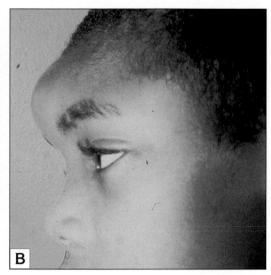

FIGURE 4-24 Pott's puffy tumor. **A** and **B**, A 13-year-old boy presented with a 10-day history of respiratory symptoms and headache. His fever had been low-grade. The headache was not relieved by acetaminophen. During the last 3 days, his forehead had become tender to touch. On physical examination, the middle of his forehead was swollen, tender, and fluctuant. This is an example of Pott's puffy tumor—subperiosteal abscess of the frontal bone, secondary to frontal sinusitis.

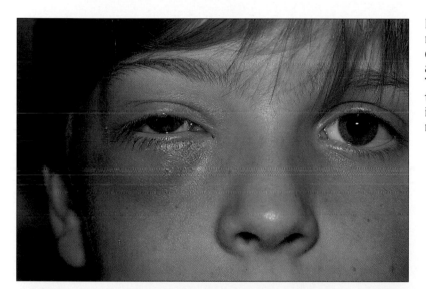

FIGURE 4-25 Inflammatory edema. A boy with infection of his right ethmoid and maxillary sinuses. On occasion, when the ethmoid sinus is completely congested, periorbital swelling occurs around the ipsilateral eye due to impedance of venous drainage. This condition is referred to as inflammatory edema, or sympathetic effusion. Although this does not represent an actual orbital infection, it may progress to a subperiosteal abscess and should be regarded as more serious than a case of uncomplicated sinusitis.

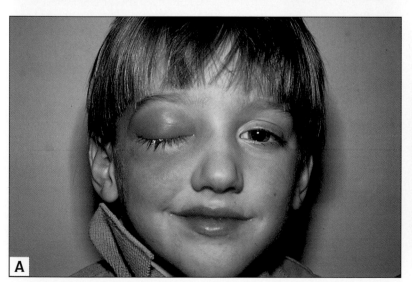
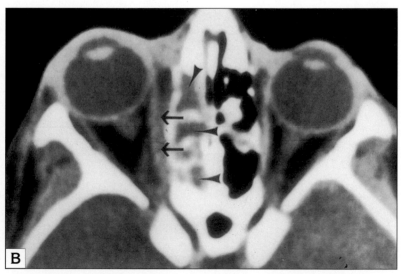

FIGURE 4-26 Right-sided subperiosteal abscess. A 6-year-old boy had a cold for 9 days. Two days before presentation, his right eye began to hurt, but it appeared normal. **A**, One day previously, his eye became swollen and erythematous. On physical examination, he was afebrile. When his lids were everted, there was minimal anterior displacement of his right globe and an impairment of upward gaze. **B**, The axial computed tomography scan shows complete filling of the right ethmoids (*arrowheads*). The slight anterior displacement of the right globe can be seen. The *arrows* indicate some inflammatory tissue between the medial rectus and the lateral wall of the ethmoid. Because this was not a well-demarcated subperiosteal abscess, he was treated medically with high-dose antibiotics and responded well.

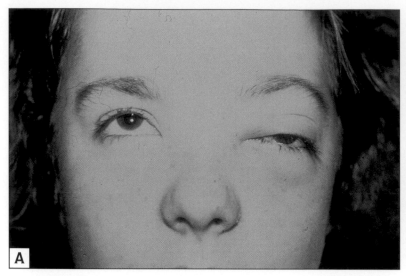

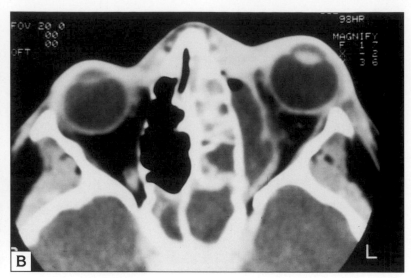

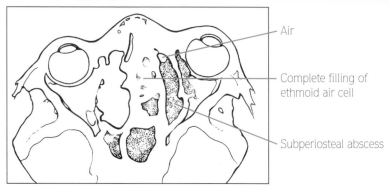

Air

Complete filling of ethmoid air cell

Subperiosteal abscess

FIGURE 4-27 Left-sided subperiosteal abscess. True orbital infections are almost always characterized by anterior displacement of the globe and an impairment of extraocular eye movements, most often upward gaze. **A,** A 25-year-old woman had an upper respiratory tract infection for 1 week. For the previous 2 days, she had progressive swelling of her left eye and a headache. On physical examination, her left eye was displaced anteriorly and laterally. She was unable to elevate her left eye. (*Courtesy of* M. Casselbrant, MD.) **B,** An axial computed tomography scan demonstrates complete filling of the left ethmoid air cells, both anteriorly and posteriorly. There is a large subperiosteal abscess along the lateral wall of the left ethmoid bone (lamina papyracea). The air within the abscess cavity indicates that there is a dehiscence of the lateral ethmoid bone.

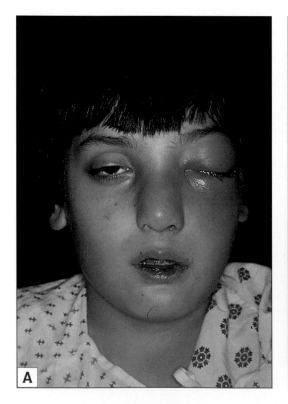

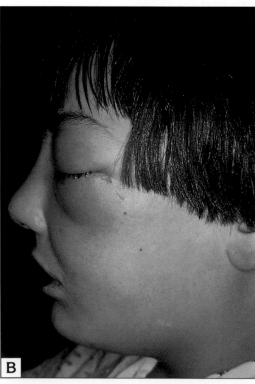

FIGURE 4-28 Intra- and extraorbital suppurative complications of sinusitis. **A** and **B,** A 10-year-old boy had long-standing allergic symptoms, including chronic nasal discharge and congestion. For 3 days, he had left-sided facial pain and headache, with progressive swelling of his left eye. On physical examination, he was febrile to 38.4° C (101.2° F). When his lids were mechanically everted, his left globe was frozen and there was intense chemosis of the conjunctiva. (*continued*)

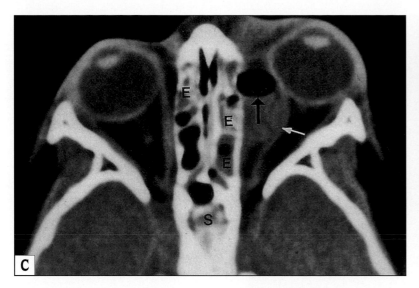
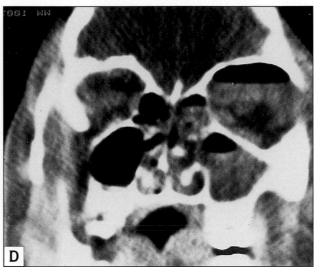

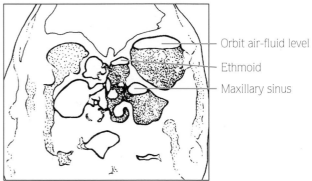

FIGURE 4-28 (*continued*) **C** and **D,** An axial computed tomography (CT) scan shows anterior and lateral displacement of his left eye. There is an air-fluid level (*black arrow*) in the area between the lateral border of the left ethmoid and the medial rectus of his left eye (*white arrow*). The coronal CT shows air-fluid levels in his orbit, ethmoid sinus, and maxillary sinus. (E—ethmoid air cells; S—sphenoid sinus.)

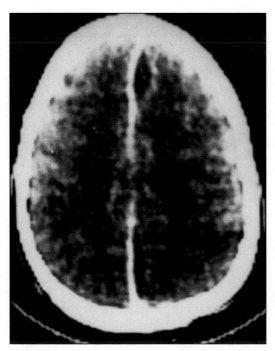

FIGURE 4-29 Parafalcine epidural abscess. An axial computed tomography scan of the head demonstrates an epidural collection of fluid in the parafalcine area. This was obtained from an 18-year-old with frontal sinusitis, severe headache, and photophobia. (*From* Wald ER, Pang D, Milmoe GJ, *et al.*: Sinusitis and its complications in the pediatric patient. *Pediatr Clin North Am* 1981, 28:777–796; with permission.)

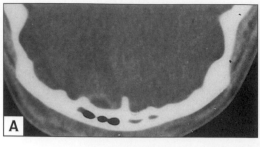
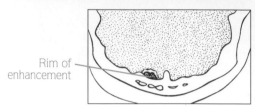
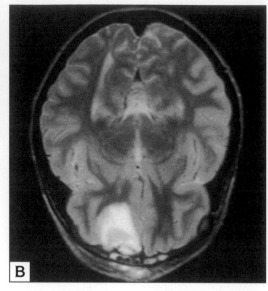
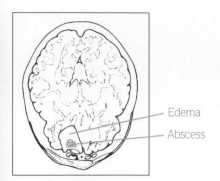

FIGURE 4-30 Epidural abscess. A 30-year-old man had nasal congestion and headache for 1 month. During the last 3 days, the headache became extremely intense; he was vomiting daily and developed a low-grade fever. On physical examination, he appeared very uncomfortable. His face was tender to touch, especially over his brow.

Computed tomography (CT) scan and magnetic resonance (MR) imaging were done. **A**, The CT scan demonstrates a faint rim of enhancement of an epidural abscess on the right side. **B**, The MR also demonstrates the abscess and a large area of edema posterior to it in the right frontal area.

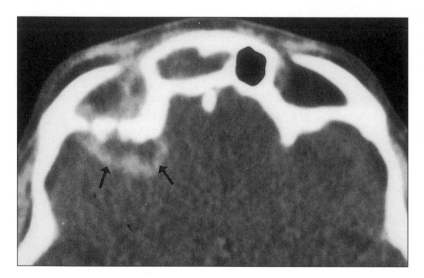

FIGURE 4-31 Frontal sinusitis and epidural abscess. An axial computed tomography (CT) scan in a plane above the orbits in a 25-year-old woman with long-standing allergic symptoms. She had a headache for 2 weeks, which was unrelieved by treatment with acetaminophen with codeine. On physical examination, she was afebrile with bilateral papilledema. A CT scan revealed frontal sinusitis and an epidural abscess (*arrows*). The superior portion of the orbit on the side of the abscess also demonstrates some inflammatory reaction.

SELECTED BIBLIOGRAPHY

Lusk RP, Tychsen L, Park TS: Complications of sinusitis. *In* Lusk RP (ed.): *Pediatric Sinusitis*. New York: Raven Press; 1992.

Rabuzzi DD, Hengerer AS: Complications of nasal and sinus infections. *In* Bluestone CB, Stool SE (eds.): *Pediatric Otolaryngology*, 2nd ed. Philadelphia: W.B. Saunders; 1990.

Wald ER: Sinusitis in children. *N Engl J Med* 1992, 326:319–323.

Wald ER: Rhinitis and acute and chronic sinusitis. *In* Bluestone CB, Stool SE (eds.): *Pediatric Otolaryngology*, 2nd ed. Philadelphia: W.B. Saunders; 1990.

Zinreich J: Imaging of inflammatory sinus disease. *Immunol Allergy Clin North Am* 1994, 14:17–30.

CHAPTER 5

Infectious Diseases of the Oral Cavity

Marlin E. Gher, Jr
George Quintero

HEALTH

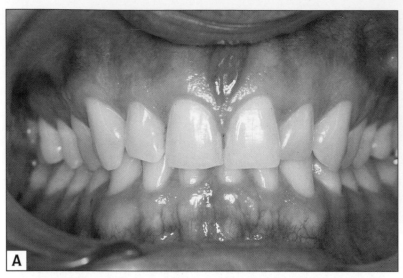

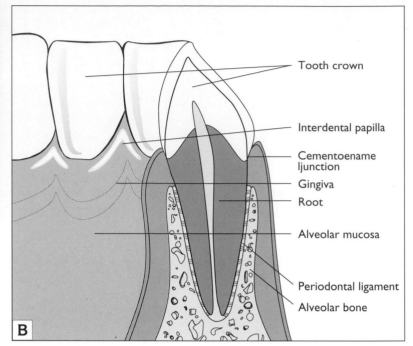

FIGURE 5-1 Oral tissues in health. **A**, The normal dentition is free from extensive hypocalcifications or carious lesions and ranges in color from white to gray or yellow. The teeth are well positioned in the arch and free from bacterial plaque deposits. The masticatory gingival tissue is keratinized and a coral-pink color, with a potential melanin pigmentation in persons of African or Mediterranean heritage. It extends from the free gingival margin to the mucogingival junction and varies in width from 1–9 mm. The free gingival margin should be located at or coronal to the cementoenamel junction of the teeth. The interproximal (interdental) papillae fill the embrasure space between adjacent teeth and are firm, noninflamed, and well adapted to the teeth. Apically, the masticatory gingiva is usually well demarcated from the loosely anchored and movable alveolar mucosa by the mucogingival junction. The alveolar mucosa extends to the vestibular fornix and joins with the buccal and labial mucosa. An anastomosing capillary network is easily discernible in the alveolar mucosa. In health, the alveolar, buccal, and labial mucosas are more red in color than the gingiva due to the thin, nonkeratinized, and translucent epithelium. It is free from ulcerations and induration and maintains a consistent surface integrity. **B**, The normal periodontium is characterized by the following. The alveolar bone surrounds the root and extends to within 1–2 mm of the cementoenamel junction (CEJ). A periodontal ligament, composed principally of dense collagen fibers, joins the root to the bone. Gingival fibers insert into the cementum of the root in the area coronal to the alveolar bone and apical to the CEJ and serve to attach the gingiva to the tooth. A thin probe, when placed in the sulcus between the free gingiva and crown, should not penetrate past the CEJ, indicating that there is no attachment loss. (Panel 1B *adapted from* Rateitschak KH, Rateitschak EW, Wolf HF, Hassel TM: *Color Atlas of Periodontology.* New York: Thieme; 1985.)

DISEASES OF BACTERIAL ETIOLOGY

Gingivitis

Gingivitis

Plaque-associated gingivitis
  Acute inflammatory gingivitis
  Chronic gingivitis
Acute necrotizing ulcerative gingivitis
Gingivitis associated with systemic conditions or medications
  Hormone-influenced gingivitis
  Drug-induced gingivitis
  Linear gingival erythema (HIV gingivitis)
Gingival manifestations of systemic diseases and mucocutaneous lesions
  Bacterial, viral, or fungal infection
  Blood dyscrasias
  Mucocutaneous disease
Other gingival changes

FIGURE 5-2 Gingivitis. Gingivitis is a nonspecific inflammatory reaction of the gingiva to a variety of irritants. Bacterial plaque is the most common etiologic agent, with a wide variety of microorganisms able to stimulate an acute or a chronic gingivitis. Gingivitis is a reversible disease, which rapidly responds to the removal of accumulations of bacterial plaque and improved oral hygiene. Marginal gingivitis that does not respond to proper oral hygiene may indicate the presence of another etiology, such as chronic mouth breathing, mechanical trauma, chemical or thermal trauma, and allergic reactions. Gingivitis may be exacerbated by systemic factors such as hormonal changes (pregnancy gingivitis), infections (HIV-associated gingivitis), neoplasms, blood dyscrasias, mucocutaneous diseases, or metabolic diseases (diabetes mellitus–associated gingivitis).

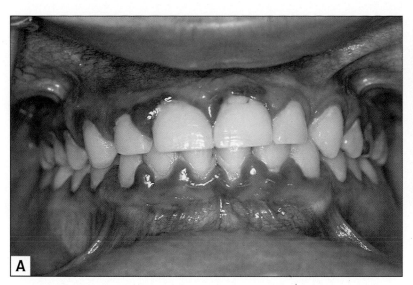

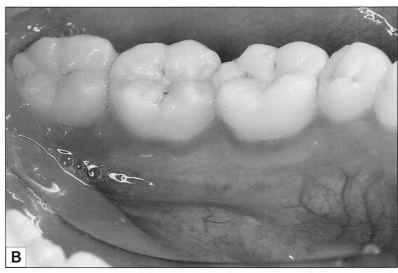

FIGURE 5-3 Acute inflammatory and chronic gingivitis. **A,** Acute gingivitis is characterized by an intense inflammatory response to direct injury or acute infection. The gingival tissue is highly erythematous and edematous and has varying levels of discomfort. Bleeding from the gingival crevicular area may be easily elicited or even spontaneous. A differential diagnosis includes necrotizing ulcerative gingivitis, primary herpetic gingivostomatitis, desquamative gingivitis, infectious mononucleosis, acute leukemia, agranulocytosis, and secondary syphilis. **B,** Chronic gingivitis is a more common form of gingivitis and is characterized by erythema, edema, and hypertrophy of the gingival tissues. Ulceration of the sulcular epithelium and proliferation into the corneum, a marked inflammatory infiltrate, and increased vascularity of the tissue are demonstrated clinically as bleeding on minimal manipulation of the gingival tissues. After a prolonged low-grade bacterial insult, the gingival tissue may become fibrotic, giving the appearance of normal gingival tissue. Chronic gingivitis is detectable by the presence of bleeding after gentle probing of the sulcus.

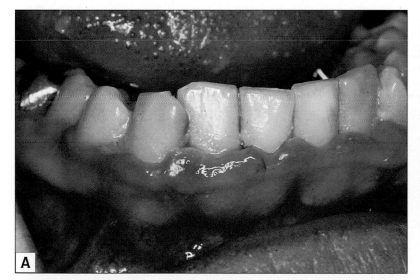

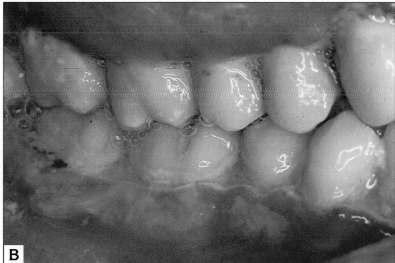

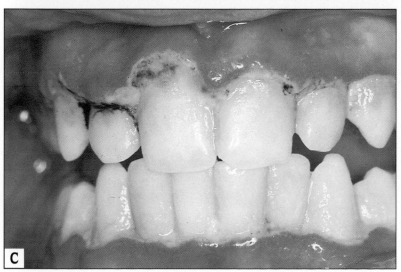

FIGURE 5-4 Acute necrotizing ulcerative gingivitis (ANUG). Also termed *Vincent's infection* and *trench mouth*, ANUG is a severe form of gingivitis associated with infection by spirochetes, fusiform bacteria, and *Prevotella intermedia*. This rapidly progressing infection is characterized by acute fiery-red gingivitis, soft-tissue necrosis with formation of a necrotic surface layer (referred to as a pseudomembrane), severe pain, fetid odor, and, at times, malaise, lymphadenopathy, and low-grade fever. The hallmark sign of ANUG is necrosis and cratering of the interproximal papillae, referred to as "punched-out papillae." **A–C,** ANUG may be localized (*panel 4A*), generalized (*panel 4B*), or generalized severe (*panel 4C*) in its presentation.

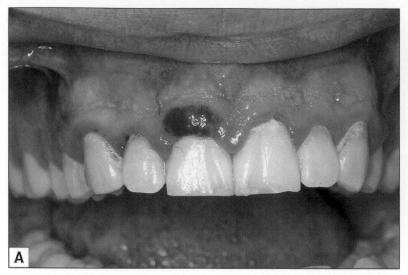

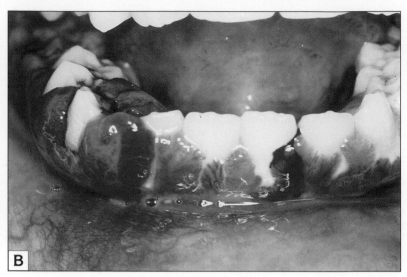

FIGURE 5-5 Hormone-influenced gingivitis (pregnancy gingivitis). An exaggerated growth of bacterial plaque may occur in response to hormonal changes associated with pregnancy, puberty, or menopause. Gingival changes start as a mild marginal inflammation, progressing to include interproximal and attached gingiva. Gingival bleeding on tooth brushing, flossing, or mechanical manipulation is common due to vascular hyperemia. This condition is generally reversible with meticulous oral hygiene and the return to normal hormone levels. **A** and **B**, Gingival hyperplasia, presenting clinically as a localized pyogenic granuloma (*panel 5A*) or generalized hyperplasia (*panel 5B*), can result as a long-term sequelae. Hyperplastic gingival enlargement may not be reversible and may require surgical intervention to reestablish normal contours.

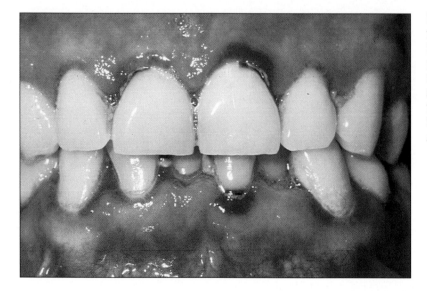

FIGURE 5-6 Linear gingival erythema (HIV gingivitis). An acute form of gingivitis can be seen in HIV infection. The microorganisms associated with such gingivitis are those common in bacterial plaque and associated with chronic gingivitis. The exaggerated response is an overreaction due to the immune-incompetent status of the patient. A distinctive linear erythematous pattern follows the free gingival margin, but the hallmark of HIV gingivitis is its resistance to conventional therapy. (*Courtesy of* D.A. Assad, DDS.)

Periodontitis

Periodontitis
Adult periodontitis
Early-onset periodontitis
Prepubertal (generalized or localized)
Juvenile (generalized or localized)
Rapidly progressive
Periodontitis associated with systemic disease
Necrotizing ulcerative periodontitis
Refractory periodontitis
Periapical periodontitis
Peri-implantitis

FIGURE 5-7 Periodontitis. Periodontitis is a group of microorganism-induced inflammatory diseases that lead to destruction of the supporting structures of the teeth, including the alveolar bone, periodontal ligament, and adjacent soft tissues. These diseases differ in etiology, clinical progression, and response to therapy. Adult periodontitis results from chronic bacterial infection that causes progressive destruction of the supporting structures of the teeth. Early-onset periodontitis is associated with underlying host immune defects and is seen in age groups ranging from children through adults. Systemic disease can predispose to more rapid progression of periodontitis.

Disease Stage	Signs and Symptoms	Presentation
Normal	Healthy coral-pink-colored gingiva Gingival margin tightly adapted to the teeth with a knife-edge margin Gingival papillae fill the interproximal space No loss of attachment; probe stops at the cementoenamel junction Shallow, 1–3 mm, sulcus depth	
Gingivitis	Bleeding on brushing, flossing, or gentle probing Gingiva inflamed and edematous with darker red color of papillae and marginal tissues No loss of connective tissue attachment	
Early periodontitis	Slight loss of connective tissue attachment to the tooth leading to 3–4-m pockets between the teeth and gingiva Slight bone loss on radiographs Inflammation and edema of gingiva with bleeding and possible suppuration	
Moderate periodontitis	Moderate horizontal and/or angular bone loss that may extend to involve furcation of multirooted teeth Attachment loss with 4–5-mm pockets between teeth and gingiva noted on probing Bleeding or suppuration from depths of pockets on probing Gingiva may appear inflamed or fibrotic Gingival recession may occur with exposure of roots	
Advanced periodontitis	Severe horizontal and/or angular bone loss that commonly extends to involve furcations of multirooted teeth Attachment loss and pockets >5 mm between the teeth and gingiva Teeth become mobile and may migrate out of normal position Gingiva may appear inflamed or fibrotic Gingival recession usually occurs with exposure of roots	

A

FIGURE 5-8 Adult periodontitis. **A**, Adult periodontitis results from a chronic bacterial infection that causes progressive destruction of the supporting tissues of the teeth. Gram-negative anaerobic microorganisms are considered etiologic agents of this disease and include (but are not limited to) *Actinobacillus actinomycetemcomitans*, *Porphyromonas gingivalis*, *Prevotella intermedia*, *Eikenella corrodens*, *Fusobacterium nucleatum*, *Wolinella recta*, and spirochetes. Subclassification of adult periodontitis as early, moderate, and advanced is based on the amount of bone and soft tissue lost to disease. (*continued*)

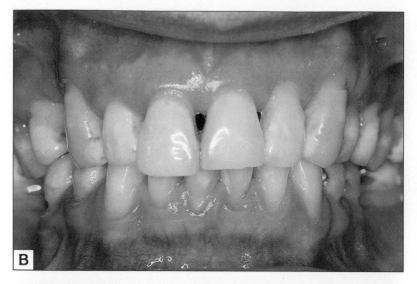

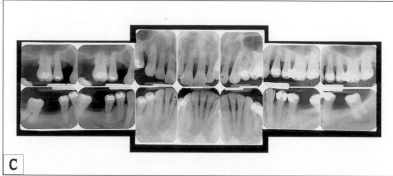

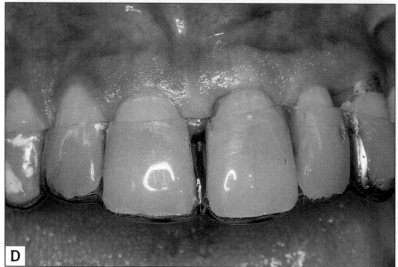

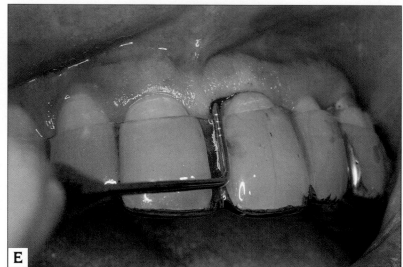

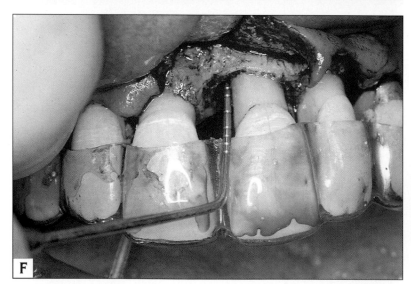

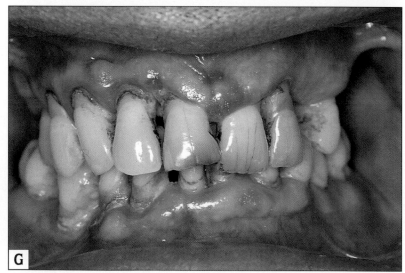

FIGURE 5-8 (*continued*) **B,** Most commonly, progression of the disease may not be clinically evident because little or no pain is involved, and the gingival tissues may become fibrotic and show little evidence of inflammation or recession while bone loss is continuing. **C,** Radiographic examination and probing of the periodontal pocket (shown in *panel 8B*) to evaluate the level of gingival attachment and bone support are required to provide early diagnosis of this disease. **D,** Clinically, the gingival tissue adjacent to the maxillary central incisors appears to be within normal limits.

E, However, when a 10-mm periodontal probe is used, attachment loss of 6–7 mm can be demonstrated. **F,** Upon surgical reflection of the gingiva, an obvious osseous defect is seen on the mesial of the maxillary left central incisor and intact alveolar bone on the maxillary right central incisor. **G,** Periodically, periodontitis may present with severe gingival recession, osseous loss, and mobile teeth in an obviously unclean state. (Panels 8B and 8C *courtesy of* T.A. Lafferty, DDS.)

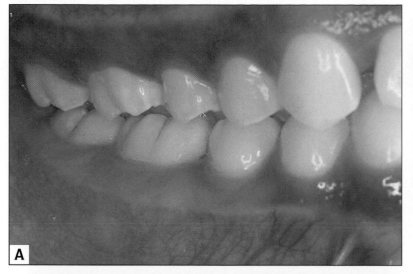

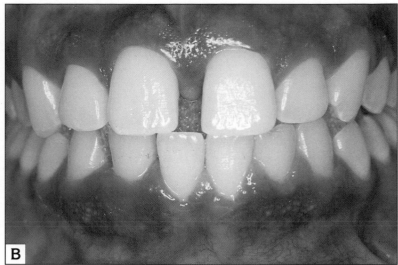

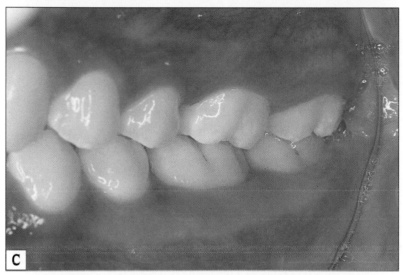

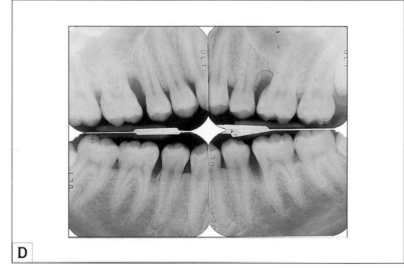

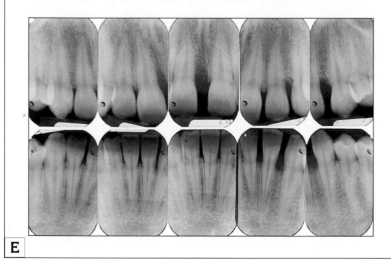

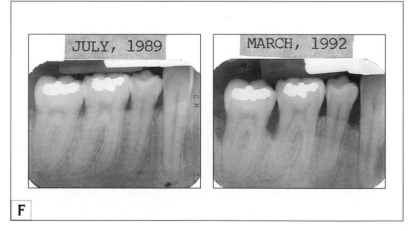

JULY, 1989   MARCH, 1992

FIGURE 5-9 Early-onset periodontitis. Early-onset periodontitis includes prepubertal, juvenile, and rapidly progressive forms. These forms are associated with varying degrees of host immune defects generally related to deficiency in leukocyte chemotaxis and phagocytosis. The most severe immune problems are encountered in patients with prepubertal periodontitis, which leads to tooth loss soon after eruption. **A–C,** Juvenile periodontitis is characterized by its association with minimal plaque accumulation and relative lack of clinically evident gingival inflammation. **D** and **E,** Bone loss in patients with juvenile periodontitis is first evident around puberty and may be generalized to all teeth or localized most commonly to the first molars and incisors. Severe bone loss can lead to tooth loss within a few years. Rapidly progressive periodontitis is a disease of young adults, through the third to fourth decades, which can present as an acute infection with severe gingival inflammation, rapid bone loss, malaise, elevated temperature, and tooth loss. **F,** Extensive osseous loss occurs over a relatively short time. (Panels 9A–9E *courtesy of* D.A. Assad, DDS.)

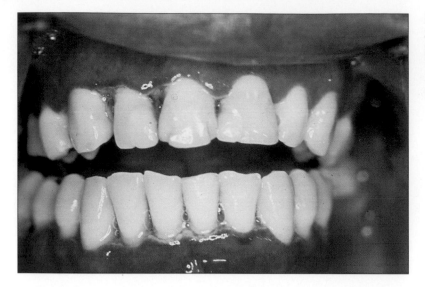

FIGURE 5-10 Periodontitis associated with systemic disease. Systemic disease may predispose an individual to more rapid progression of periodontitis. Such diseases include diabetes, HIV infection (as pictured), and any disease that decreases the immune system's ability to function effectively. (*Courtesy of D.A. Assad, DDS.*)

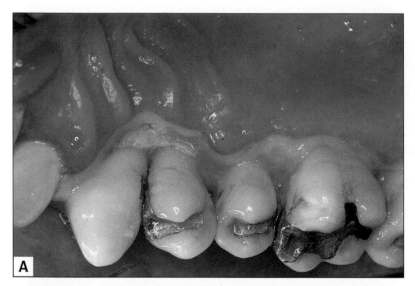

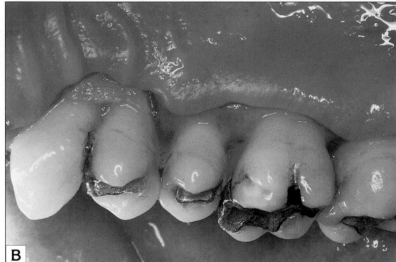

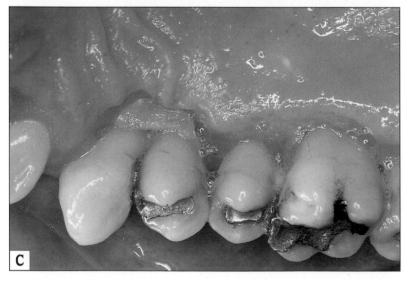

FIGURE 5-11 Necrotizing ulcerative periodontitis. **A**, Necrotizing ulcerative gingivitis, if untreated, progresses to an advanced stage with destruction of the supporting tissues of the teeth, including the alveolar bone and periodontal ligament. **B** and **C**, With periodontal therapy, the condition will resolve; after 3 days of therapy, the gingival tissues start to resolve (*panel 11B*), and at 3 weeks, gingival tissues progress with healing, but necrotic bone persists (*panel 11C*). This infection, if left untreated, rapidly leads to necrosis and loss of alveolar bone and ultimately to the loss of the affected teeth. The most severe form of this disease, usually seen in debilitated patients, is termed *noma* and can be life-threatening.

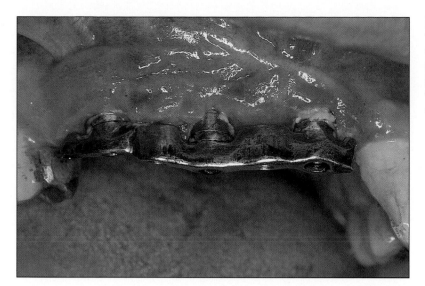

FIGURE 5-12 Peri-implantitis. Inflammation of the tissues adjacent to a dental implant due to the presence of bacterial plaque is termed *peri-implantitis*. This condition leads to hyperplastic gingivitis, bone loss, and, without treatment, loss of the dental implant. The bone loss noted in peri-implantitis must be differentiated from bone loss associated with occlusal trauma to permit effective treatment.

Abscesses

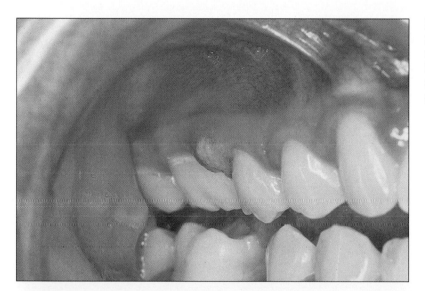

FIGURE 5-13 Gingival abscess. A localized acute infection of the marginal or interdental gingiva is usually caused by the impaction of a foreign object (*ie*, popcorn hull, peanut husk, toothbrush bristle, or toothpick splinter) that initiates the infection. Local debridement of dental plaque and removal of the foreign body are sufficient to abort the infection and permit healing.

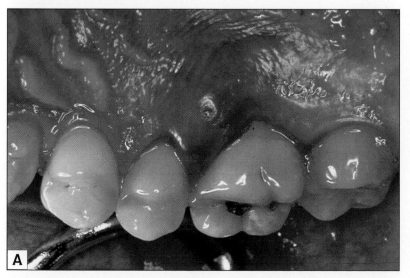

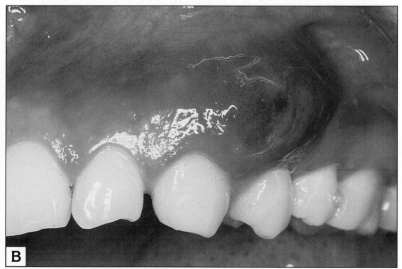

FIGURE 5-14 Periodontal abscess. A periodontal abscess is a localized purulent inflammatory process, which is initiated by the pathogenic organisms associated with periodontitis and involves the subgingival periodontal structures. Comprehensive evaluation of the patient usually shows generalized periodontal disease in conjunction with the periodontal abscess. Often, the abscess is associated with root surface accretions and deep tortuous periodontal pockets. Clinically, patients present with pain and percussion sensitivity, mobility, and slight elevation of the involved tooth, or with a feeling of "pressure in the gums." **A–C**, The periodontal abscess may present interproximally (*panel 14A*) or buccally (*panel 14B*) or in the furcation areas (*panel 14C*). (*continued*)

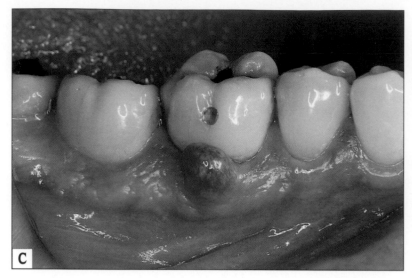

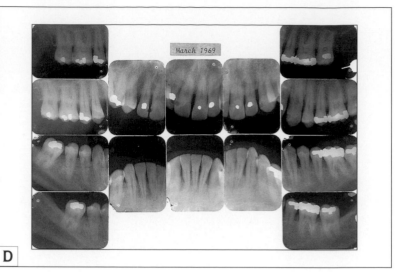

FIGURE 5-14 (*continued*) The periodontal abscess must be differentiated from abscesses resulting from necrosis of the dental pulp to ensure proper treatment. Clinical and radiographic evaluation combined with tests to determine the pulp vitality of the affected tooth help differentiate these lesions. **D**, Radiographically, the periodontal abscess is indistinguishable from the surrounding generalized osseous loss. Debridement of the affected root surface aborts the acute symptoms and leads to healing if the area is maintained plaque-free. The use of systemic antibiotics is rarely indicated.

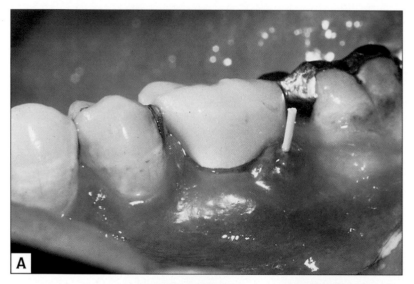

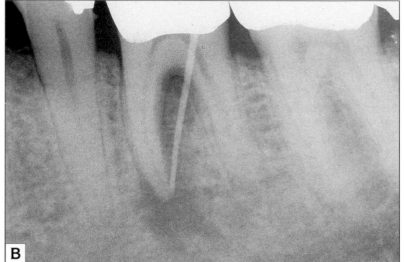

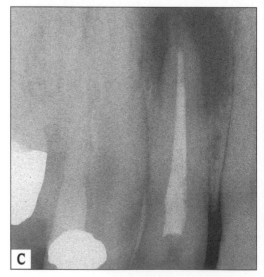

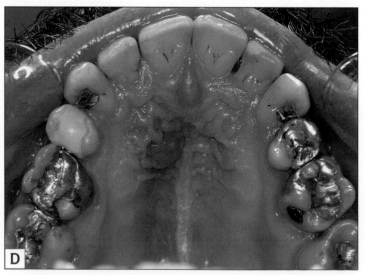

A and **B**, To diagnose, an opaque gutta-percha point may be inserted into the parulis (*panel 15A*), and a radiograph will demonstrate from which root apices the abscess is emanating (*panel 15B*). Removal of the necrotic pulp, debridement of the pulp canal, and filling the pulp canal with an occlusive material are required for healing. Untreated lesions become chronic and lead to localized osteomyelitis, cyst, or granuloma formation. **C** and **D**, Infrequently, a periapical abscess will not resolve following therapy (*panel 15C*), and the parulis will persist (*panel 15D*). Endodontic surgery is necessary in these cases. (Panels 15A and 15B *courtesy of* J.W. Hutter, DDS.)

FIGURE 5-15 Periapical abscess. Infection of the dental pulp, primarily due to caries, leads to pulpal necrosis and production of a purulent exudate, which drains through the root apex. This results in abscess formation with concurrent destruction of periapical bone. Severe pain associated with the affected tooth, which is relieved when the abscess is drained, is a hallmark of this lesion. The abscess may drain through the bone into the soft tissues to form a raised fluctuant boil (parulis) or perforate the tissue to form a sinus tract.

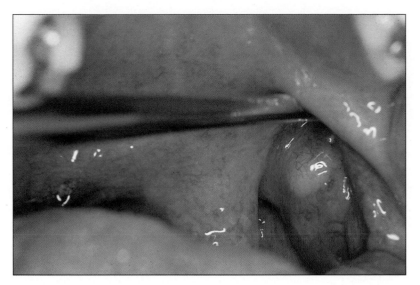

FIGURE 5-16 Peritonsillar abscess. Formation of a peritonsillar abscess may occur as a complication of acute tonsillitis caused by β-hemolytic streptococci. Acute abscess formation may cause pain, tonsillar swelling, and dysphagia. Extension of the infection to deeper structures of the neck can be life-threatening. The infection may be treated with penicillin or erythromycin once viral infections (such as mononucleosis or primary herpetic gingivostomatitis) have been ruled out.

Dental Caries

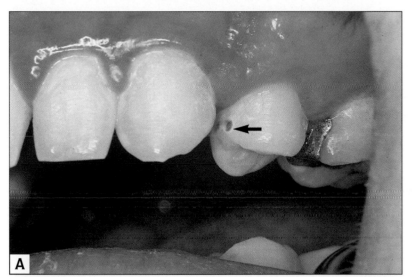

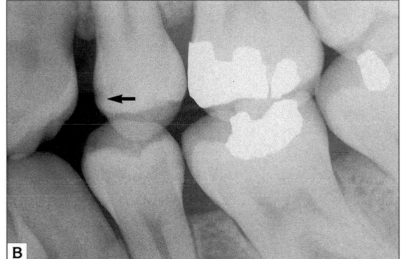

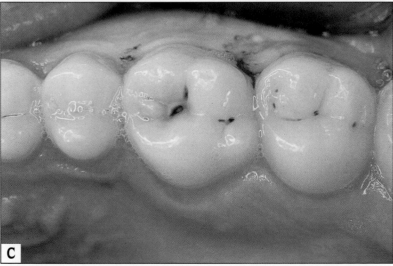

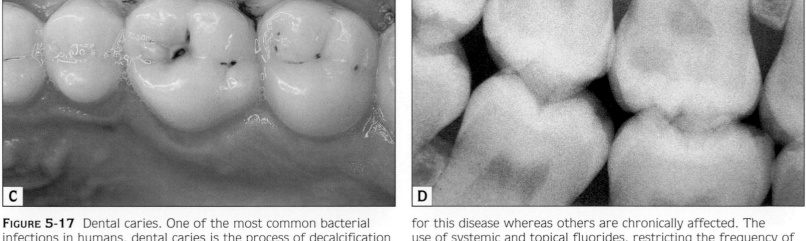

FIGURE 5-17 Dental caries. One of the most common bacterial infections in humans, dental caries is the process of decalcification of the inorganic portion of the tooth, followed by disintegration of the organic portion leading to cavitation. This disease is caused by the *Lactobacillus* and *Streptococcus mutans* class of acid-producing bacteria, which metabolize carbohydrates that have been ingested into the mouth and produce lactic acid, which in turn dissolves the mineralized portion of the tooth. Though this is considered a life-long disease, there are varying degrees of susceptibility within population groups. Some individuals remain at low risk for this disease whereas others are chronically affected. The use of systemic and topical fluorides, restricting the frequency of sucrose intake, and the removal of bacterial plaque are the major preventive measures used to control dental caries. **A–H,** Dental caries is subclassified principally by location, recurrence, and severity as coronal (smooth surface, *panels 17A* and *17B* [dental caries, *arrows*]; and fissure, *panels 17C* and *17D*), cervical and root (*panels 17E* and *17F*), recurrent (at the margins of dental restorations, *panel 17G*), (*continued*)

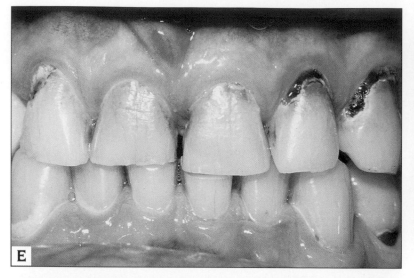

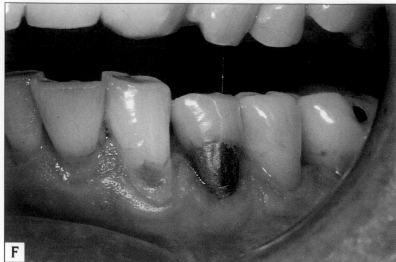

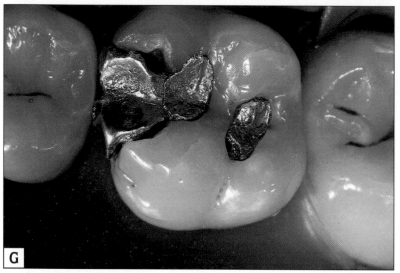

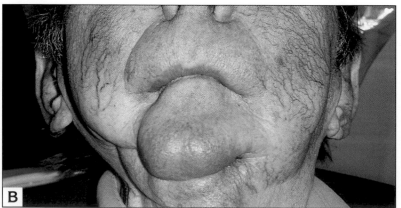

FIGURE 5-17 (*continued*) and rampant caries (*panel 17H*). Root caries increases in prevalence with age due to gingival recession, which exposes the root surface and makes it susceptible to colonization by caries-producing organisms. The etiology of root caries is similar to coronal caries, with the addition of *Actinomyces* sp. as causative organisms. Rampant caries is seen principally in young individuals with high sucrose intake and high lactobacillus counts and in xerostomic individuals. (Panels 17E, 17F, and 17H *courtesy of* J.C. Meiers, DDS; panel 17G *courtesy of* H. St. Germain, DDS.)

Oral Manifestations of Systemic Bacterial Diseases

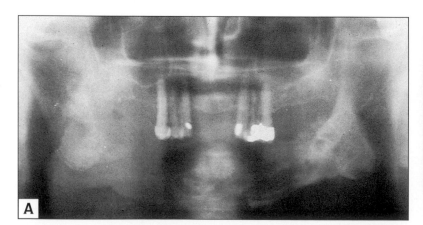

FIGURE 5-18 Osteomyelitis. Osteomyelitis is an infection of the bone, caused by pyogenic bacteria, which may remain localized or spread to the periosteum, cancellous and cortical bone, and marrow. **A**, On radiographs, the affected bone of the mandible has lost its normal trabeculation and demonstrates a mottled and inconsistent bony pattern. Osseous sequestra also may be discerned. Although this infection may be seen with periapical lesions associated with disease of the dental pulp, it most commonly occurs in patients with systemic disease or those who have received large doses of radiation therapy to the affected area. Radiation therapy causes fibrosis and decreased vascularity that becomes progressively more severe with time. Therefore, patients with a history of high-dose radiation therapy should be considered permanently predisposed to this infection. **B**, This patient, who previously received 6,000 rads for a squamous cell carcinoma of the retromolar pad, later developed osteomyelitis and clinically demonstrates chronic orocutaneous draining fistulas. (*continued*)

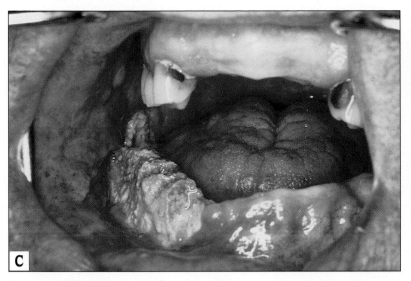

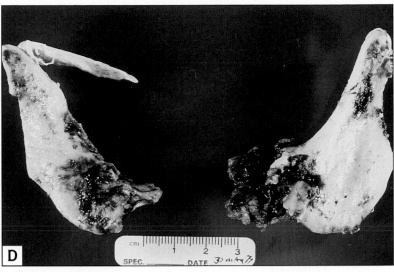

FIGURE 5-18 (*continued*) **C**, Intraorally, necrotic bone is sequestrating out of the gingival tissues. Therapy includes localized debridement, antibiotics, and use of hyperbaric oxygen. **D**, In advanced cases, surgical resection is necessary; a resected specimen demonstrates necrotic bone with a lack of vascular integrity. (*Courtesy of* D.P. Golden, DDS.)

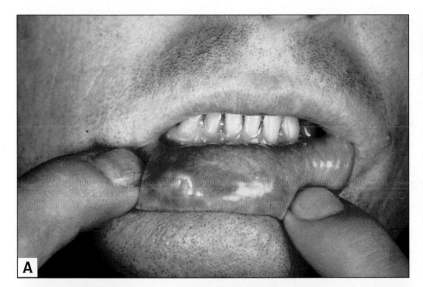

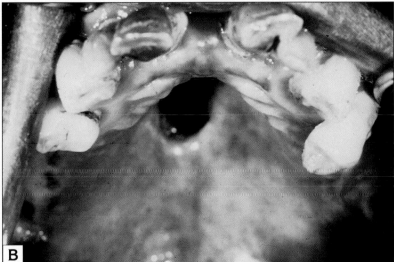

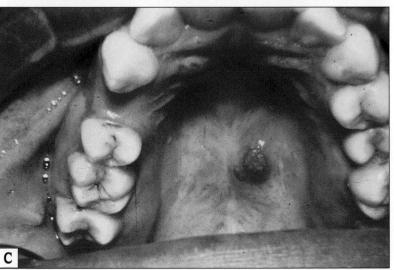

FIGURE 5-19 Syphilis. **A**, Syphilis, a venereal disease caused by a motile spirochete *Treponema pallidum*, is characterized by its primary lesion, the chancre. The chancre, an ulcerative indurated lesion with a slightly raised border and reddish-brown base, can occur on any of the oral mucous membranes. It occurs at the site of inoculation acquired by direct contact with a lesion of an infected individual. Secondary lesions of syphilis, which are highly infectious, include macules, papules, and mucous patches. **B** and **C**, Tertiary syphilis may give rise to atrophic glossitis, interstitial glossitis, and palatal perforation (*panel 19B*) resulting from a gumma (*panel 19C*). (*Courtesy of* G.R. Warnock, DDS.)

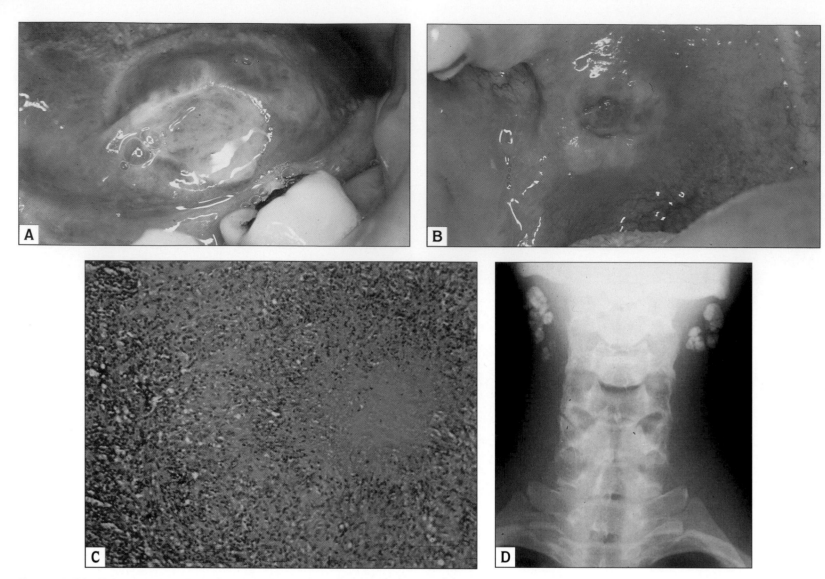

FIGURE 5-20 Tuberculosis. Oral tuberculosis is rare and usually secondary to well-established pulmonary tuberculosis. Dissemination of the *Mycobacterium tuberculosis* bacilli from the lungs to the oral cavity is via infected sputum, and the lesions are most commonly seen on the dorsum of the tongue, followed by the commissure of the lips. **A** and **B**, Lesions may be seen in other locations, such as the lateral border of the tongue (*panel 20A*) or the soft palate (*panel 20B*). Clinically, the lesion is an ulceration with a depressed, yellowish-gray necrotic center and a well-demarcated, undermined margin. The peripheral region is undulating and lumpy, sometimes described as "cobblestoned." **C**, Diagnosis is made by the isolation of the acid-fast *M. tuberculosis*, and histologically, the characteristic coalescent granulomas with central caseation and Langhans' giant cells are present. **D**, Radiographically, after healing, the lymph node lesions may calcify and are identified as the "Ghon complex." The primary lung lesion is treated with streptomycin and isoniazid. (*Courtesy of* D.P. Golden, DDS.)

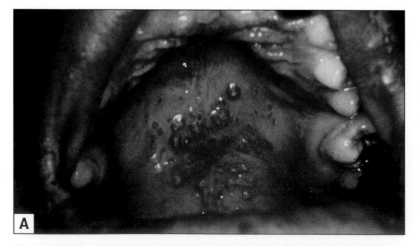

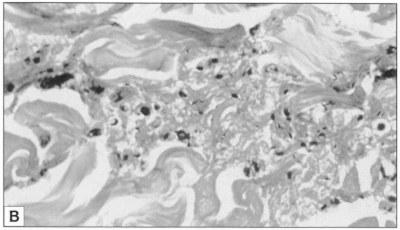

FIGURE 5-21 Leprosy. A slightly contagious granulomatous infection, leprosy is caused by an acid-fast bacillus, *Mycobacterium leprae*. Three forms of leprosy exist—lepromatous, dimorphous, and tuberculoid. **A**, Orally, the lesions (lepromas) appear as raised nodules, which have a tendency to ulcerate and are primarily located on the tongue, hard palate (shown here), and lips. **B**, Histologically, a granulomatous nodule demonstrates a fibrous stroma filled with lymphocytes and epithelioid cells and lepra cells, which are vacuolated macrophages containing the *M. leprae* bacilli. (*Courtesy of* G.R. Warnock, DDS.)

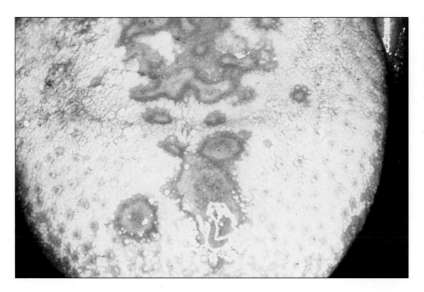

FIGURE 5-22 Gonorrhea. Gonorrhea is a venereal disease caused by *Neisseria gonorrhoeae* transmitted to the oral cavity either by urogenital sexual contact or by a gonococcemia in the bloodstream. Erosive vesiculobullous lesions may affect any of the oral tissues. Diagnosis is established by cultures. Oral lesions are infectious.

Actinomycosis

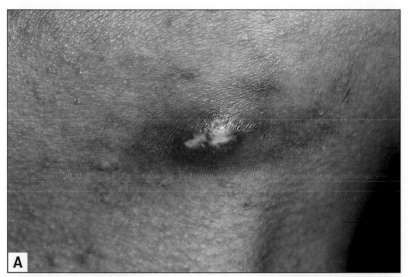

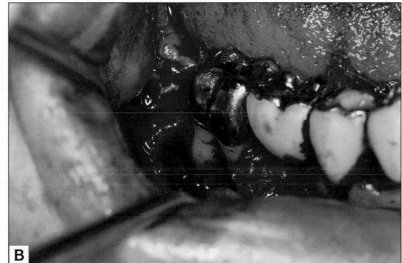

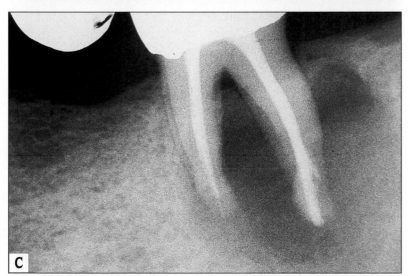

FIGURE 5-23 Actinomycosis. Actinomycosis is a suppurative and granulomatous infectious disease caused by *Actinomyces israelii* (called the "ray fungus" due to its histologic appearance of a central mass with raylike filaments). *A. israelii* is considered a constituent of the normal oral flora, with infection being endogenous in origin. Infection leads to suppuration, necrosis, and granulomatous tissue formation at the affected site. **A**, Most actinomycotic infections occur in the cervicofacial area. **B** and **C**, Clinical presentation may be as a nonhealing extraction site, severe bone loss around a tooth (*panels 23B and 23C*), multiple draining sinus tracts involving the alveolus, a nonhealing periapical infection, or as an indurated swelling of the tongue. (*continued*)

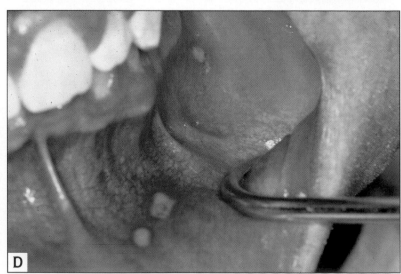

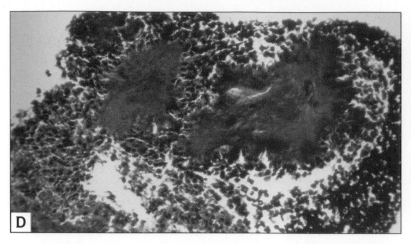

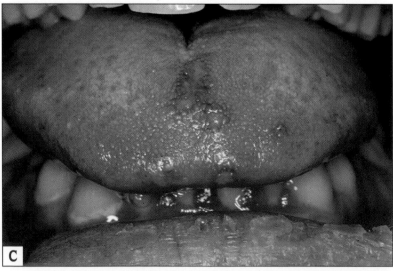

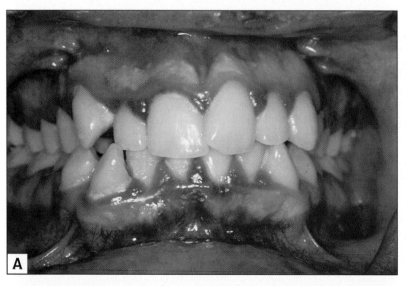

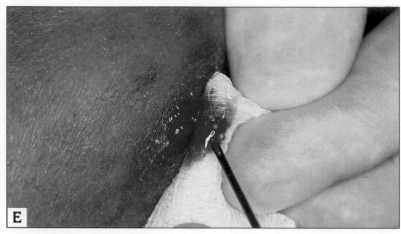

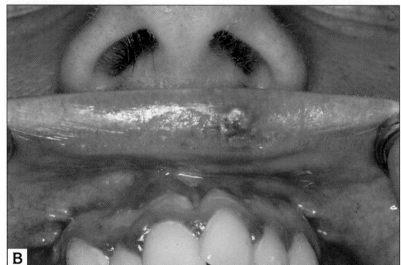

FIGURE 5-23 (*continued*) **D** and **E**, Diagnosis is based on identification of the organism histologically in tissue samples and the presence of "sulfur granules" in the suppurative exudate.

Treatment is generally protracted, including surgical debridement and antibiotic therapy. (Panels 23A and 23E *courtesy of* M.D. Callihan, DDS; panel 23C *courtesy of* G.R. Warnock, DDS.)

DISEASES OF VIRAL ETIOLOGY

FIGURE 5-24 Primary herpetic gingivostomatitis. Primary herpetic gingivostomatitis is a contagious disease caused by the herpes simplex virus type 1 and, less frequently, type 2. It may be subclinical or acute, affecting all of the soft tissues of the mouth including the gingiva, mucosa, tongue, lips, pharynx, and palate. **A–D**, Clinical signs include fiery red, swollen, and bleeding gingiva (*panel 24A*) and formation of clusters of small vesicles that burst to form yellowish ulcers with a circumscribing red halo (*panels 24B–24D*). The small ulcers may coalesce to form large ulcers. Symptoms include fever, malaise, and localized pain associated with ulceration. This phase of the infection usually regresses spontaneously in 10–14 days. Supportive treatment includes the use of a liquid diet, topical anesthetics, and acyclovir in severe cases. (*continued*)

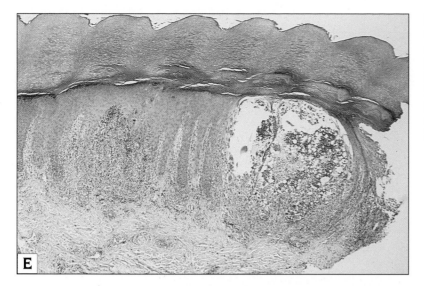

FIGURE 5-24 (*continued*) **E,** Histologically, the herpetic vesicle demonstrates intraepithelial splitting and cellular ballooning degeneration. Eosinophilic intranuclear inclusions (Lipschötz bodies) are characteristically present. Following the primary infection, the patient continues to harbor the virus, which can later reactivate causing recurrent herpes simplex lesions. Primary herpetic gingivostomatitis should be clinically differentiated from erythema multiforme, which can produce similar appearing oral lesions. (Panel 24E *courtesy of* G.R. Warnock, DDS.)

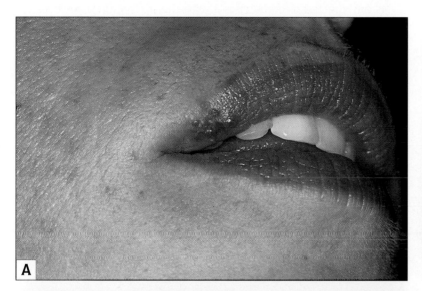

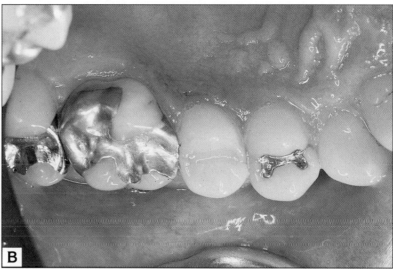

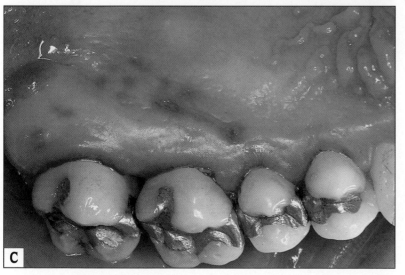

FIGURE 5-25 Recurrent herpes simplex (fever blister, cold sore). A secondary infection is caused by the reactivation of the dormant herpes simplex virus (HSV), which was retained following the primary viral infection. Reactivation of the virus is thought to occur due to precipitating events such as exposure to trauma, sunlight, heat, stress, or immunosuppressive therapy. A prodromal period, characterized by itching or burning in the area, precedes the formation of clusters of small vesicles, which then rupture to leave coalescing ulcers. Repeated occurrence at the same site is due to retention of HSV in nerve ganglia that innervate the affected area. **A–C,** The ulcerations are generally limited to the keratinized tissues of the lip (*panel 25A*), gingiva (*panel 25B*), and hard palate (*panel 25C*). Immunosuppressed patients may have more widespread recurrence of the disease. Autoinoculation from infected sites can occur as herpetic whitlow (finger), keratoconjunctivitis, and genital herpes. Therapy may include sunscreens to prevent recurrence, and the use of lysine, vitamin C, and acyclovir for frequent recurrences or in immunosuppressed patients.

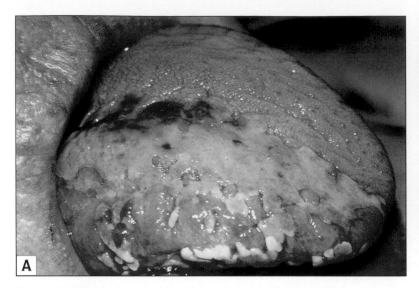

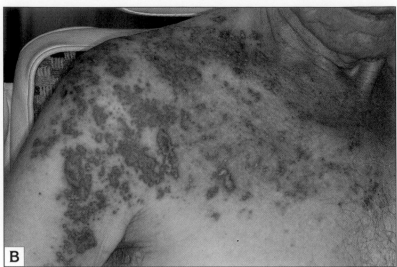

FIGURE 5-26 Herpes zoster. Herpes zoster ("shingles") is a recurrent infection by the varicella-zoster virus, which is the causative agent of chickenpox. **A,** Intraoral herpes zoster presents as vesicular and ulcerative lesions with a red border, which are distributed along the involved nerve pathway. **B,** The face and trunk are most commonly involved, with lesions ending abruptly at the midline. Prior to vesicle formation, patients may present with prodromal signs of itching and burning or paresthesia. Intense pain, malaise, fever, and distress are associated with the formation of the vesicular and ulcerative lesions. Healing occurs without scarring in approximately 3 weeks. Pain (posttherapeutic neuralgia) may persist for 6 months to 1 year after the lesions have healed. Therapy is principally supportive. (Panel 26A *courtesy of* C.L. Hatch, DDS.)

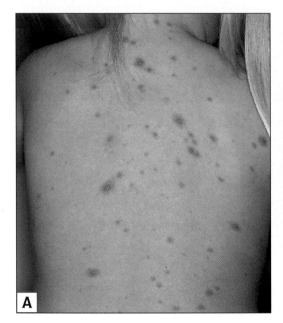

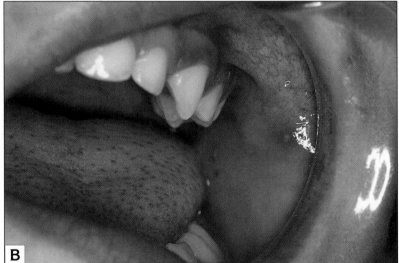

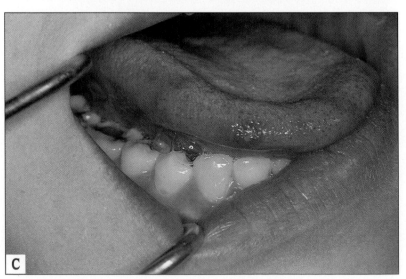

FIGURE 5-27 Chickenpox. Chickenpox, caused by the varicella-zoster virus, represents the primary infection by the virus whereas "shingles" is recognized as a recurrent infection by the same virus. The infection occurs generally in children in the winter and spring. **A,** A pruritic rash followed by vesicle and pustule formation involves the head, neck, trunk, and extremities. **B** and **C,** Intraoral lesions are usually limited to a few isolated vesicles on the soft palate or buccal mucosa, which rupture to form ulcers with erythematous borders. Patients present with fever, chills, musculoskeletal aches, and malaise. Healing occurs in 7–10 days. Therapy is supportive.

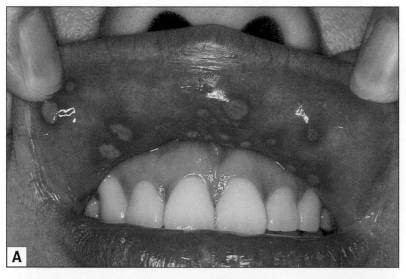

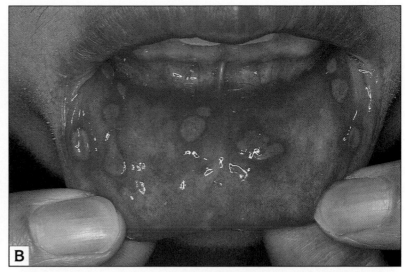

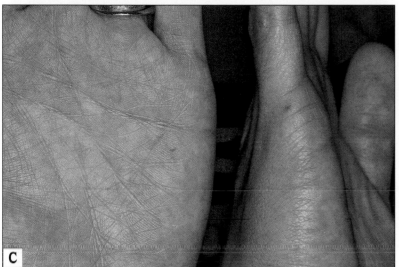

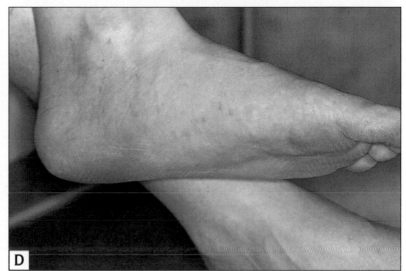

FIGURE 5-28 Hand, foot, and mouth disease. Hand, foot, and mouth disease is a viral infection caused by a number of coxsackie A and B viruses. This disease of young adults usually occurs in the spring and summer. **A–D**, It presents as ulcerative lesions of the mouth and lips (*panels 28A* and *28B*), with an associated rash on the hands and feet (*panels 28C* and *28D*). Ulcerative areas repre- sent multiple pinpoint vesicles that rupture to form coalescent ulcers. Intraorally, the tongue, palate, and buccal and labial mucosa and pharynx are the most commonly involved areas. Patients present with pain, malaise, elevated temperature, and lymphadenopathy. Healing occurs in about 10 days. (Panels 28A–28C *courtesy of* R. Holderman, DDS.)

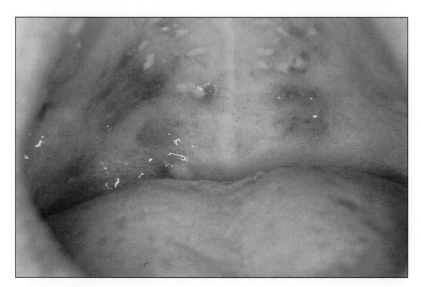

FIGURE 5-29 Herpangina. Herpangina is a highly contagious disease of children and young adults caused primarily by retro- viruses, coxsackie B, or ECHO viruses. Intraoral vesicles, which rupture to form multiple ulcers with erythematous borders, are seen limited to the soft palate and uvula, anterior pillars of the fauces, and tonsils. Patients may present with a painful sore throat, fever, lymphadenopathy, and malaise. The lesions are active for 3–5 days, followed by rapid healing. Treatment is supportive. (*Courtesy of* R. Holderman, DDS.)

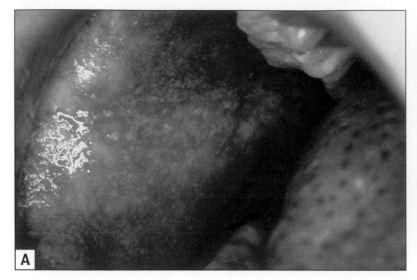

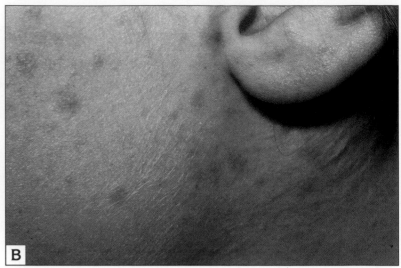

FIGURE 5-30 Measles. Measles is a common, contagious, acute viral infection primarily affecting children. Following an incubation period of approximately 9 days, initial clinical symptoms include fever, malaise, conjunctivitis, photophobia, cough, and eruptive lesions on the oral mucosa and skin. **A,** The oral lesions (Koplik's spots) precede the dermal lesions by 2–3 days and are pathognomonic for this disease. They usually occur on the buccal mucosa and appear as small irregularly shaped macules with a bluish-white center and a bright red margin. Within days, they coalesce to form small erythematous patches. **B,** The dermal lesions are initially small erythematous macules, which coalesce to form blotchy irregular lesions. The lesions initially and characteristically appear on the hairline of the head and behind the ears and then spread to the rest of the body. (*Courtesy of* F.J. Kratochvil, III, DDS.)

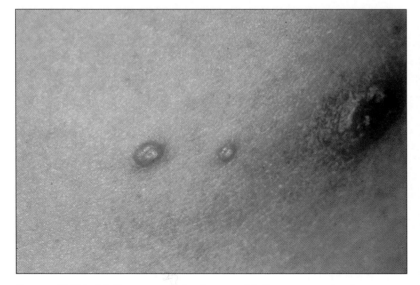

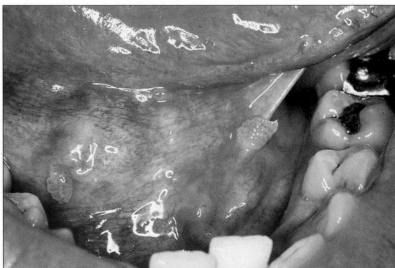

FIGURE 5-31 Molluscum contagiosum. Molluscum contagiosum presents on the skin as isolated or multiple small waxy papules with depressed centers. Lesions, most commonly seen on the inner thigh and external genitalia, are the result of epithelial proliferation in response to viral infection. Intraoral lesions, as seen here on the lingual frenum, are rare but have been reported on the lips, buccal mucosa, and other oral areas. Diagnosis is by clinical evaluation supplemented with scraping or biopsy and histologic examination to identify molluscum bodies. Treatment is unnecessary because most lesions resolve spontaneously in 1–3 months.

FIGURE 5-32 Condyloma acuminatum. Condyloma acuminatum (venereal warts) appear clinically identical to the intraoral papilloma (*see* Fig. 5-34). Clinically, they present initially as multiple small nodules, which proliferate and coalesce to form soft sessile or pedunculated papillary lesions. The human papillomavirus types 6 and 11 are considered the etiologic agents. A history of orogenital sexual contact between similarly infected individuals, particularly with multiple recurrences, helps to confirm the diagnosis. Treatment is by complete excision. (*Courtesy of* F.J. Kratochvil, III, DDS.)

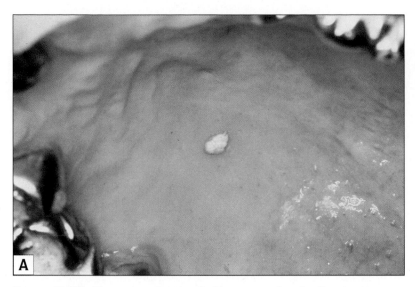

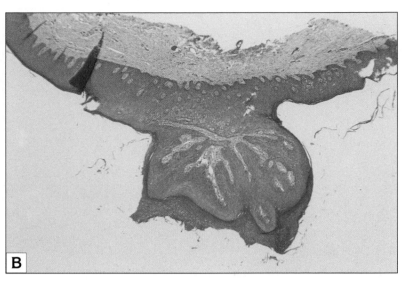

FIGURE 5-33 Verruca vulgaris. **A**, Verruca vulgaris, the common wart, is a benign exophytic growth, which intraorally presents with the same surface characteristics as the papilloma (*see* Fig. 5-34), *ie*, as a pedunculated mass with a surface that can vary from smooth, pink, and pebbly to one with multiple white feathery projections. It is thought to be caused by the human papillomavirus type 2 or 4. It can occur anywhere on the skin but is most common on the hands. Intraoral verruca may occur as a result of autoinoculation. **B**, Histologically, verruca vulgaris has a wider and thicker connective tissue base and viral inclusion bodies not present in the papilloma. Treatment is by complete excision including the base or by freezing with liquid nitrogen. (Panel 33B *courtesy of* G.R. Warnock, DDS.)

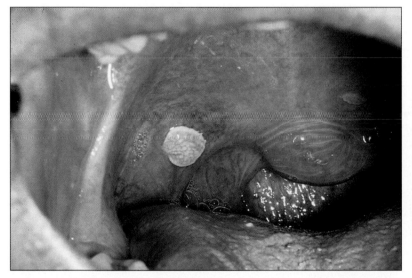

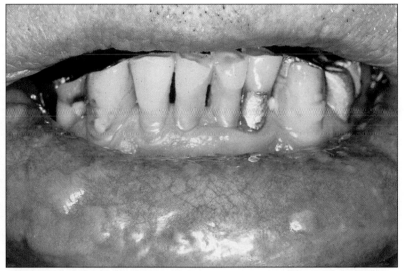

FIGURE 5-34 Papilloma. Papilloma is a common benign neoplasm of the oral cavity thought to be caused by human papillomavirus (HPV) types 6 and 11. It presents as a slow-growing pedunculated mass with a surface that can vary from smooth, pink, and pebbly to one with multiple white feathery projections. Papillomas are most frequently seen on the hard and soft palate but are also common to the tongue, lips, gingiva, and buccal mucosa. Treatment is by complete excision including the base. Differentiation from other HPV-induced lesions, such as condyloma acuminatum, focal epithelial hyperplasia (Heck's disease), and verruca vulgaris requires histologic evaluation.

FIGURE 5-35 Focal epithelial hyperplasia (Heck's disease). Focal epithelial hyperplasia is thought to be caused by human papillomavirus type 13 or 32 and is seen most often in North American Eskimos and Indians and South American Indians aged 3–18 years. The lesions present as multiple sessile-based nodules that are 1–5 mm in diameter. They are whitish in color and occur primarily on the mandibular labial mucosa or buccal mucosa and almost never occur on the palate or floor of the mouth. No treatment is necessary as the lesions undergo spontaneous remission in 4–6 months.

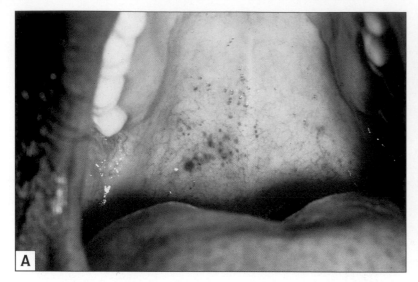

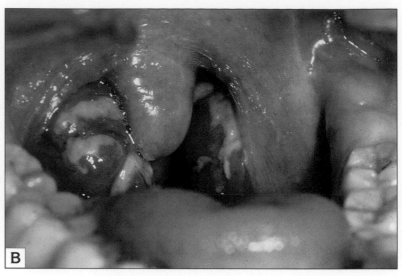

FIGURE 5-36 Infectious mononucleosis. Infectious mononucleosis is an infection, principally of children and young adults, caused by the Epstein-Barr virus. The disease is mildly contagious, with outbreaks noted in closed communities. **A** and **B**, Intraoral lesions present as red palatal petechiae located at the junction of the hard and soft palates (*panel 36A*), ulcerative gingivitis, pharyngeal ulcerations, and an erythematous exudative tonsillitis (*panel 36B*).

Bilateral lymphadenopathy of the posterior cervical lymph nodes is the most consistent diagnostic sign. Mild debilitation, fever, malaise, pharyngitis, and stomatitis are common clinical symptoms. Treatment is supportive and should include rest, soft diet, analgesics, and antipyretics. Healing and recovery from other symptoms usually occurs in 1–2 months. (Panel 36A *courtesy of* C.L. Hatch, DDS.)

DISEASES OF FUNGAL ETIOLOGY

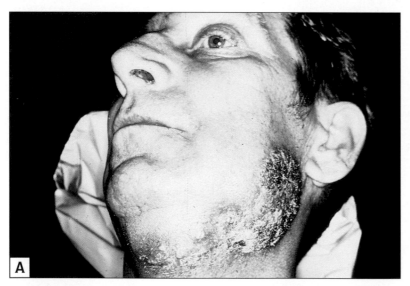

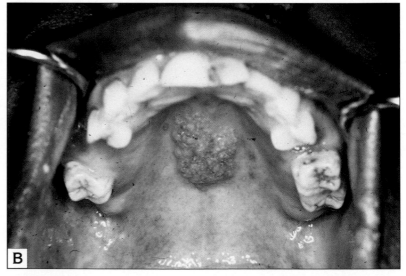

FIGURE 5-37 North American blastomycosis. Blastomycosis is caused by *Blastomyces dermatitidis*, which can grow in a yeast or mycelial phase. This infection is prevalent in the mid-Atlantic and southeastern United States but is also found in Central and South America. **A**, It generally occurs as a pulmonary or systemic infection, with spreading to the skin. **B**, Intraorally, the infection presents as a chronic nonhealing ulcer with a warty surface. Oral

lesions (25%) are secondary to the primary pulmonary infection, which can be chronic with mild symptoms that inhibit detection. Diagnosis involves biopsy to identify pseudoepitheliomatous hyperplasia that resembles malignant changes, combined with chest radiography to identify pulmonary lesions. Treatment involves the use of antifungal agents. (*Courtesy of* G.R. Warnock, DDS.)

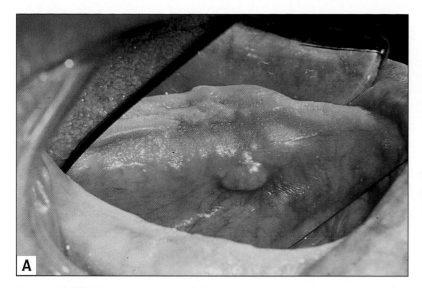

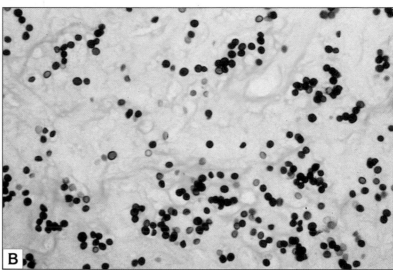

FIGURE 5-38 Histoplasmosis. Histoplasmosis is caused by *Histoplasma capsulatum*, a yeast-type fungus transferred in the excrement of birds and bats. **A**, Oral lesions may present as a papule, nodule, vegetation, or ulcer and are usually secondary to a pulmonary infection. Untreated lesions progress from papule to nodule to an enlarging ulceration resembling squamous cell carcinoma. **B**, Diagnosis is by biopsy or culture to identify the yeast organism. Treatment is with antifungal agents. (*Courtesy of* G.R. Warnock, DDS.)

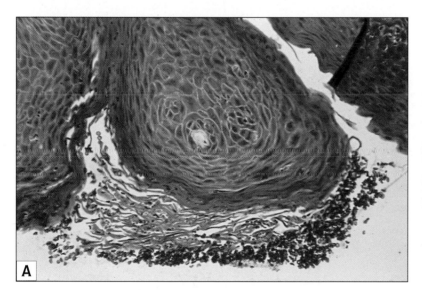

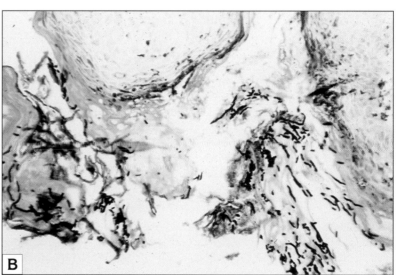

FIGURE 5-39 Candidiasis. Candidiasis is caused by various *Candida* species, which are yeastlike fungi. **A** and **B**, *Candida albicans* is the most commonly isolated species, histologically demonstrating budding yeast cells (*panel 39A*) and pseudohyphae (*panel 39B*). Candida has been identified as an isolate from a variety of clinical lesions, including pseudomembranous candidiasis (thrush), angular cheilitis, antibiotic sore mouth, denture stomatitis, and chronic hyperplastic candidiasis (candida leukoplakia). It is a normal member of the oral flora that is low in virulence and is considered an opportunistic pathogen. Infection by candida usually indicates a lowering of the host's resistance or a change in the oral flora that permits candida to predominate. Its presence as a secondary infection in lesions such as angular cheilitis and erythema multiforme may mask the underlying disease process. Factors that may precipitate candida infections include prolonged use of broad-spectrum antibiotics, chemotherapy, immunosuppressive drugs, irradiation, steroid therapy, and systemic or local disease that affects the patient's immune response. Treatment involves the use of a variety of topical and systemic antifungal medications. (*Courtesy of* G.R. Warnock, DDS.)

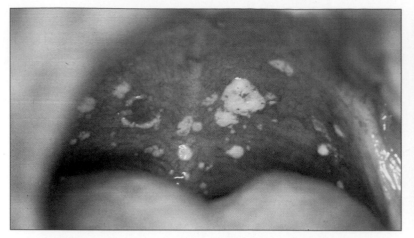

FIGURE 5-40 Pseudomembranous candidiasis (thrush). Thrush presents clinically as white patches on the oral mucosa, which wipe off to reveal a red or ulcerated area. Diagnosis is made by clinical appearance and demonstration of the organism on a stained smear from the lesion.

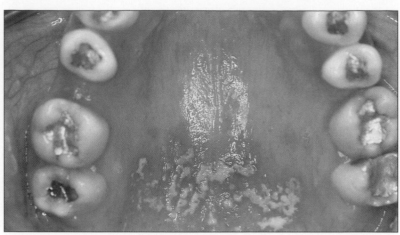

FIGURE 5-41 Chronic hyperplastic candidiasis. The condition presents clinically as a white, pebbly surfaced, slightly raised plaque or leukoplakia. Scattered erythematous areas may be noted. The plaque represents a hyperplastic response by the epithelium to the invading organism. The plaque will not wipe off as with pseudomembranous candidiasis. Biopsy and periodic acid–Schiff stain help make the diagnosis.

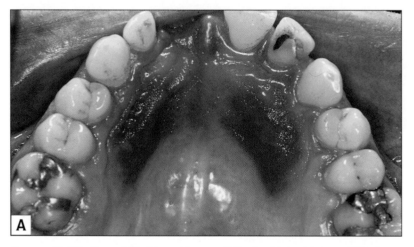

A

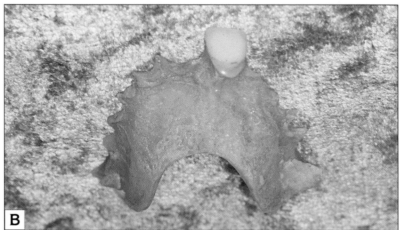

B

FIGURE 5-42 A and **B**, Atrophic candidiasis. Atrophic candidiasis presents clinically as an erythematous area under a denture base and is clinically diagnosed as denture stomatitis caused by an ill-fitting denture. Trauma from the denture is suspected as a precipitating or perpetuating factor for a candidal infection.

HIV-RELATED ORAL LESIONS

HIV-related oral lesions: Group I

Candidiasis
  Pseudomembranous candidiasis (thrush)
  Erythematous candidiasis
  Hyperplastic candidiasis
  Angular cheilitis
Oral hairy leukoplakia
Recurrent herpes simplex
Condyloma acuminatum
Linear gingival erythema (HIV gingivitis)
Kaposi's sarcoma
Acute necrotic ulcerative gingivitis
Necrotizing ulcerative periodontitis (HIV periodontitis)

FIGURE 5-43 HIV-related infections of the oral cavity include fungal, viral, bacterial, and neoplastic diseases. These infections may be frequent, severe, persistent, and recurrent and often are early prognosticators of the HIV infection. These oral lesions have been classified according to their relative frequency and association with HIV infections, with the most strongly associated oral lesions in group I listed here. Candidiasis is the most common oral lesion and usually the initial manifestation of symptomatic HIV infection (*see* Fig. 5-38). Pseudomembranous candidiasis is seen mostly in advanced stages of HIV infection and has a negative prognostic value (*see* Fig. 5-40). Erythematous candidiasis is an early oral manifestation of HIV infection, presenting as an erythematous area on the dorsum of the tongue and palate. Hyperplastic candidiasis (*see* Fig. 5-41) and angular cheilitis candidiasis (*see* Fig. 5-44) are candidal infections also in group I. Other noncandidal group I conditions include recurrent herpes simplex (*see* Fig. 5-25), condyloma acuminatum (*see* Fig. 5-32), linear gingival erythema (HIV gingivitis, *see* Fig. 5-6), acute necrotizing ulcerative gingivitis (*see* Fig. 5-4), necrotizing ulcerative periodontitis (HIV periodontitis, *see* Figs. 5-10 and 5-11), oral hairy leukoplakia (*see* Fig. 5-45), and Kaposi's sarcoma (*see* Fig. 5-46).

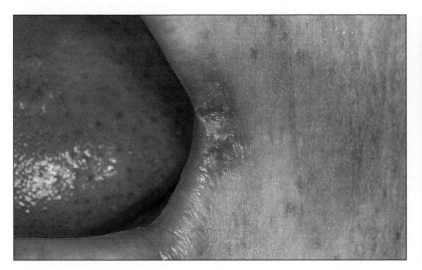

FIGURE 5-44 Angular cheilitis candidiasis (perlèche). Angular cheilitis occurs in the commissure of the mouth and consists of erythematous, possibly ulcerated, fissures with overlying white plaques. The fissures are confined to the external epithelial surfaces and do not involve the mucosal surface of the commissures inside the mouth. Angular cheilitis may occur in children and adults, and its symptoms include dryness and a burning sensation at the corners of the mouth. Theoretical etiologies include an intraoral candidal infection, overclosure of the jaws (such as in a denture patient who has lost vertical dimension), and riboflavin deficiency.

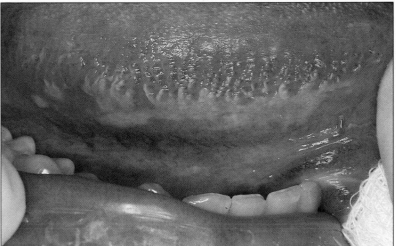

FIGURE 5-45 Oral hairy leukoplakia. A newly described oral lesion, oral hairy leukoplakia is highly predictive of the development of AIDS and indicative of the patient's immune status. It most often develops bilaterally on the lateral surfaces of the tongue, appearing as white corrugations, flat plaques, or shaggy plaques with hairlike projections, and is asymptomatic to the patient. Histologically, hyperparakeratosis, hyperplastic acanthosis, hairlike keratin projections, and ballooning cytopathic alterations of the spinous layer are seen. Its etiology is unclear but is thought to involve either Epstein-Barr virus or human papillomavirus. It does not respond to antifungal therapy. Because it is asymptomatic and not associated with complications, treatment is not indicated.

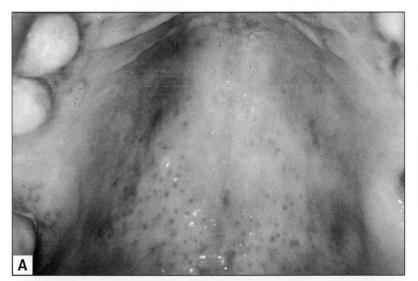

A

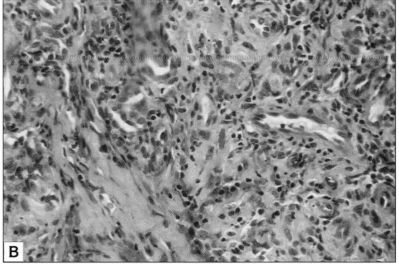

B

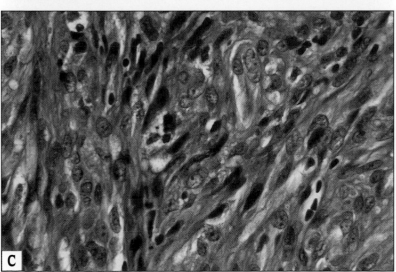

C

FIGURE 5-46 Kaposi's sarcoma. The most common malignancy associated with HIV infection, Kaposi's sarcoma affects approximately 20% of all AIDS patients. It is a tumor of vascular proliferation affecting the mucosal and cutaneous tissues; orally, it occurs primarily on the palate followed by the gingiva and buccal mucosa. **A,** The initial lesion is an asymptomatic red macule that enlarges to a red-blue plaque. The advanced lesion presents as lobulated, blue-violet nodules that ulcerate and cause pain. **B,** Histologically, the early Kaposi's lesion resembles a pyogenic granuloma, with a proliferation of perivascular immature spindle cells. (*Courtesy of* G.R. Warnock, DDS.) C, The advanced lesion is characterized by an increased spindle-cell cellularity, resembling a fibrosarcoma with numerous slitlike vascular spaces. Radiation and chemotherapy treatments are only palliative. (*Courtesy of* F.J. Kratochvil, III, DDS.)

DISEASES OF UNKNOWN ETIOLOGY (SUSPECTED INFECTIOUS)

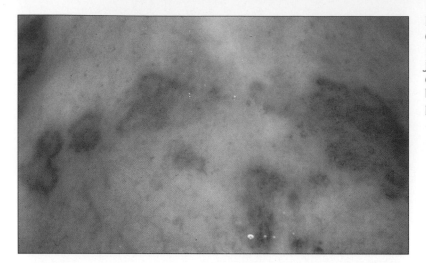

FIGURE 5-47 Reiter's syndrome. Reiter's syndrome is of unknown etiology, but HLA-B27 is present in 80% to 98% of the patients. It is a tetrad, manifesting a nonspecific urethritis, arthritis, conjunctivitis, and mucocutaneous lesions. Oral lesions are painless, erythematous, slightly elevated vesicles that have white circinate borders. They occur on the buccal mucosa, lips, gingiva, and palate. Treatment consists of antibiotic and corticosteroid therapy.

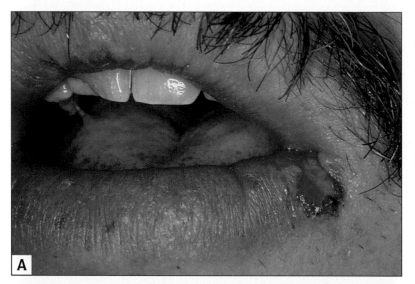

A

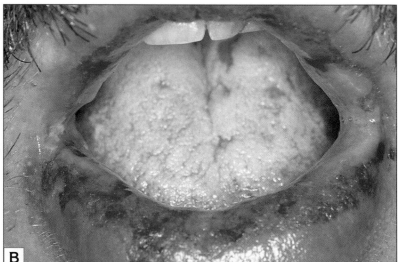

B

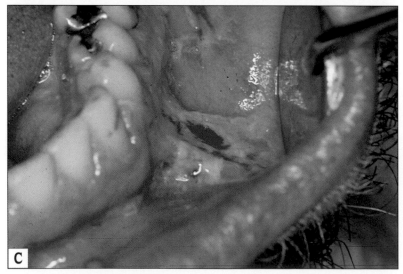

C

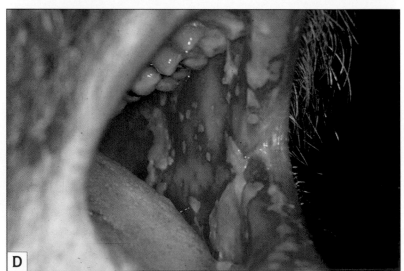

D

FIGURE 5-48 Erythema multiforme. Erythema multiforme is an acute disease affecting the oral tissues and skin, which is thought to represent an immune reaction to a wide variety of bacterial, viral, and fungal infections and to other antigens, including food and drugs. However, in most cases the causative agent cannot be determined. Clinically, patients present with very rapid onset of ulceration, severe pain, fever, malaise, and dysphagia. **A,** In this patient, the initial lesion was located at the commissure of the lip. **B,** Two days later, the ulcerations encompassed the entire mandibular and maxillary lips. **C** and **D,** Intraorally, the disease presents as multiple vesicles or bullae that rupture to leave a raw exudative crusting surface. Target lesions on the skin and cytologic smear for herpesvirus help to differentiate this disease from primary herpetic gingivostomatitis. Treatment involves supportive therapy with analgesics, topical anesthetic mouthwash, and a soft or liquid diet. Severe cases may require intravenous fluid therapy and short-term high-dose steroids. Extension of lesions to involve skin, mouth, eyes, and genitalia is called Stevens-Johnson syndrome.

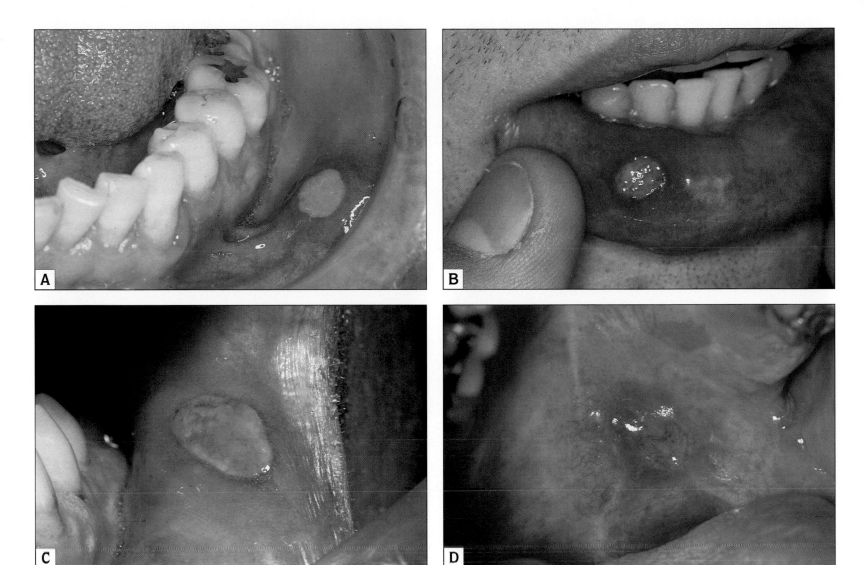

FIGURE 5-49 Recurrent aphthous stomatitis. **A** and **B**, Recurrent aphthous stomatitis clinically presents as single or multiple painful ulcerations of the buccal and labial mucosa. It is considered to be an immune reaction to oral bacteria, particularly *Streptococcus sanguis* 2A. Up to six recurrences per year are common. Minor lesions are 0.3–1.0 cm in diameter and heal within 10–14 days of onset. **C** and **D**, Major aphthae range in size from 1.0–5.0 cm (Sutton's disease, periadenitis mucosa necrotica recurrens) and can be disabling due to their frequent recurrences, severe pain, and prolonged duration of months. This disease may actually represent a spectrum of diseases that ranges from minor aphthae to major aphthae to Behçet's disease, which presents as ulcerative lesions of the oral cavity, eyes, and genitals. Treatment includes analgesics and topical corticosteroids for minor aphthae and topical tetracycline and steroid mouthrinse or lozenges in refractory cases of major aphthae.

SUGGESTED BIBLIOGRAPHY

Ficarra G, Shillitoe EJ: HIV-related infections of the oral cavity. *Crit Rev Oral Biol Med* 1992, 3:207–231.

Langlais RP, Miller CS: *Color Atlas of Common Oral Diseases*. Philadelphia: Lea & Febiger; 1992.

Lynch MA, Brightman VJ, Greenberg MS: *Burket's Oral Medicine*, 9th ed. Philadelphia: J.B. Lippincott Co.; 1994.

Pindborg JJ: *Atlas of Diseases of the Oral Mucosa*, 5th ed. Copenhagen: Musksgaard; 1992.

Wood NK, Goaz PW: *Differential Diagnosis of Oral Lesions*, 4th ed. St. Louis: C.V. Mosby; 1991.

CHAPTER 6

Pharyngotonsillitis

Harris R. Stutman

ETIOLOGY

A. Etiologic agents of pharyngotonsillitis: Bacteria

	Common (> 10%)	Uncommon (< 5%)	Rare (< 1%)
Bacteria	GABHS	*Arcanobacterium hemolyticum*	*Neisseria gonorrhoeae* *Neisseria meningitidis* *Corynebacterium diphtheriae* *Bacillus pertussis* *Francisella tularensis* *Treponema pallidum*

GABHS—group A β-hemolytic streptococci.

B. Etiologic agents of pharyngotonsillitis: Viruses

	Common (> 5%)	Uncommon (< 5%)	Rare (< 1%)
Viruses	Epstein-Barr Adenoviruses Coxsackie A Influenza A/B	Parainfluenzae Herpes simplex CMV	Measles Rubella HHV-6

CMV—cytomegalovirus; HHV-6—human herpesvirus type 6.

C. Etiologic agents of pharyngotonsillitis: Other causes

Common	Uncommon (< 5%)	Rare (< 1%)
Mycoplasma	*Mycoplasma pneumoniae*	*Chlamydia trachomatis*
Chlamydia	*Chlamydia pneumoniae*	
Fungi	*Candida* spp.	
Others	Kawasaki disease Aphthous stomatitis	Cyclic neutropenia Stevens-Johnson syndrome

FIGURE 6-1 Etiologic agents of pharyngotonsillitis. Pharyngitis or pharyngotonsillitis ("sore throat") is an inflammatory disorder of the posterior oral cavity involving the lymphoid tissues of the posterior pharynx and lateral pharyngeal bands and is caused by several groups of microorganisms. **A**, Bacteria. The group A β-hemolytic streptococci (GABHS) are the most important of the bacterial infections, with *Streptococcus pyogenes* causing approximately 15% to 30% of all cases of pharyngitis. **B**, Viruses. Most cases of pharyngotonsillitis are of viral etiology and occur as part of common colds or influenzal syndromes due to common respiratory viruses. Adenovirus and herpes simplex virus pharyngitis, although less common, are notable for their clinical severity. **C**, Other causes. *Mycoplasma pneumoniae* and *Chlamydia trachomatis* are less common causes of pharyngotonsillitis. Noninfectious causes also may be responsible for some cases.

Common causes of pharyngotonsillitis

Group A β-hemolytic streptococci
Epstein-Barr virus
Adenovirus
Influenza A or B virus
Coxsackie A viruses
Parainfluenzae viruses

FIGURE 6-2 Common causes of pharyngotonsillitis. Although many microorganisms are associated with pharyngitis and pharyngotonsillitis syndromes, over 90% of documented infections are due to a few organisms: *Streptococcus pyogenes* (GABHS), Epstein-Barr virus, adenovirus, influenzae A or B virus, coxsackie A viruses, and *Mycoplasma pneumoniae*. There are clearly many other etiologic agents, including possibly noninfectious ones. Specific epidemiologic, historical, and clinical findings may prioritize some of these as possible diagnoses.

A. Clinical clues to the etiology of pharyngotonsillitis: Historical findings

Historical findings	
Seasonal	GABHS, influenza
Age	GABHS (rare in persons < 2 yrs of age)
	Arcanobacterium hemolyticum (rare in persons < 13 yrs of age)
Sexually active	*Neisseria gonorrhoeae, Treponema pallidum, Chlamydia trachomatis*
Animal contacts	*Francisella tularensis, Coxiella burnetii*
Antibiotic usage	*Candida albicans*

GABHS—group A β-hemolytic streptococci.

B. Clinical clues to the etiology of pharyngotonsillitis: Clinical findings

Clinical findings	
Conjunctivitis	Adenoviruses
Influenzal syndrome	Influenza A and B, *mycoplasma*
Exanthemata	GABHS, *Arcanobacterium hemolyticum*
Common cold symptoms	Measles, rubella (in children)
	Viral (not GABHS)
	Respiratory

GABHS—group A β-hemolytic streptococci.

C. Clinical clues to the etiology of pharyngotonsillitis: Pharyngeal findings

Pharyngeal findings	
Exudates	GABHS, Epstein-Barr virus (less commonly *Candida albicans, Francisella tularensis*)
Petechiae	GABHS, Epstein-Barr virus, measles
Follicular lesions	Adenoviruses
Ulcerative lesions	Enteroviruses (herpangina), herpes simplex

GABHS—group A β-hemolytic streptococci.

FIGURE 6-3 Clinical clues to the etiology of pharyngotonsillitis. Among the clues to the causes of pharyngeal syndromes are historical, clinical, and specific pharyngeal findings. It should be noted that GABHS are the most common cause of pharyngitis and, especially in season (October to April), need to be considered in any patient with this infection. **A**, Historical findings. Sexual activity should raise suspicions of sexually transmitted pathogens, such as the gonococcus, chlamydia, or treponemes. **B**, Clinical findings. Clinical features such as rash, conjunctivitis, or systemic symptoms can be very useful. **C**, Pharyngeal findings. The appearance of the pharynx and the types of lesions can differ among the various pathogenic agents.

PATIENT EXAMINATION

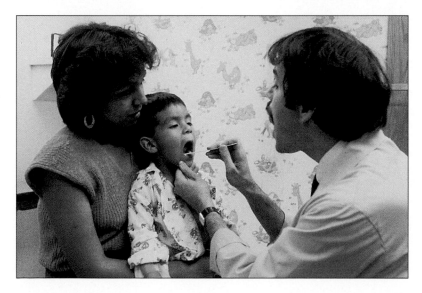

FIGURE 6-4 Patient examination. A wealth of differential diagnostic information can be gained by a thorough examination of the palate, pharynx, and tonsillar fossa. The patient must be cooperative (or adequately restrained), the tongue appropriately deflected from obscuring the examiner's vision, and the light source adequate to inspect the posterior palate for vesicles or petechiae, the pharynx for follicular or ulcerative changes, and the tonsils for exudate. This examination is also important for excluding findings of complicated disease, such as peritonsillar abscess, retropharyngeal abscess, Vincent's stomatitis, or the pseudomembranes of diphtheria.

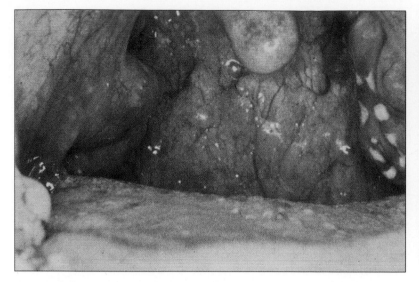

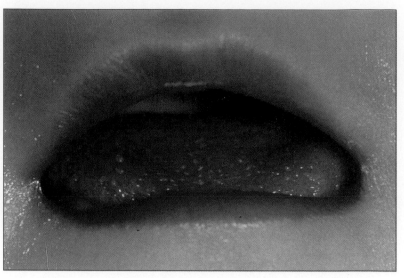

FIGURE 6-5 Marked pharyngeal erythema with edema. Marked pharyngeal erythema with edema and bilaterally enlarged and boggy tonsils with whitish or whitish-yellow exudate are the most characteristic features of pharyngitis due to GABHS. Although these features are occasionally seen in infectious mononucleosis, other pathogens producing this picture (diphtheria, tularemia, and candidiasis) are much less common. Uvulitis is also typical for streptococcal etiologies. Because *Haemophilus influenzae* type b may also rarely be a cause, coincident epiglottitis should be considered in cases in which uvulitis is seen without pharyngitis.

FIGURE 6-6 Strawberry tongue. An erythematous tongue with prominent papillae (strawberry tongue) is often seen in patients with streptococcal pharyngitis with or without a scarlatiniform rash. In patients with this feature, Kawasaki disease, adenovirus or influenza virus infection, and Stevens-Johnson syndrome should be included in the differential diagnosis.

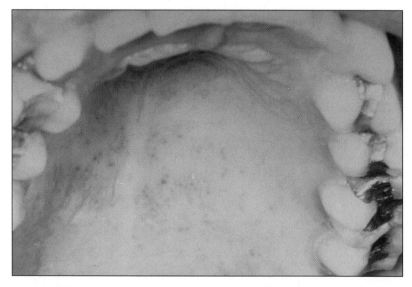

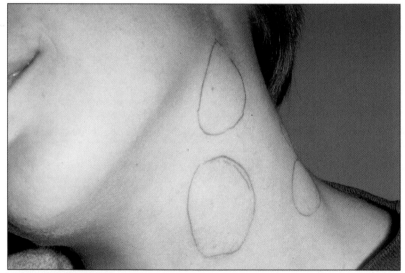

FIGURE 6-7 Palatal petechiae. Palatal petechiae are most commonly seen in streptococcal rather than viral pharyngitis. However, Epstein-Barr virus infections and childhood exanthems—particularly measles and rubella—may be associated with this finding, especially on the soft palate.

FIGURE 6-8 Cervical adenopathy. Cervical adenopathy or lymphadenitis is frequently seen in conjunction with pharyngeal infections. When it is seen in association with acute pharyngitis, GABHS and Epstein-Barr virus infection should be the major considerations. Other possibilities include adenoviruses, human herpesvirus type 6, childhood exanthems, tularemia, and, rarely, syphilis. Rare conditions that merit some consideration include Kawasaki disease, HIV infection, and candidiasis. *Staphylococcus aureus* is a frequent cause of cervical adenitis but is rarely associated with coincident pharyngitis.

BACTERIAL INFECTIONS

Bacterial causes of acute pharyngitis

Pathogen	Manifestations	Pharyngeal signs	Frequency
Streptococcus pyogenes (GABHS)	Pharyngitis Scarlet fever	Erythema Exudate Follicular changes Petechiae	Common
Group C streptococci	Pharyngotonsillitis	Erythema Exudate Follicular changes Petechiae	Uncommon
Neisseria gonorrhoeae	Pharyngitis	Erythema Exudate (occasional)	Rare
Corynebacterium diphtheriae	Pharyngitis (diphtheria)	Erythema Exudate (gray pseudomembranes)	Rare
Francisella tularensis	Pharyngotonsillitis (tularemia)	Erythema Exudate	Rare
Yersinia enterocolitica	Pharyngitis	Erythema	Rare
Treponema pallidum	Pharyngitis (secondary syphilis)	Erythema Follicular changes	Rare
Arcanobacterium hemolyticum	Pharyngitis Scalatina-like rash	Erythema Exudate	Uncommon
Mixed flora (anaerobic)	Gingivitis, pharyngitis (Vincent's angina) Peritonsillitis (quinsy)	Erythema Exudate	Rare

GABHS—group A β-hemolytic streptococci.

FIGURE 6-9 Bacterial causes of acute pharyngitis. Among bacterial causes of pharyngitis, GABHS are clearly the most common. The clinical presentation of GABHS infection with exudative pharyngitis associated with follicular erythematous changes and palatal and pharyngeal petechiae is typical. Group C streptococci can produce similar manifestations in outbreak situations but has not been associated with cyclical endemic disease as has GABHS. All other bacterial etiologies are uncommon and lack typical features, save the grayish pharyngeal pseudomembranes of diphtheria.

Group A β-Hemolytic Streptococci

Defining characteristics of streptococcal pharyngitis

Acute onset
Fever > 38.5° C
Headache, sore throat, malaise
Exudative pharyngitis
Cervical adenopathy
Absence of common cold symptoms

FIGURE 6-10 Defining characteristics of streptococcal pharyngitis. The acute onset of a pharyngeal infection associated with fever, cervical adenopathy, and tonsillar exudate strongly suggests GABHS infection. The absence of common cold symptoms is also a key factor suggesting this diagnosis, the most common of the infectious etiologies. However, even with a typical picture, the positive predictive value of clinical assessment seldom exceeds 75%. (Poses RM, Cebul RD, Collins M, Fager SS: The accuracy of experienced physicians' probability estimates for patients with sore throats: Implications for decision making. *JAMA* 1985, 16:925–929.)

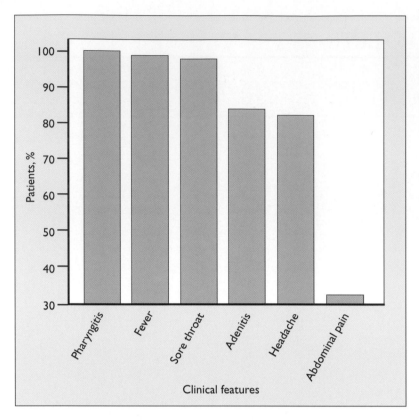

FIGURE 6-11 Frequency of clinical features in streptococcal pharyngitis. The defining characteristics of culture-proven streptococcal pharyngitis are fever, sore throat, and exudative pharyngitis. In a study by Gerber and colleagues, cervical adenitis or adenopathy and headache were also seen in over three quarters of the patients. Abdominal pain was the most common of the nonpharyngeal symptoms. Less than 10% of patients had common cold symptoms, supporting the negative predictive value of this observation. (Gerber MA, Randolph MF, DeMeo K, *et al.*: Failure of once-daily penicillin V therapy for streptococcal pharyngitis. *Am J Dis Child* 1989, 143:153–155.)

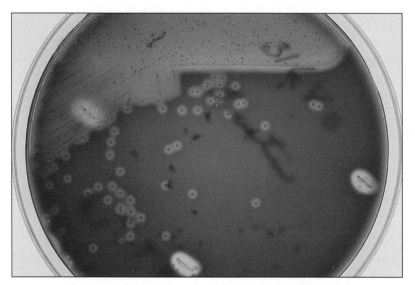

FIGURE 6-12 Throat culture. The diagnosis of GABHS pharyngotonsillitis is made by the isolation and identification of typical small gray-white β-hemolytic colonies on throat culture. A cotton pledget is vigorously swabbed across the tonsils and posterior pharynx and then is streaked onto 5% sheep blood agar using the "four-quadrant" technique. Stabbing the inoculating loop into the agar may enhance growth in the zones of hemolysis.

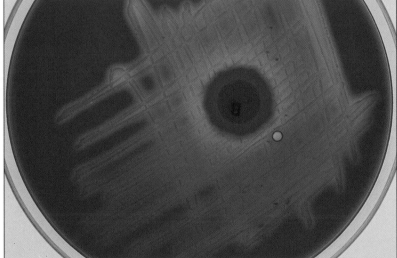

FIGURE 6-13 Bacitracin inhibition. GABHS are almost universally inhibited by bacitracin and thus differentiated from other β-hemolytic streptococci (*eg*, some group B strains) and *Staphylococcus aureus*, which rarely cause pharyngitis but may be found as components of upper respiratory flora. In office laboratories without easy access to typing antisera, bacitracin inhibition is an acceptable method to identify these organisms.

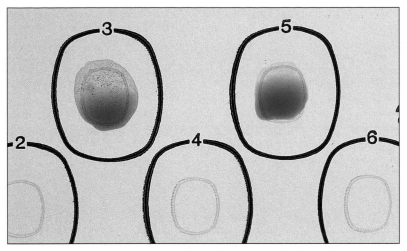

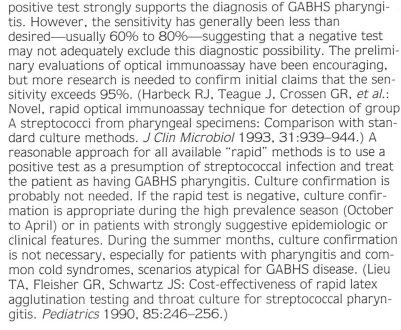

FIGURE 6-14 Rapid streptococcal screening methods. Rapid streptococcal screening methods, to detect GABHS antigens in ≤ 30 minutes, have become popular. Available methods include coagglutination (illustrated here), enzyme immunoassay, or optical immunoassay. Almost all of these tests are highly specific; a

positive test strongly supports the diagnosis of GABHS pharyngitis. However, the sensitivity has generally been less than desired—usually 60% to 80%—suggesting that a negative test may not adequately exclude this diagnostic possibility. The preliminary evaluations of optical immunoassay have been encouraging, but more research is needed to confirm initial claims that the sensitivity exceeds 95%. (Harbeck RJ, Teague J, Crossen GR, *et al.*: Novel, rapid optical immunoassay technique for detection of group A streptococci from pharyngeal specimens: Comparison with standard culture methods. *J Clin Microbiol* 1993, 31:939–944.) A reasonable approach for all available "rapid" methods is to use a positive test as a presumption of streptococcal infection and treat the patient as having GABHS pharyngitis. Culture confirmation is probably not needed. If the rapid test is negative, culture confirmation is appropriate during the high prevalence season (October to April) or in patients with strongly suggestive epidemiologic or clinical features. During the summer months, culture confirmation is not necessary, especially for patients with pharyngitis and common cold syndromes, scenarios atypical for GABHS disease. (Lieu TA, Fleisher GR, Schwartz JS: Cost-effectiveness of rapid latex agglutination testing and throat culture for streptococcal pharyngitis. *Pediatrics* 1990, 85:246–256.)

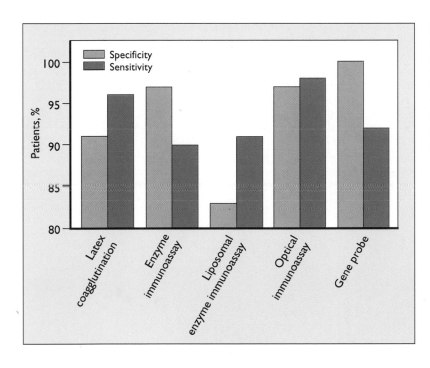

FIGURE 6-15 Sensitivity and specificity of rapid streptococcal screening tests. Rapid detection methods for GABHS have variable sensitivity and specificity. Typically, the published results derive from optimal research conditions—well-trained technologists, no time constraints, and optimal specimen acquisition and preparation—that may not reflect the usual office or clinic setting. Hence, these results are often not attainable in the typical office and should be considered as the best possible rather than routinely attainable values.

Treatment of Group A β-Hemolytic Streptococci Pharyngitis

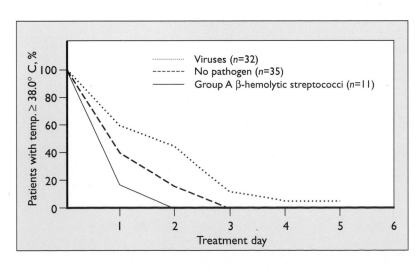

FIGURE 6-16 Resolution of fever in pharyngitis during penicillin treatment. With penicillin treatment, patients with GABHS pharyngitis become afebrile 24 to 48 hours earlier than those with documented viral etiologies. The reason for a more rapid response to penicillin in patients without documented pathogens is unclear but may relate to immune factors, undiagnosed GABHS infection, or other penicillin-susceptible causal bacteria not distinguishable from normal flora. (Pichichero ME, Disney FA, Talpey WB, et al.: Adverse and beneficial effects of immediate treatment of group A beta-hemolytic streptococcal pharyngitis with penicillin. *Ped Infect Dis J* 1987, 6:635–643.)

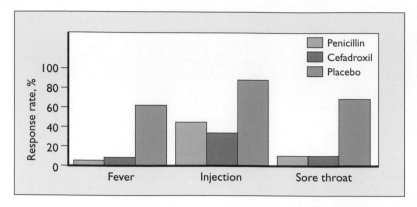

FIGURE 6-17 Effect of antibiotic therapy in streptococcal pharyngitis. There has been a prolonged controversy concerning the benefit of penicillin or other antibiotics on the acute course of GABHS pharyngitis. More recent studies, such as that by Randolph and colleagues, have provided strong evidence that compared with placebo, penicillin and other antibiotics do shorten the febrile course and alleviate other acute symptoms more rapidly. These differences are statistically significant ($P < 0.05$). However, their importance—a febrile course shortened by 1 to 2 days—must be balanced against the costs of therapy. (Randolph MF, Gerber MA, DeMeo KK, Wright L: Effect of antibiotic therapy on the clinical course of streptococcal pharyngitis. *J Pediatr* 1985, 106:870–875.)

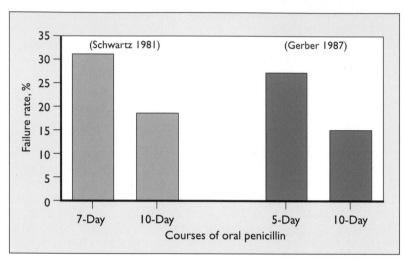

FIGURE 6-18 Duration of penicillin therapy for GABHS pharyngitis. Intramuscular penicillin therapy is considered the gold-standard therapy for GABHS pharyngitis. It is clear that 10-day courses of oral

penicillin are equivalent to intramuscular penicillin in their effects on acute symptoms (the possible difference in prevention of rheumatic fever has not been studied). However, both Schwartz and Gerber have found courses of oral penicillin < 10 days to yield more microbiologic failures (as shown) and poorer clinical results than does the recommended 10-day course. Whether these data apply to other antibiotics, such as cephalosporins or macrolides, requires further study. A possible explanation for the greater bacteriologic efficacy of cephalosporins (clindamycin and amoxicillin-clavulanic acid) in GABHS pharyngitis is their effect on β-lactamase–producing flora. Although GABHS do not produce β-lactamase, other oral flora, such as *Staphylococcus aureus*, *Prevotella* spp., *Haemophilus influenzae*, and *Fusobacterium* spp., may coexist with GABHS and may inactivate penicillin by enzymatic means before it can act on susceptible GABHS. (Schwartz RH, Wientzen RL Jr, Pedreira F, *et al.*: Penicillin V for group A streptococcal pharyngotonsillitis: A randomized trial of seven vs ten days' therapy. *JAMA* 1981, 246:1790–1795. Gerber MA, Randolph MF, Chanatry J, *et al.*: Five vs ten days of penicillin V therapy for streptococcal pharyngitis. *Am J Dis Child* 1987, 141:224–227.)

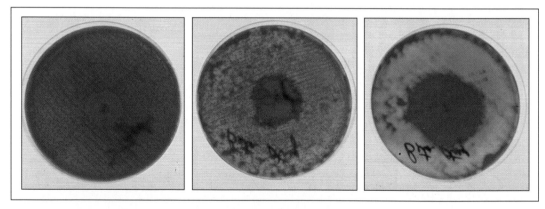

FIGURE 6-19 Effect of *Staphylococcus aureus* on susceptibility of GABHS to penicillin. To demonstrate the proposed effect of *S. aureus* on the ability of penicillin to eradicate GABHS, a simple experiment is performed. When GABHS and *S. aureus* are coincubated (*middle panel*), *S. aureus* inactivates the penicillin, presumably through elaboration of penicillinase (*left panel*), permitting GABHS to remain viable in a zone of penicillin diffusion which exhibits bactericidal activity when exposed alone (*right panel*). Similar events are proposed to occur in the pharynx where *S. aureus* and GABHS may be coresident. (*From* Brook I: *Anaerobic Infections in Children.* St. Louis: Mosby; 1989; with permission.)

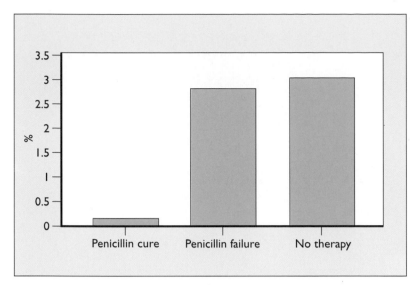

FIGURE 6-20 Incidence of rheumatic fever following penicillin treatment of GABHS pharyngitis. The initial studies of Wannamaker and colleagues confirmed that a course of penicillin that resulted in microbiologic cure of GABHS pharyngitis—defined as a negative throat culture at 10 days—was associated with a 90% reduction in the incidence of rheumatic fever in military recruits. Unfortunately, no similar data exist for oral macrolides or cephalosporins. It has been assumed that antibiotics resulting in similar microbiologic cures will also result in reductions in rheumatic fever rates. (Wannamaker LW, Rammelkemp CH Jr, Denny FW, *et al.*: Prophylaxis of acute rheumatic fever. *Am J Med* 1951, 10:673–695.)

Antimicrobials in treatment of GABHS tonsillitis

| | Acute | Recurrent or carrier |
First line	Alternative	state
Penicillin	Cephalosporins (first or second generation)	Clindamycin
Amoxicillin	Amoxicillin-clavulanate Macrolides	Penicillin plus rifampin Amoxicillin-clavulanate

GABHS—group A β-hemolytic streptococci.

FIGURE 6-21 Antimicrobials in treatment of GABHS tonsillitis. Numerous studies and meta-analyses have shown bacteriologic and clinical outcomes for the treatment of streptococcal pharyngitis to be superior with cephalosporin than with penicillin therapy. Nevertheless, because these differences, though statistically significant, may not be clinically important (5% to 15%), penicillin or amoxicillin remains the usual therapy of choice. These latter agents are inexpensive, well tolerated, and usually sufficient. In cases in which they have failed or allergy or other circumstances dictate alternative choices, cephalosporins, β-lactamase inhibitor compounds, or macrolides are suggested. It should be noted that resistance rates for macrolides against GABHS in the United States vary between 2% and 8%, whereas β-lactam resistance rates are < 1%. When conditions mandate treatment of carriers, antibiotics with high penetration into mucosal secretions—such as clindamycin or rifampin—are strongly suggested. β-Lactam compounds are unlikely to be useful in the management of carriers.

Complications of Group A β-Hemolytic Streptococci Pharyngitis (Scarlet Fever and Rheumatic Fever)

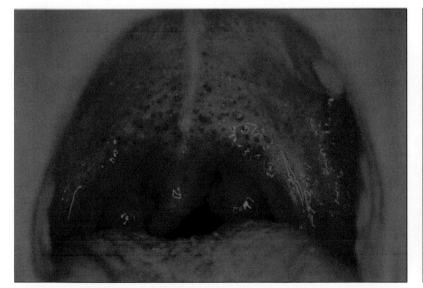

FIGURE 6-22 Marked petechial stippling of the soft palate in scarlet fever. The typical appearance of the pharynx—severe erythema with exudate and palatal petechiae—does not differ in patients with GABHS pharyngitis with rash (scarlet fever) and those without rash. (*From* Stillerman M, Bernstein SH: Streptococcal pharyngitis: Evaluation of clinical syndromes in diagnosis. *Am J Dis Child* 1961, 101:476–489; with permission.)

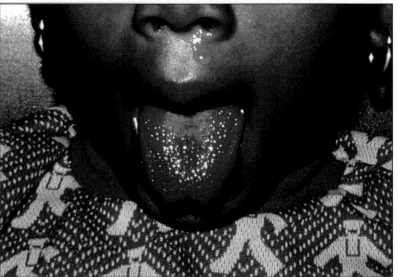

FIGURE 6-23 Circumoral pallor and strawberry tongue in scarlet fever. Patients with streptococcal pharyngitis often have circumoral pallor and a strawberry tongue. The circumoral pallor is relative to the facial flushing and labial erythema often seen in this infection. The tongue is often erythematous with prominent papillation, giving a strawberry-like appearance. These features are often more noteworthy in patients with scarlet fever than those without.

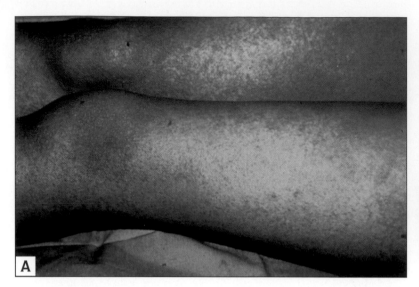

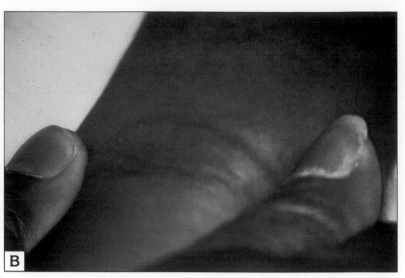

A

B

Figure 6-24 Scarlatiniform rash in scarlet fever. The scarlatiniform rash of scarlet fever is due to an erythrogenic toxin produced by some strains of GABHS that results in a macular or maculopapular rash that is dry and sandpapery. This rash usually begins within 2 days of disease onset, is most prominent on the trunk and proximal extremities, and is accentuated in the flexor creases (Pastia's lines). **A,** Macular rash is evident on the patient's legs. **B,** Pastia's lines are seen in the skin creases of the patient's elbow.

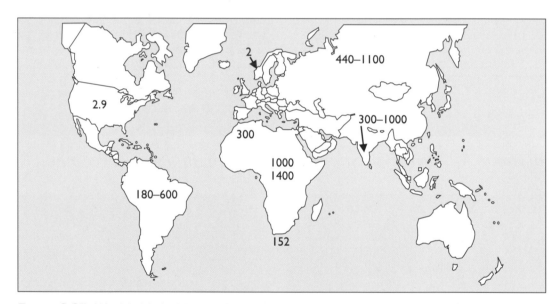

Figure 6-25 Worldwide incidence of rheumatic fever (per 100,000 population). The most common nonsuppurative complication of streptococcal pharyngitis remains rheumatic fever. Although the incidence of rheumatic fever has decreased significantly in the United States in the past four decades, it continues to be a major problem worldwide. Poor socioeconomic conditions and crowding (increased number of household members per room) are significant risk factors for rheumatic fever, and these conditions are obviously more common in developing, as compared with developed, countries. Despite a substantial decrease in the incidence of rheumatic fever in the United States in the 1960s and 1970s, there has been a resurgence here apparently related to periodic variation in the strains of *Streptococcus pyogenes* in circulation. Certain *S. pyogenes* serotypes (M1, 3, 5, 6, 18) are much more likely to be rheumatogenic, and regardless of other risk factors, when these strains are in circulation, the incidence of rheumatic fever is likely to rise.

Modified Jones criteria for rheumatic fever		
Major manifestations	**Minor manifestations**	**Supporting evidence of antecedent group A streptococcal infection**
Carditis	Clinical findings	Positive throat culture or rapid streptococcal antigen test
Polyarthritis	Arthralgia	
Chorea	Fever	Elevated or rising streptococcal antibody titer
Erythema marginatum	Laboratory findings	
Subcutaneous nodules	Elevated acute-phase reactants (ESR, C-reactive protein)	
	Prolonged PR interval	

ESR—erythrocyte sedimentation rate.

FIGURE 6-26 Modified Jones Criteria for rheumatic fever. Because there is no single pathognomonic feature for the diagnosis of rheumatic fever, a set of diagnostic guidelines were developed by Jones in 1944, and these have been updated regularly by the American Heart Association, most recently in 1992. The diagnosis of an initial attack of acute rheumatic fever is strongly suggested in patients with two major or one major and one minor criteria and documentation of recent streptococcal infection (positive throat culture or elevated serum streptococcal antibodies). When major and minor criteria are used in concert, they may not refer to the same organ system; *eg*, if carditis is a major criterion, then prolonged PR interval cannot be a minor criterion to satisfy the diagnostic definitions. (Special Writing Group of the Committee on Rheumatic Fever, Endocarditis, and Kawasaki Disease, Council on Cardiovascular Disease in the Young, American Heart Association: Guidelines for the diagnosis of rheumatic fever: Jones criteria, 1992 update. *JAMA* 1992, 268:2069–2073.)

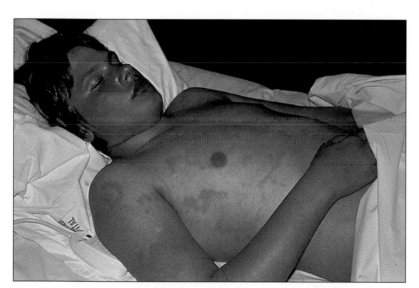

FIGURE 6-27 Erythema margination in rheumatic fever. Of all the major criteria for acute rheumatic fever, erythema marginatum is the most clearly pathognomonic. This serpentine, raised rash occurs in 3% to 13% of patients with rheumatic fever. Carditis and arthritis are more common features, each occurring in 30% to 50% of affected patients, but are not specific for the diagnosis.

Other Bacterial Infections

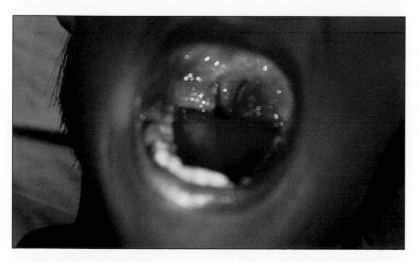

FIGURE 6-28 *Arcanobacterium haemolyticum* pharyngitis. *A. haemolyticum* (formerly *Corynebacterium haemolyticum*) is an occasional bacterial cause of pharyngitis, especially in adolescents and young adults. The pharynx is typically erythematous, although a slight exudate may be present. A maculopapular rash, reminiscent of scarlet fever (although usually less prominent or diffuse) may be present and initially confuse the diagnosis. This organism is easily cultured if the clinical laboratory is notified of its possibility in an adolescent with pharyngitis, rash, and a negative streptococcal screen.

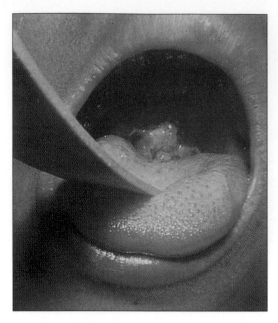

FIGURE 6-29 Pseudomembrane of diphtheria. Diphtheria is now a rare cause of exudative pharyngitis in the United States, but outbreaks continue to occur in underimmunized countries and regions. The pharyngitis has an acute onset, is characterized by severe dysphagia, and is accompanied by a thick, tenacious, gray-white exudate on the tonsils, uvula, and pharynx. As the exudate coagulates, it forms a so-called pseudomembrane, which may result in respiratory obstruction.

VIRAL INFECTIONS

Viral causes of acute pharyngitis

Pathogen	Manifestations	Pharyngeal signs	Frequency
Adenovirus	Pharyngitis Conjunctivitis	Erythema Follicular changes	Common
Epstein-Barr virus	Pharyngitis Mononucleosis	Erythema Exudate	Uncommon
Coxsackie A virus	Pharyngitis Herpangina Hand-foot-mouth disease	Erythema Vesicles	Uncommon
Herpes simplex virus	Gingivostomatitis Pharyngitis	Erythema Vesicles Ulcers	Uncommon
Influenza (A,B,C)	Pharyngitis Influenza	Erythema	Uncommon (except outbreaks)
Parainfluenza	Common cold Laryngotracheitis	Erythema	Uncommon
Rhinoviruses	Common cold	Erythema	Common
Coronaviruses	Common cold	Erythema	Common
Exanthematous viruses	Exanthems (rubella, rubeola, exanthema subitum)	Erythema	Rare (except outbreaks)
Cytomegavirus	Pharyngitis Mononucleosis	Erythema	Rare

FIGURE 6-30 Viral causes of acute pharyngitis. Infection by a number of viral agents will present with pharyngitis as an early feature. In most cases, these syndromes occur with nasopharyngitis as part of a common cold presentation. Only Epstein-Barr virus commonly presents with tonsillar exudate, and only adenovirus presents with prominent follicular changes. Enteroviruses and herpes simplex viruses may produce pharyngitis with vesicles or ulcers on the soft palate or pharynx.

Clinical characteristics of Epstein-Barr virus pharyngitis

Pharyngeal exudate

Cervical adenopathy

Older child (school age or adolescent)

Hepatosplenomegaly

Rash with ampicillin

Lymphocytosis, atypical lymphocytes

Moderately elevated liver enzymes

FIGURE 6-31 Clinical characteristics of Epstein-Barr virus (EBV) pharyngitis. Although exudative pharyngitis with cervical adenopathy may suggest EBV or GABHS infection, the other features of EBV infection are reasonably differentiating.

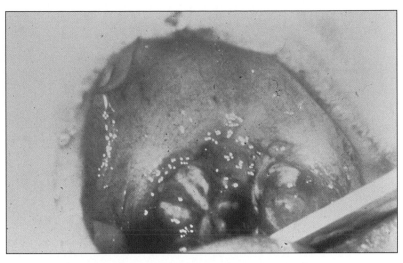

FIGURE 6-32 Pharyngeal findings in mononucleosis. The pharynx in patients with mononucleosis, usually due to EBV infection, typically demonstrates significant erythema without ulcers, vesicles, or follicular changes. Tonsillar exudate is common and can easily be confused with GABHS infection. It should be noted that EBV and GABHS can coexist, and the clinician should consider this possibility in selected cases.

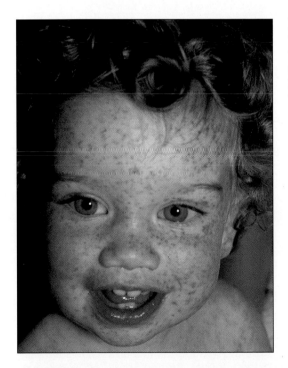

FIGURE 6-33 Ampicillin rash in EBV infection. Patients with EBV infection often respond to ampicillin challenge with a diffuse, nonpruritic, maculopapular rash, which may superficially resemble measles. The rash does not have the dry texture or Pastia's lines typical of scarlet fever and should not be confused with that exanthem. Similarly, patients do not have other features of measles, and the morbilliform appearance should not more than transiently suggest this diagnosis.

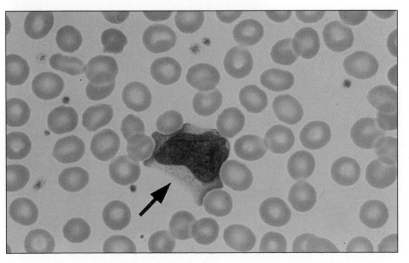

FIGURE 6-34 Downey cell in infectious mononucleosis. Patients with EBV pharyngitis usually show the hematologic changes of mononucleosis: relative neutropenia and lymphocytosis with atypical forms. A large atypical lymphocyte (Downey cell) characteristic of infectious mononucleosis is pictured. The abundant cytoplasm and lack of bizarre nuclear changes, especially multiple nucleoli, differentiate this from the immature blast forms of hematologic malignancies.

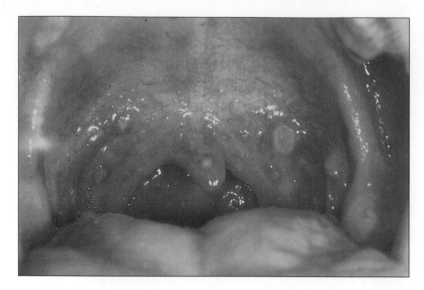

FIGURE 6-35 Herpangina (enteroviral stomatitis). Enteroviruses are not uncommon causes of pharyngitis during the summer months. Coxsackie A virus and, less commonly, echoviruses are most frequently seen. Small ulcers (< 5 mm in diameter) with minimal surrounding erythema differentiate the stomatitis of enteroviral infection (herpangina) from that of herpes simplex. These patients may also have vesicles on the palms and soles (hand-foot-mouth syndrome). (*Courtesy of* A. Margileth, MD.)

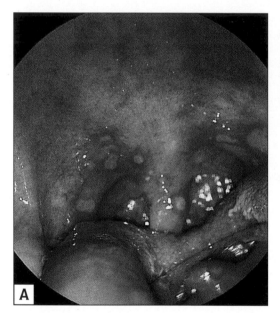

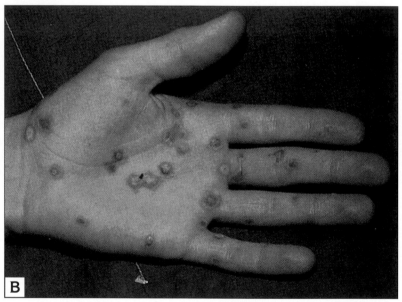

FIGURE 6-36 Hand-foot-mouth syndrome (coxsackie A virus infection). A papulovesicular rash on the palms and soles is a rare clinical finding. When seen in association with pharyngitis, or pharyngostomatitis, especially in the summer or fall, the diagnosis of hand-foot-mouth syndrome, typically due to coxsackie A viruses, is strongly suggested. **A,** Oral lesions of hand-foot-mouth syndrome on the uvula and palate. **B,** Papules and vesicles of hand-foot-mouth syndrome are seen on a patient's hand.

Associated findings in adenovirus and herpes simplex pharyngitis	
Etiology	**Features**
Adenovirus	Associated common cold symptoms
	Conjunctivitis
Herpes simplex virus (Gingivostomatitis)	Usually infant, toddler
	Ulcers on lips, gingiva, buccal mucosa, tongue
	Vesicles on skin around lips

FIGURE 6-37 Associated findings in adenovirus and herpes simplex pharyngitis. Adenoviruses and herpes simplex virus (HSV) are not infrequently associated with pharyngeal syndromes. Conjunctivitis and other cold symptoms support adenovirus etiologies, which often occur as part of local outbreaks. HSV pharyngitis is most common in young children—herpes labialis is more typical in adolescents and adults—and is an endemic infection that occurs year-round.

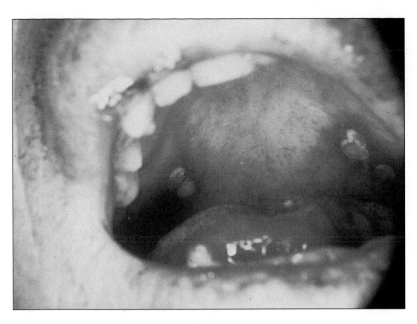

FIGURE 6-38 Herpes simplex stomatitis. In addition to pharyngitis, herpes simplex virus often causes a stomatitis with vesicles and ulcers. These lesions are typically larger than in enterovirus-related syndromes—5 to 10 mm in diameter—and have a more intense erythematous, inflammatory border. These lesions may be found on the gingiva and palate, as well as on the pharynx.

OTHER CAUSES

Miscellaneous causes of acute pharyngitis

Pathogen	Manifestations	Pharyngeal signs	Frequency
Infectious			
Chlamydia trachomatis	Pharyngitis Conjunctivitis Infantile pneumonia	Erythema	Uncommon
Chlamydia pneumoniae	Pharyngitis Bronchopneumonia	Erythema	Uncommon
Mycoplasma pneumoniae	Pharyngitis Bronchopneumonia	Erythema Follicular changes	Uncommon
Candida spp.	Gingivostomatitis Thrush	Erythema Exudate	Common (in predisposed hosts)
Noninfectious			
Kawasaki disease	Mucositis Lymphadenitis Extremity changes	Erythema	Rare
Aphthous stomatitis	Gingivostomatitis	Erythema Vesicles Ulcers	Rare
Stevens-Johnson syndrome	Mucositis Erythema multiforme	Erythema Ulcers	Rare
Cyclic neutropenia	Stomatitis	Erythema	Rare

FIGURE 6-39 Miscellaneous causes of acute pharyngitis. None of the nonbacterial, nonviral causes of acute pharyngitis are common. *Chlamydia pneumoniae* and *Mycoplasma pneumoniae* should be suspected in school-aged children to young adults with pharyngeal syndromes, especially when influenzal symptoms and lower respiratory tract signs are present. Unfortunately, the pharyngeal signs seen with these pathogens are not characteristic. *Chlamydia trachomatis* is only seen as a respiratory tract pathogen in young infants (< 6 months of age) and should be strongly suspected in those less than 6 weeks of age with conjunctivitis and afebrile pneumonia. Eosinophilia is also typical, though not universal. The features of Kawasaki disease, Stevens-Johnson syndrome, and aphthous stomatitis are all typical of the individual conditions, and pharyngitis is merely an associated manifestation.

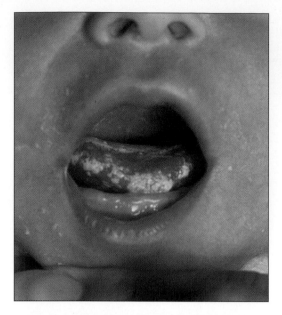

FIGURE 6-40 Oral thrush due to *Candida albicans*. Thrush is a common stomatitis, caused by *C. albicans*, involving the oral and gingival mucosa as well as the pharynx. The whitish exudates are often adherent and, when removed with gentle scraping by a tongue depressor, often result in mucosal bleeding. This infection is most commonly seen in the very young, the elderly, the immunocompromised, and those patients receiving prolonged antibiotic therapy resulting in altered colonization resistance. Therapy consists of correction of underlying factors—*eg*, discontinuing antibiotic treatment—and the use of topical or oral antifungal agents.

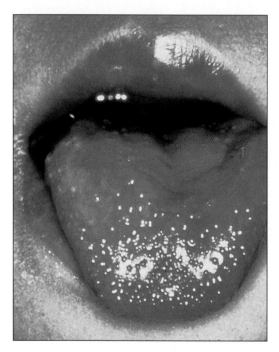

FIGURE 6-41 Kawasaki syndrome. Kawasaki syndrome is a condition of unknown etiology associated with fever, mucosal and cutaneous manifestations, swollen hands and feet, lymphadenopathy, and periungual desquamation. Prolonged fever and extreme irritability are characteristic. The oral manifestations include nonexudative pharyngitis, strawberry tongue, and swollen, red, cracked lips. This is a generalized vasculitis, and other features may include hepatitis, hydrops of the gallbladder, sterile pyuria, aseptic meningitis, and pleuritis. The most ominous feature is coronary arteritis with aneurysm formation. In some recent studies, Kawasaki disease has been a more common form of acquired heart disease in children than acute rheumatic fever. When diagnosed early, high-dose immunoglobulin therapy (2 g/kg) has proven useful in speeding resolution of acute symptoms and significantly decreasing the incidence of coronary aneurysms. (Taubert KA, Rowley AH, Shulman ST: Nationwide survey of Kawasaki disease and acute rheumatic fever. *J Pediatr* 1991, 119:279–282. Newburger JW, Takahashi M, Beiser AS, *et al.*: A single intravenous infusion of gamma globulin as compared with four infusions in the treatment of acute Kawasaki syndrome. *N Engl J Med* 1991, 324:1633–1639.)

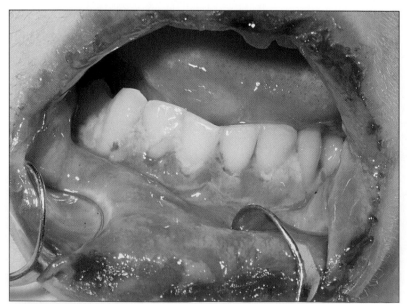

FIGURE 6-42 Stevens-Johnson syndrome. Patients with erythema multiforme major (Stevens-Johnson syndrome) have both cutaneous and mucosal findings. The mucosal inflammation may include the oral and conjunctival mucosa, pharynx, and genitourinary and perineal mucosa. The pharyngitis is nonexudative, and tonsillar involvement is unusual. The syndrome is immunologically mediated, although some infectious agents, particularly *Mycoplasma pneumoniae* and herpes simplex virus, have been associated with recurrent cases. Therapy is largely supportive, although those with large areas of involved skin may be treated in a fashion similar to burned patients.

SELECTED BIBLIOGRAPHY

Denny FW: Tonsillopharyngitis. *Pediatr Rev* 1994, 15:185–191.

Kline JA, Runge JW: Streptococcal pharyngitis: A review of pathophysiology, diagnosis, and management. *J Emerg Med* 1994, 12:665–680.

Lieu TA, Fleisher GR, Schwartz JS: Cost-effectiveness of rapid latex agglutination testing and throat culture for streptococcal pharyngitis. *Pediatrics* 1990, 85:246–256.

Peter G: Streptococcal pharyngitis: Current therapy and criteria for evaluating new agents. *Clin Infect Dis* 1992, 14(suppl 2):S218–S223.

Randolph MF, Gerber MA, Demeo KK, Wright L: Effect of antibiotic therapy on the clinical course of streptococcal pharyngitis. *J Pediatr* 1985, 106:870–875.

CHAPTER 7

Epiglottitis, Croup, Laryngitis, and Tracheitis

Debra A. Tristram

EPIGLOTTITIS

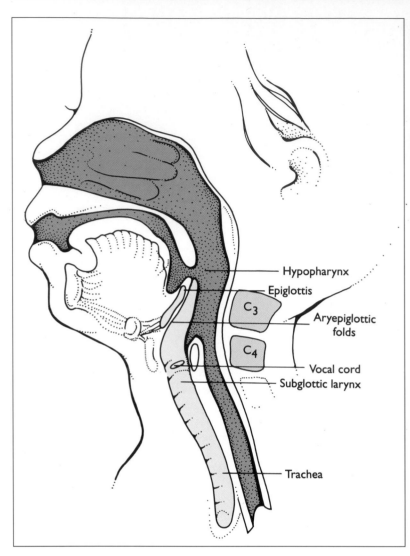

FIGURE 7-1 Normal airway, seen from the lateral neck view. The epiglottis can be located on radiographic films adjacent to the C₃ vertebra and normally is fairly slender. The area between the epiglottis to slightly below the vocal cords is the larynx but is not visualized well by radiography. The hypopharyngeal shadow is normal and usually is continuous with the lower tracheal and pharyngeal shadows.

In the diagram labels: Hypopharynx, Epiglottis, Aryepiglottic folds, Vocal cord, Subglottic larynx, Trachea, C₃, C₄

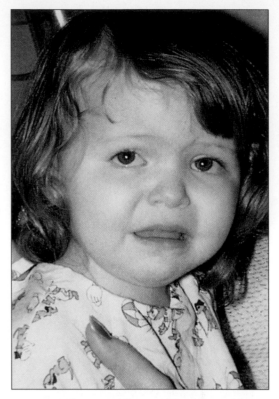

FIGURE 7-2
Early epiglottitis. A child with early epiglottitis displays an anxious appearance. Drooling and more severe airway compromise are not yet present. (*From* Riley J, Davis H: Pediatric otolaryngology. *In* Zitelli B, Davis H (eds.): *The Atlas of Pediatric Diagnosis.* St. Louis: C.V. Mosby; 1987; with permission.)

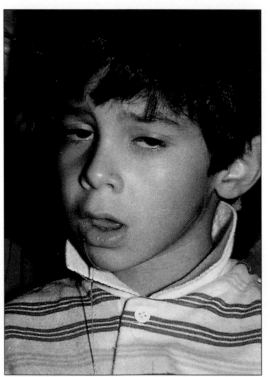

FIGURE 7-3
Severe epiglottitis. A slightly older child with more severe epiglottitis appears tired and cannot swallow his oral secretions. Mouth breathing is characteristic, as is forward extension of the chin to optimize airway size. (*From* Riley J, Davis H: Pediatric otolaryngology. *In* Zitelli B, Davis H (eds.): *The Atlas of Pediatric Diagnosis.* St. Louis: C.V. Mosby; 1987; with permission.)

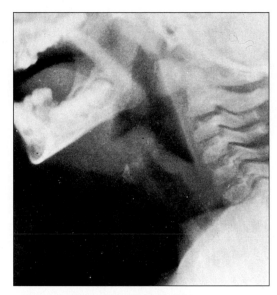
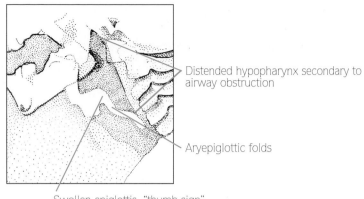

FIGURE 7-4 Lateral neck radiograph demonstrating the swollen epiglottis and aryepiglottic folds present in acute epiglottitis. Such a radiograph should not be part of the normal evaluation for suspected epiglottitis in a child, because in this emergent condition, children may have acute airway compromise at any time leading to cardiopulmonary arrest. Intubation can be extremely difficult with an acutely swollen epiglottis blocking the airway. In adults, the larger airway diameter may prevent sudden airway compromise in most, but not all, patients. Examination of the adult airway in suspected epiglottitis should also be performed in a controlled environment. (Denholm S, Rivron RP: Acute epiglottitis: A potentially lethal cause of sore throat. *J R Coll Surg Edinb* 1992, 37:333–335.)

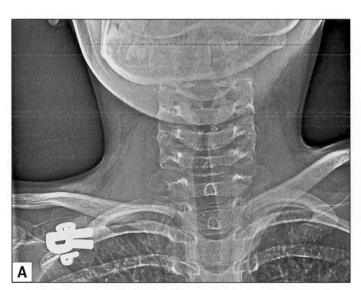
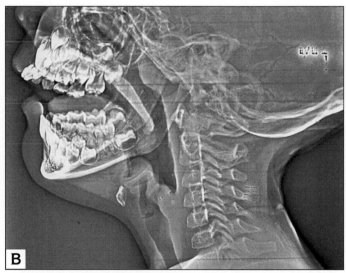
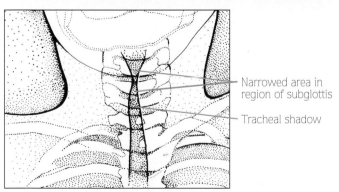
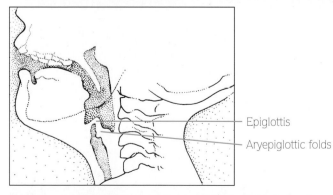

FIGURE 7-5 Epiglottitis, as seen by xeroradiography. **A,** Anteroposterior view of the neck of a child with documented epiglottitis shows narrowing in the diameter of the trachea, which can be confused with acute viral croup. The lateral neck view is preferable because it can demonstrate the enlarged epiglottis, or "thumb sign."

B, A xeroradiograph showing a lateral neck view of the same child demonstrates the acute epiglottic and aryepiglottic swelling seen in acute epiglottitis. Direct visualization in the operating room revealed a markedly swollen epiglottis.

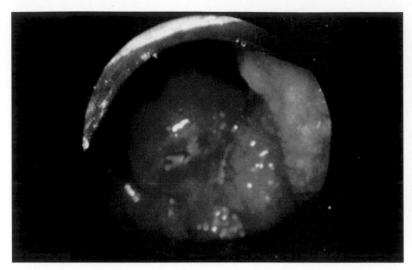

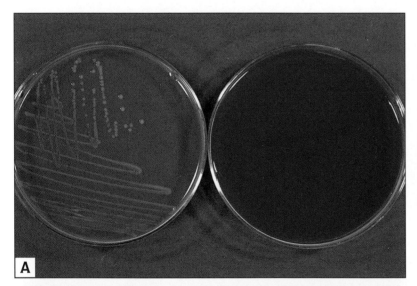

FIGURE 7-6 Epiglottitis, as seen by laryngoscopy. On direct laryngoscopy, a beefy red appearance of the epiglottis is characteristic of acute epiglottitis in children. In addition, the epiglottis may be infolded during severe swelling. This child was intubated to protect his airway during the initial 3–4 days of acute epiglottic swelling. Cultures were taken at the time of intubation and grew *Haemophilus influenzae* type B. In adults, the epiglottis may be swollen but is often pale in color. (*From* Riley J, Davis H: Pediatric Otolaryngology. *In* Zitelli B, Davis H (eds.): *The Atlas of Pediatric Diagnosis*. St. Louis: C.V. Mosby; 1987; with permission.)

Causes of acute epiglottitis

Children
  Haemophilus influenzae type B
  Diphtheria
  Staphylococcus aureus
  Streptococcus pneumoniae
  Group A streptococcus (rare)

Adults
  Same as children
  Nontypeable *Haemophilus* spp.

FIGURE 7-7 Causes of acute epiglottitis. The etiology of acute epiglottis is nearly always *Haemophilus influenzae* type B (HIB) in children. However, with the advent of an effective HIB vaccination, the incidence of epiglottitis has decreased markedly. Other less common bacterial agents are possible etiologies in both children and adults and should be sought by appropriate cultures taken at the time of intubation.

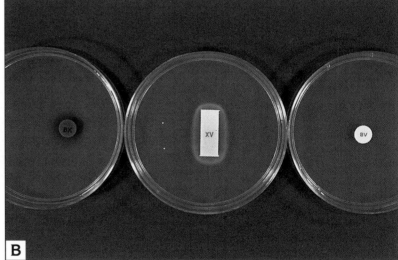

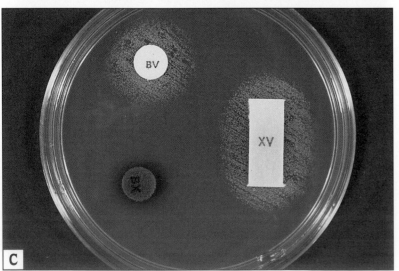

FIGURE 7-8 *Haemophilus influenzae* culture. **A,** Culture demonstrates typical colonies of *H. influenzae* on chocolate agar (*left plate*) but not blood agar (*right plate*). *H. influenzae* requires X and V factors (hemin and nicotinamide adenine dinucleotide/coenzyme 1) for growth. Disks containing X and V factors are placed on trypticase soy agar. **B,** Hazy growth of *H. influenzae* surrounds the X and V plate but not plates with X or V factors separately. **C,** *H. influenzae* can be easily distinguished from *H. parainfluenzae*, as *H. parainfluenzae* requires only the V factor for growth. Hazy growth surrounds both the V and X and V disks. (Kilian M: *Haemophilus. In* Balows A, *et al.* (eds.): *Manual of Clinical Microbiology*, 5th ed. Washington, DC: American Society for Microbiology; 1991:463–470.)

Differential diagnosis of acute obstruction in the epiglottic and laryngeal area

Foreign body aspiration
Viral croup
Spasmodic croup
Toxic ingestion (*eg,* with caustic agent such as lye)
Acute laryngitis
Acute tracheitis
Acute angioneurotic edema
Acute epiglottitis

FIGURE 7-9 Differential diagnosis of acute obstruction in the epiglottic and laryngeal area. The differential diagnosis of acute epiglottitis should include a range of entities. Expectant management of the airway should always be carried out, regardless of the underlying etiology, and manipulation of the child or adult should be limited until controlled conditions exist in the operating room. Toxic appearance and high fevers are more likely to be present in acute epiglottitis and tracheitis than in the other conditions, but these conditions should not be ruled out if the patient is afebrile or nontoxic.

Clinical features of acute epiglottitis

	Children	Adults
Age at acquisition	3–5 yrs	—
Location of pathology	Supraglottic	Supraglottic
Onset	Rapid	Most have a mild illness with prolonged course, painful dysphagia, and pharyngitis
Fever	High	Variable
Appearance	Toxic	Usually not toxic
Stridor	+++	Not usual
Cough	Not usual	—
Drooling	Often	—

FIGURE 7-10 Clinical features of acute epiglottitis. Epiglottitis is a severe respiratory disease, consisting of high fever, stridor, and acute supraglottic swelling that can lead to airway compromise and death in children if not treated. Epiglottitis can also attack adults, and despite the less severe disease course, there is a 7% mortality rate associated with adult supraglottitis. Most pediatric cases are caused by *Haemophilus influenzae* type b infection, but the incidence has decreased since the institution of effective vaccines against this bacteria.

Management of epiglottitis

Do not attempt to visualize epiglottis, especially in agitated child
Have caretaker administer O$_2$ if child remains calm during administration
Do not send child for neck radiographs
Contact operating room and special medical team
Most experienced medical personnel should accompany child to operating room
In operating room, direct visualization and intubation are performed
Obtain blood culture and swab of epiglottis for culture
Administer antibiotics directed against *H. influenzae,* streptococci, and staphylococci (*eg,* ceftriaxone or β-lactam penicillins)
Transfer to intensive care unit; consider paralyzation or strong restraints so that child does not remove airway accidentally
Maintain intubation for 2–4 days until epiglottic swelling has subsided

FIGURE 7-11 Management of epiglottitis. Clinical suspicion of epiglottitis is a medical emergency. A medical team should be assembled that consists of otolaryngologists, anesthesiologists, or other medical personnel skilled in the management of acute airway compromise and difficult intubation or emergency tracheostomy. The same procedure should be considered for adults, who may not look as toxic as children but still may have acute airway compromise necessitating intubation or tracheostomy.

CROUP

Clinical features of croup

Occurs mostly in children 3 mos—3 yrs of age
Subglottic location of pathology
Slow onset, often with upper respiratory prodrome
Low-grade or no fever
Appearance not toxic
Stridor + to +++
"Barky" cough
Drooling possible

FIGURE 7-12 Clinical features of croup. Croup (also called acute laryngotracheobronchitis) is a common viral disease in children < 3 years of age. It is characterized by low-grade fever, variable upper respiratory tract prodrome, and acute onset of respiratory distress consisting of barky, seallike coughing and stridor. Occasionally, croup associated with parainfluenzae virus 3 infection can result in a high fever to 39° C.

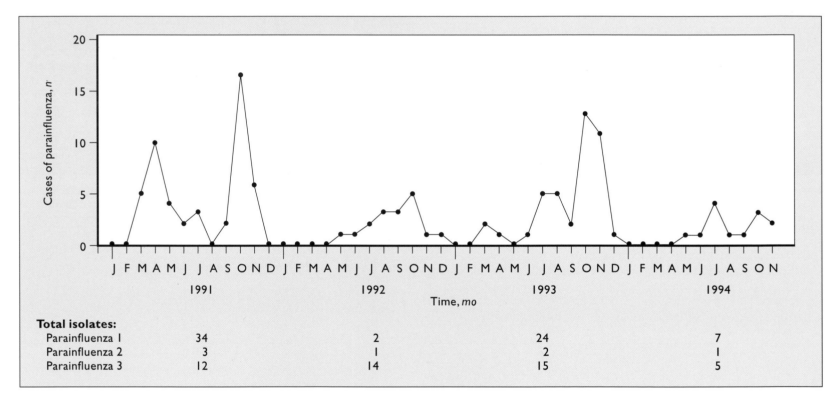

Total isolates:			
Parainfluenza 1	34	2	24	7
Parainfluenza 2	3	1	2	1
Parainfluenza 3	12	14	15	5

FIGURE 7-13 Seasonal occurrence of parainfluenza. Parainfluenza has a seasonal predilection for the fall, which is when the majority of croup cases are diagnosed. In any season there is usually a predominant type of parainfluenza virus, but more than one type may be active in the community during an outbreak. Parainfluenza type 4 has been recently identified as a separate virus, but rapid fluorescent antibody testing for it is not yet widely available.

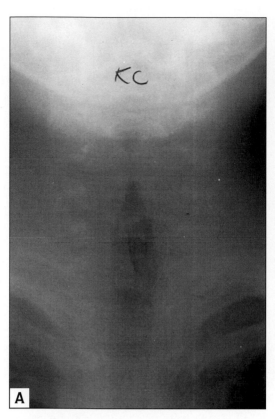

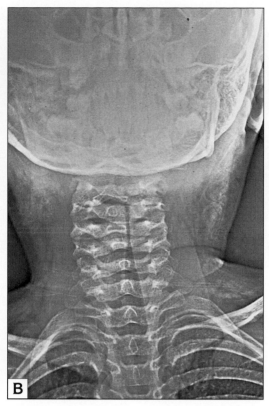

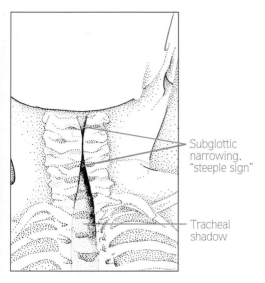

Subglottic narrowing, "steeple sign"

Tracheal shadow

FIGURE 7-14 Croup, radiographic views. **A** and **B**, An anteroposterior radiograph of the neck (*panel 10A*) and a xeroradiograph of the neck (*panel 10B*) demonstrate a long area of narrowing extending well below the normal anatomic narrowing seen at the level of the larynx. This finding is called the *steeple sign* and is characteristic of children with croup. However, this finding is occasionally seen in cases of epiglottitis as well.

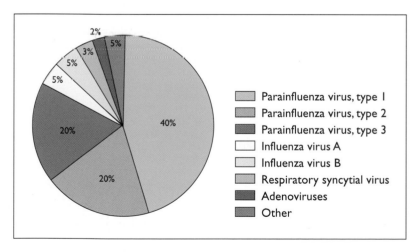

- Parainfluenza virus, type I
- Parainfluenza virus, type 2
- Parainfluenza virus, type 3
- Influenza virus A
- Influenza virus B
- Respiratory syncytial virus
- Adenoviruses
- Other

FIGURE 7-15 Viral causes of acute croup in infants and children. Commonly, a seasonal pattern is noted, with clustering of cases in the fall and a secondary peak in the late winter and early spring. Parainfluenza viruses are most often isolated in cases of clinical croup. Other less common pathogens include rubeola virus, enteroviruses, adenoviruses, and *Mycoplasma pneumoniae*.

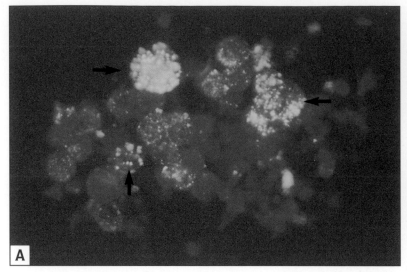

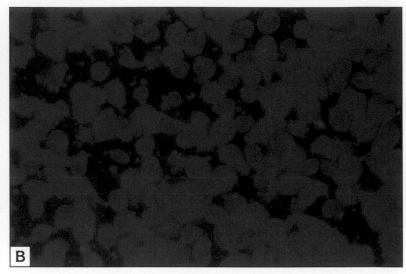

FIGURE 7-16 Parainfluenza 3 (PI3) virus grown in MRC5 cell culture. **A** and **B**, PI3-specific fluorescent monoclonal antibody is applied to the cell culture after the characteristic cytopathic effects are noted. The infected cells (*arrows*) show a green-yellow granular fluorescence pattern (*panel 16A*) as compared with uninfected cell culture (*panel 16B*). This technique can also be applied to respiratory specimens containing infected cells obtained from nasopharyngeal or endotracheal aspirates. Other respiratory viruses, such as respiratory syncytial and influenza viruses, can also be identified by rapid immunofluorescent methods. (Leland DS, French MLV: Virus isolation and identification. *In* Lennette EH, Halonen P, Murphy FA (eds.): *Laboratory Diagnosis of Infectious Diseases: Principles and Practice*, vol II. New York: Springer-Verlag; 1988.)

Management of croup

Initial home management if child is not in severe respiratory distress
    Place child in cool, moist air (*eg*, fill bathroom with steam and open window to let in cool air)
    Maintain good hydration
If home measures are not successful, consider hospitalization
    Place child in humidified oxygen tent
    Administer racemic epinephrine via aerosol
    Administer steroids

FIGURE 7-17 Management of croup. Most children can be managed as outpatients with cool-mist humidifiers. Very severe cases may require hospitalization and administration of aerosolized racemic epinephrine. Because of rebound swelling after racemic epinephrine, it should not be used in an outpatient setting. The use of steroids is still a controversial issue; some recommend their use for severe croup to decrease subglottic swelling, whereas others do not think steroids are useful. Intubation is rarely necessary. For severe airway compromise, tracheostomy may be necessary but is rarely needed. Antibiotics are not indicated except for bacterial complications. Antivirals are not yet useful as the majority of croup cases are caused by parainfluenza viruses.

LARYNGITIS

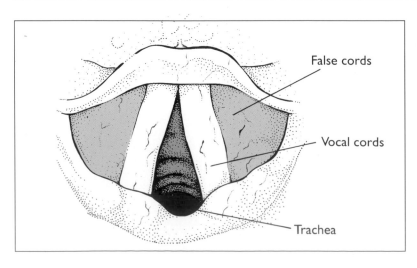

FIGURE 7-18 Acute infectious laryngitis. Marked swelling and pale edema of the true vocal cords and the false cords are common. Viruses are the most common pathogens isolated from patients with acute laryngitis. Often, laryngitis is only one area of involvement in the respiratory tree and may be overshadowed by more prominent upper respiratory tract symptoms or serious lower respiratory disease.

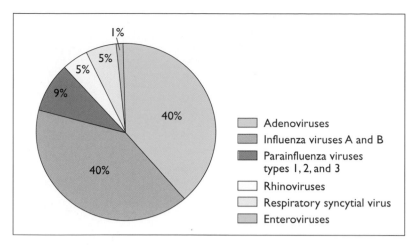

FIGURE 7-19 Causes of acute laryngitis in children and adults. Most of the viral causes of laryngitis produce seasonal epidemics, with peak incidence in the late fall and winter. The exception is the enterovirus group, which predominates in the summer and early fall. Although most enteroviruses produce gastrointestinal symptoms, coxsackie viruses may produce respiratory symptoms, including laryngitis.

Differential diagnoses of laryngitis

Viral (acute edema and erythema)
Bacterial
  Streptococcal (membranous or exudative appearance)
  Mycobacterial (granulomatous appearance)
Neoplasm
  Benign
  Malignant
Chronic or recurrent
  Secondary to sinusitis with postnasal drainage
  Allergy
  Overuse syndromes (*eg*, singers)

FIGURE 7-20 Differential diagnoses of laryngitis. Acute viral laryngitis is a self-limited condition and easily recognizable. Chronic or recurrent laryngitis may either represent numerous acute viral episodes or an underlying problem such as polyps, infection of the sinuses, or other progressive conditions and should be investigated by direct visualization of the larynx.

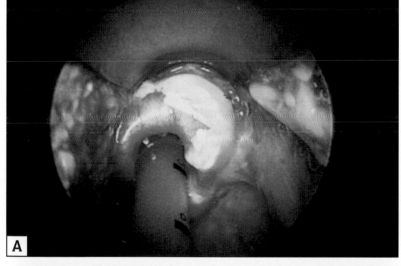

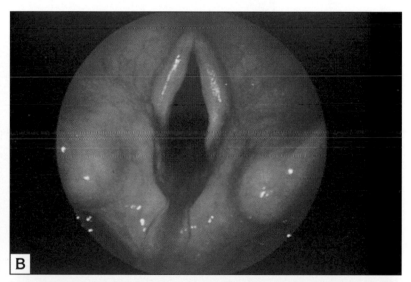

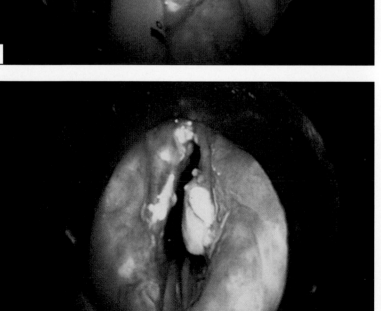

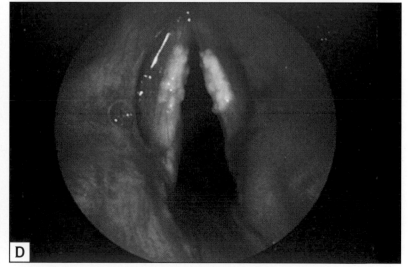

FIGURE 7-21 Examination of the larynx. **A,** Lye burns of the supraglottic structures and epiglottis in a 4-year-old. **B,** Chronic laryngitis with substantial edema. **C,** Squamous cell carcinoma suggesting a granulomatous lesion. **D,** Fungal laryngitis, which occurred in an adolescent on long-term steroid therapy for asthma. (*From* Benjamin BNP: *Diagnostic Laryngology: Adults and Children.* Philadelphia: W.B. Saunders; 1990; with permission.)

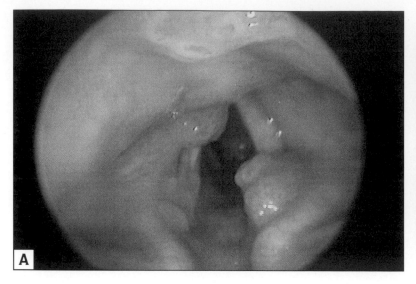

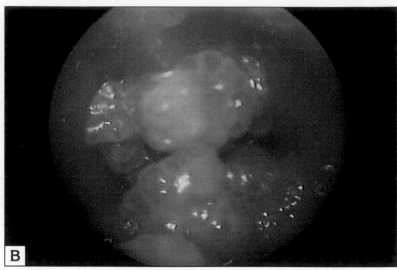

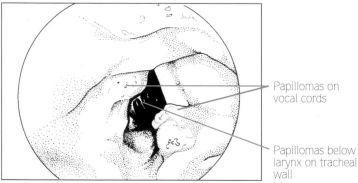

Papillomas on
vocal cords

Papillomas below
larynx on tracheal
wall

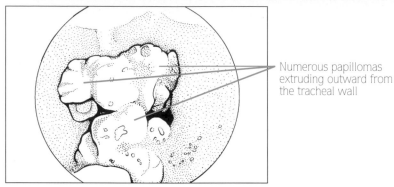

Numerous papillomas
extruding outward from
the tracheal wall

FIGURE 7-22 Laryngeal and tracheal papillomatosis. **A,** Laryngeal papillomatosis is a rare cause of laryngitis. A bronchoscopic view of the larynx shows fleshy growths on the vocal cords. This child presented with increasing laryngitis and shortness of breath. **B,** More severe narrowing of the trachea is seen on lower-level bronchoscopy of the same child. Such lesions commonly occur on the vocal cords, but other sites in the respiratory tract have been documented as well (nose, trachea, lungs, oral cavity). The majority of such papillomas are caused by human papillomaviruses type 6 and 11. These are the most common isolates from exophytic genital condylomata and are thought to be acquired at the time of vaginal delivery in patients with juvenile onset of papillomas. Most cases are seen in children < 10 years of age, but papillomas can occur in adulthood as well. Although these growths can be removed surgically, they often recur. Viral genome is present in normal epithelium adjacent to the papillomas and is believed to account for latency and recurrence of such lesions. (Shah KV, Howley PM: Papillomaviruses. *In* Fields BN, Knipe DM, *et al.* (eds.): *Virology*. New York: Raven Press; 1990:1651–1676.) (*Courtesy of* M. Volk, MD.)

FIGURE 7-23 Management of laryngitis.

Management of laryngitis
Symptomatic relief with decongestants and antipyretics Treatment of bacterial complications if they develop

TRACHEITIS

Historical and clinical features of acute bacterial tracheitis

Antecedent history of trauma to trachea (*eg*, viral disease, prolonged intubation, caustic ingestions)

Any age can be affected

Hoarseness

Expiratory stridor

Fever

Toxic appearance

FIGURE 7-24 Historical and clinical features of acute bacterial tracheitis. Acute bacterial tracheitis is often a medical emergency and should be managed by a team similar to that for epiglottitis (*see* Fig. 7-11). Antecedent history of tracheal trauma is helpful to differentiate tracheitis from acute epiglottitis.

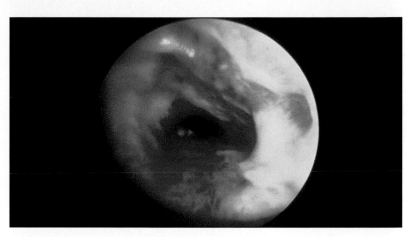

FIGURE 7-25 Acute bacterial tracheitis. Bronchoscopy of a patient with worsening airway compromise reveals marked narrowing, erythema, and edema of the trachea. Pus is easily removed from the walls of the trachea. (*Courtesy of* L. Brodsky, MD.)

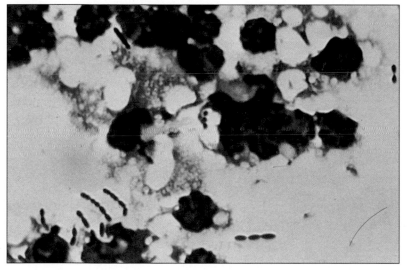

FIGURE 7-26 Gram stain from a patient with acute bacterial tracheitis. Inflammatory cells, shed epithelial cells, and chains of gram-positive cocci are seen on a gram-stained smear. Cultures from this patient subsequently grew *Streptococcus pneumoniae*. Most cases of bacterial tracheitis are caused by upper respiratory tract bacteria, such as staphylococci, streptococci, or *Haemophilus*.

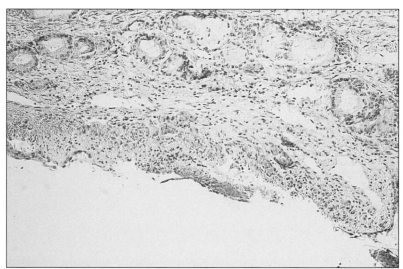

FIGURE 7-27 Tracheal specimen showing bacterial tracheitis. An autopsy specimen from patient with prolonged endotracheal intubation demonstrates loss of normal respiratory epithelium. Prolonged intubation, aspirated foreign bodies, caustic chemical aspirations and ingestions, and viral infections may predispose patients to bacterial tracheitis by disrupting the normal mucosal barrier present in the healthy respiratory tract and leading to bacterial overgrowth.

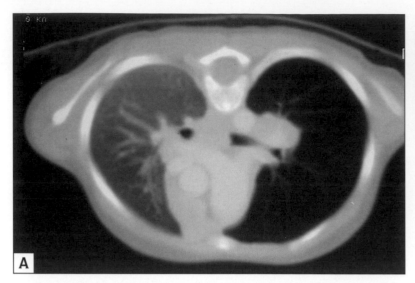

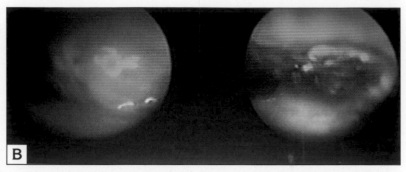

FIGURE 7-28 Unusual case of tracheitis. **A,** A computed tomographic scan of the chest in a 2-year-old child who presented with intermittent wheezing and tachypnea and was thought to have aspirated a foreign body. Hyperinflation of the left lung with volume loss of the right lung is clearly demonstrated. A narrowed area of the left mainstem bronchus is noted, as well as hilar adenopathy. She underwent diagnostic/therapeutic bronchoscopy.

B, A bronchoscopic view of the left mainstem bronchus just below the tracheal bifurcation shows a large mass with a somewhat irregular surface (*left view*). The lesion was visualized and excised by laser (*right view*). On histopathologic examination, this lesion was found to be a granulomatous lymph node. However, acid-fast staining and modified silver staining failed to reveal any organisms. Purified protein derivative testing of the child and family were negative, but atypical mycobacterial skin testing was strongly positive for *Mycobacterium avium intracellulare*, which subsequently grew from the cultured lymph node. Although an unusual cause of tracheitis/bronchitis, such lymph nodes may rupture into the airway, causing tracheitis or tracheobronchitis. (Starke JR: Nontuberculous mycobacterial infections in children. *Adv Pediatr* 1992, 7:123–159.)

Management of tracheitis

Maintain airway with intubation
Obtain cultures at time of intubation
Chest radiograph to diagnose associated pneumonia
Antibiotic administration directed against staphylococci,
  Haemophilus, streptococci (β-lactam penicillins,
  cephalosporins)

FIGURE 7-29 Management of tracheitis. Acute airway compromise may simulate epiglottitis. Initial management should be similar to that for epiglottitis until an etiology is established.

SELECTED BIBLIOGRAPHY

Baker AS, Behlau I, Tierney M: Infections of the pharynx, larynx, epiglottis, trachea, and thyroid. *In* Gorbach SL, Bartlett JG, Blacklow NK (eds.): *Infectious Diseases*. Philadelphia: W.B. Saunders; 1992:450–454.

Barrow HN, Vastola AP, Wang RC: Adult supraglottitis. *Otolaryngol Head Neck Surg* 1993, 109:474–477.

Chanock RM, McIntosh K: Parainfluenza viruses. *In* Fields BN, Knipe DM, *et al.* (eds.): *Virology*, 2nd ed. New York: Raven Press; 1990:963–988.

Cressman WR, Myer CM: Diagnosis and management of croup and epiglottitis. *Pediatr Clin North Am* 1994, 41(2):265–276.

Custer JR: Croup and related disorders. *Pediatr Rev* 1993, 14:19–29.

CHAPTER 8

Cervical Lymphadenopathy

Andrew M. Margileth

DIFFERENTIAL DIAGNOSIS

Infectious causes of cervical lymphadenopathy	
Bacterial	Pharyngitis (streptococcal group A)
	Lymphadenitis (*Staphylococcus aureus*)
	Bartonellosis (Oroya fever)
	Brucellosis
	Dental infections (anaerobes)
	Cat scratch disease (*Bartonella henselae*)
	Tuberculosis
	Nontuberculous mycobacterial disease
	Tularemia
	Actinomycosis
	Diphtheria
	Plague (*Yersinia pestis*)
	Yersinia pseudotuberculosis infection
Spirochaeta	Syphilis
	Lyme disease
Viral	Adenovirus infection
	Coxsackievirus herpangina
	Cytomegalovirus infection
	Infectious mononucleosis
	Herpes simplex gingivostomatitis
	Herpes zoster
	Roseola infantum
	Rubella
	Varicella
	HIV
	Dengue
Fungal	Histoplasmosis
Parasitic	Toxoplasmosis
	American trypanosomiasis (Chagas' disease)
	African trypanosomiasis (sleeping sickness)
Unknown	Kawasaki disease

FIGURE 8-1 Infectious causes of cervical lymphadenopathy. Various diseases manifest lymphadenopathy primarily in the neck, although adenopathy may also occur at other anatomic sites or may be generalized with or without hepatosplenomegaly. The different microbial diseases usually associated with acute and/or chronic cervical lymphadenopathy are noted.

Noninfectious causes of cervical lymphadenopathy or neck masses	
Immunologic diseases	Systemic lupus erythematosus
	Serum sickness
	Drug reactions (phenytoin, hydralazine, allopurinol, silicone implants)
	Angioimmunoblastic lymphadenopathy
Malignant diseases	Hematologic
	Hodgkin's disease
	Acute T, B, myeloid, and monocytoid cell leukemias and lymphomas
	Chronic T, B, myeloid, and monocytoid cell leukemias and lymphomas
	Malignant histiocytosis
	Metastatic tumors to lymph nodes
	Melanoma
	Kaposi's sarcoma
	Neuroblastoma
	Seminoma
	Tumors of lung, breast, prostate, kidney, head and neck, gastrointestinal tract
Lipid storage disease	Niemann-Pick disease
Congenital conditions	Branchial cleft
	Thyroglossal duct cyst
	Cystic hygroma
Benign tumors	Lipoma
	Salivary glands
	Neurofibroma
Miscellaneous or unknown causes	Sinus histiocytosis
	Dermatopathic lymphadenitis
	Sarcoidosis
	Kikuchi's histiocytic necrotizing lymphadenitis

FIGURE 8-2 Noninfectious causes of cervical lymphadenopathy or neck masses. Various diseases and syndromes manifest cervical lymphadenopathy or neck masses as part of their symptom complex. These conditions should be considered when evaluating the patient presenting with lymphadenopathy. (*Adapted from* Haynes BF: Enlargement of the lymph nodes and spleen. *In* Isselbacher KJ, *et al.* (eds.): *Harrison's Principles of Internal Medicine*, 13th ed. New York: McGraw Hill; 1994:324; with permission.)

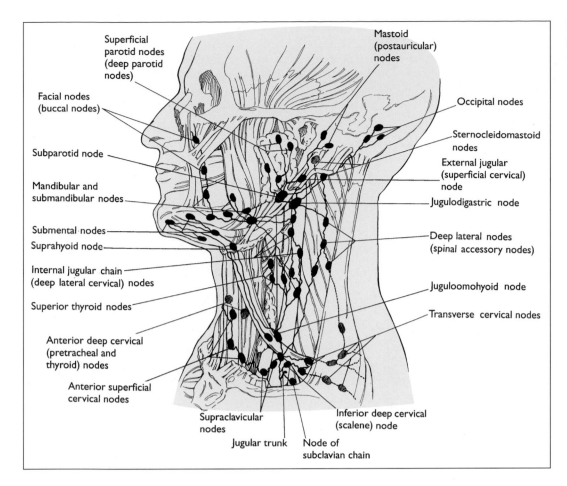

FIGURE 8-3 Lymph nodes of the head and neck. (*Adapted from* Netter FH: *Atlas of Human Anatomy*. Summit, NJ, Ciba-Geigy, 1989; with permission.)

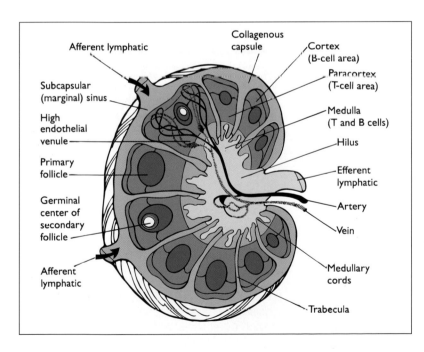

FIGURE 8-4 Lymph node structure. Beneath the collagenous capsule is the subcapsular sinus, which is lined by phagocytic cells. Lymphocytes and antigens (if present) pass into the sinus via the afferent lymphatics from surrounding tissue spaces or adjacent nodes. The cortex contains aggregates of B cells (primary follicles), most of which (secondary follicles) have a site of active proliferation (germinal centers). The paracortex contains mainly T cells, many of which are found near the interdigitating cells (antigen-presenting cells). Each node has its own arterial and venous supply, and lymphocytes enter the node from the circulation through the specialized high endothelial venules in the paracortex. The medulla contains both T and B cells and most of the lymph node plasma cells organized into cords of lymphoid tissue. Lymphocytes can only leave the node through the efferent lymphatics.

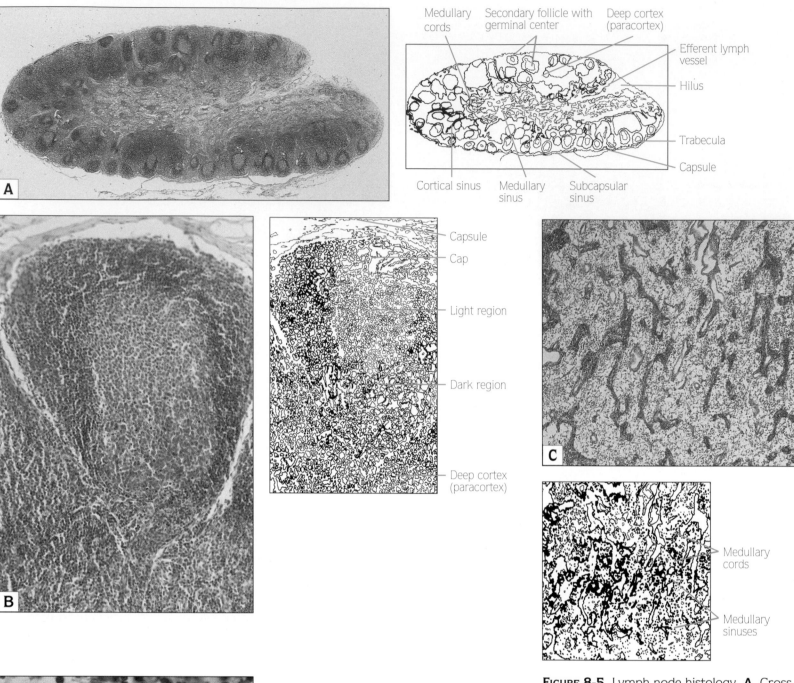

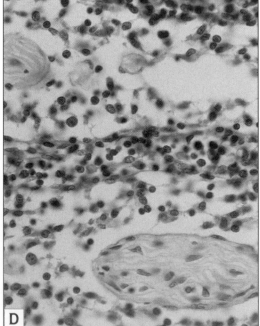

FIGURE 8-5 Lymph node histology. **A**, Cross-section of a human lymph node. The lymph node is surrounded by a connective tissue capsule and organized into three main areas: cortex (B-cell area), paracortex (T-cell area), and medulla, which contains cords of lymphoid tissue (T- and B-cell area). (Hematoxylin-eosin stain, × 15.) **B**, Section of lymph node cortex, showing a germinal center. (Hematoxylin-eosin stain, × 135.) **C** and **D**, Low- and high-power views of lymph node medulla, showing typical plasma cells in the medullary cords and sinuses. (*panel 5C*, Van Gieson stain, × 45; *panel 5D*, Hematoxylin-eosin stain, × 440.) (*continued*)

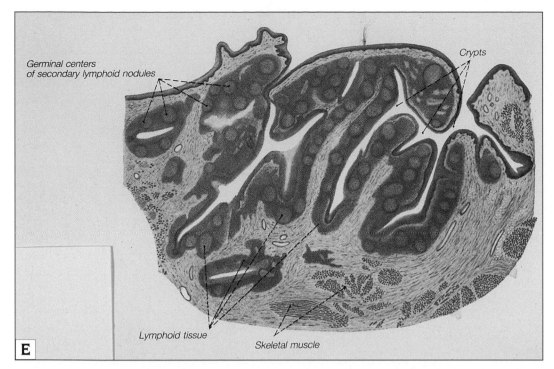

Germinal centers
of secondary lymphoid nodules

Crypts

Lymphoid tissue

Skeletal muscle

E

FIGURE 8-5 (*continued*) **E**, Section of human tonsil showing deep invaginations. Human tonsils contain abundant lymphoid tissue, frequently with many large germinal centers. (Camera lucida drawing. Hematoxylin-eosin stain, × 8.) (Panels 5A–D *from* Geneser F: *Color Atlas of Histology*. Philadelphia: Lea & Febiger; 1986:120; with permission. Panel 5E *from* Hammersen F: *Sobotta/Hammersen Histology: Color Atlas of Microscopic Anatomy*, 3rd ed. Baltimore: Urban & Schwarzenberg; 1985:80–83; with permission.)

Mechanisms of lymph node enlargement

Mechanism	Manifestation
Increase in number of lymphocytes and macrophages during response to antigens	Lymphadenopathy, transient (2–3 wks)
Infiltration by inflammatory cells in infections of the lymph nodes	Lymphadenitis (2 wks to months)
In situ proliferation of malignant lymphocytes and macrophages	Hodgkin's or other malignant disease
Infiltration of node by metastatic malignant cells	Regional tumor metastases (skin, lung, breast, gastrointestinal, etc.)
Infiltration of node by metabolite-laden macrophages in lipid-storage disease	Niemann-Pick disease

FIGURE 8-6 Mechanisms of lymph node enlargement. In normal immune responses, antigen stimulation results in increased blood flow through the affected lymph node. In stimulated nodes, lymphocytes accumulate due to increased traffic through the node, decreased egress of lymphocytes from the node, and proliferation of responding T and B cells, with the size of the node increasing up to 15 times within 5–10 days after antigen stimulation. In general, in all patients, new nodes > 1 cm require investigation. Important factors in the evaluation include patient age, physical characteristics of the node (*ie*, tenderness, mobility, size, consistency, discreteness), node location, and clinical setting. (Haynes BF: Enlargement of the lymph nodes and spleen. *In* Isselbacher KJ, *et al.* (eds.): *Harrison's Principles of Internal Medicine*, 13th ed. New York: McGraw Hill; 1994:325.)

BACTERIAL INFECTIONS

Streptococcal Infections

A. Pharyngitis: Clinical features, diagnosis, and treatment

Etiology	Streptococcus group A
Onset	Abrupt, 2–3 days
Site of adenopathy	Anterior cervical, bilateral
Clinical features	Pharyngitis or tonsillopharyngitis
	Headache
	Abdominal pain
	Occasional palate petechiae and/or scarlatiniform rash
Lab findings	Positive throat culture for group A β-hemolytic streptococcus
	Leukocytosis
Diagnostic tests	Throat culture and/or aspiration of node
	Penicillin or benzathine penicillin G intramuscularly
Treatment	Aspiration(s) of node (esp. if abscessed)

B. Spectrum of streptococcal infections manifesting pharyngitis

Tonsillopharyngitis and/or uvulitis
Nasopharyngitis in young children < 3 yrs old
Scarlet fever
Impetigo or pyoderma
Cellulitis
Toxic shock syndrome
Bacteremia

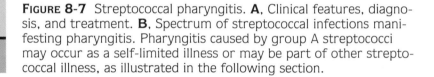

FIGURE 8-7 Streptococcal pharyngitis. **A,** Clinical features, diagnosis, and treatment. **B,** Spectrum of streptococcal infections manifesting pharyngitis. Pharyngitis caused by group A streptococci may occur as a self-limited illness or may be part of other streptococcal illness, as illustrated in the following section.

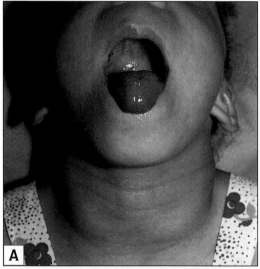

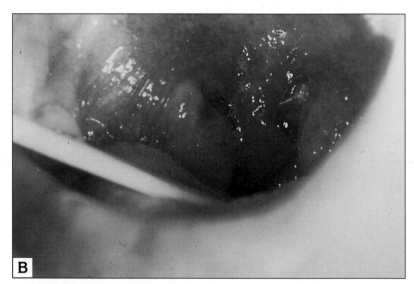

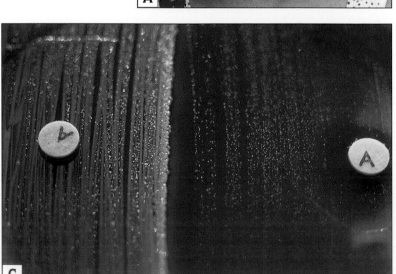

FIGURE 8-8 Scarlet fever. Scarlet fever, although uncommon today, typically presents with fever, a generalized maculopapular rash, and Pastia's lines on the neck or antecubital skin folds (dark red lines in the skinfolds). **A,** Cervical adenopathy is evident in a 5-year-old girl, as are the characteristic Pastia's lines on her neck. **B,** Red swollen tonsils and petechiae on her palate are noted. Penicillin therapy for 10 days brought prompt improvement. **C,** Diagnosis is confirmed by a throat culture positive for group A β-hemolytic streptococci. Blood agar plates show *Staphylococcus aureus* (*left panel*) and group A β-hemolytic streptococcus (*right panel*). Inhibition of bacterial growth around the bacitracin taxose A disk confirms a group A streptococcal etiology.

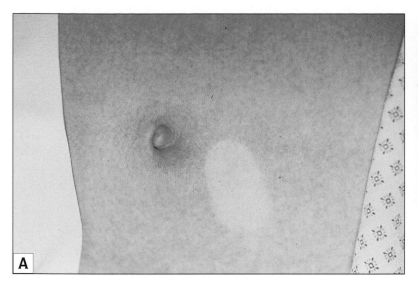

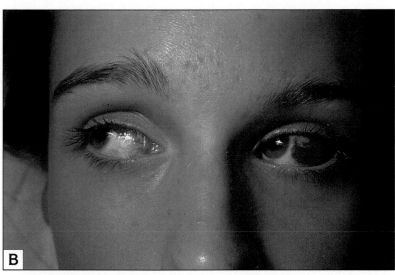

FIGURE 8-9 Streptococcal toxic shock syndrome. **A** and **B**, Sudden onset of high fever (to 40° C, 104° F), erythroderma, petechial rash (*panel 9A*), conjunctival hemorrhages (*panel 9B*), pharyngitis, and abdominal pain is typical of toxic shock syndrome, as seen in this 13-year-old girl 6 hours after onset. Shock may develop along with hypotension, very poor capillary filling, marked malaise, lethargy, and jaundice. In this patient, a throat culture was positive for group a β-hemolytic streptococcus, and her antistreptolysin titer was elevated to 1:1360 (although most cases of toxic shock syndrome are due to *Staphylococcus aureus*). Desquamation of her fingers and toes developed after 3–7 days on antibiotic therapy, with recovery following.

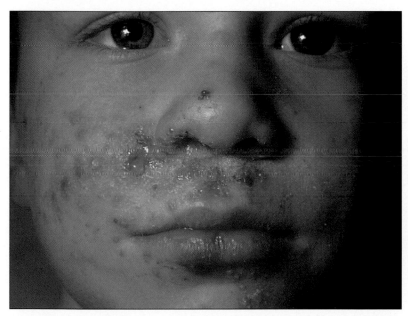

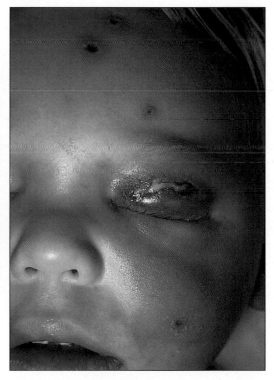

FIGURE 8-11 Cellulitis. Orbital and facial cellulitis developed in a 2-year-old child 3 days after the onset of chickenpox. The patient presented with fever (41.1° C, 106° F), grand mal seizures, and a generalized pruritic vesiculopustular exanthem, with cultures of blood and skin pustules positive for group A β-hemolytic streptococcus. Penicillin therapy was effective.

FIGURE 8-10 Impetigo. Serous, oozing, honey-yellow crusts below the nares and pustules below the lips are apparent in this 5-year-old child with classic impetigo 3 days after its onset. Culture yielded a group A β-hemolytic streptococcus.

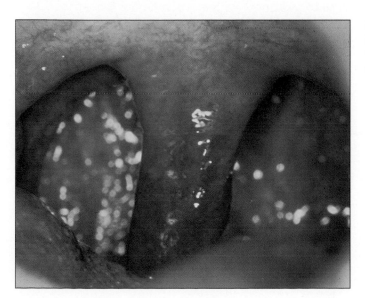

FIGURE 8-12 Uvulitis. Acute, severe uvulitis is seen in a 28-year-old pediatric resident. She had tender cervical nodes, and a throat culture was positive for group A β-hemolytic streptococcus. Note the moderate edema of the uvula and the normal-appearing pharynx. (*Courtesy of* R. Lampe, MD.)

Staphylococcal Infections

A. Lymphadenitis: Clinical features, diagnosis, and treatment	
Etiology	*Staphylococcus aureus*
Onset	Abrupt, 2–3 days
Site of adenopathy	Cervical, regional, rarely axillary or inguinal
Clinical features	Pharyngitis, usually mild
Lab findings	Leukocytosis
Diagnostic tests	Aspiration and culture of node
Treatment	Cephalexin
	Repeated aspirations of node
	Dicloxacillin
	Incision and drainage, if needed

B. Spectrum of staphylococcal infections manifesting lymphadenitis

Superficial infections
  Folliculitis
  Furuncle and/or carbuncle
  Impetigo
Toxin-mediated syndromes
  Staphylococcal scalded skin syndrome
  Toxic shock syndrome
Invasive infections
  Cutaneous abscesses in immunocompromised host
  Wound infections
  Septicemia and/or bacteremia

FIGURE 8-13 Staphylococcal lymphadenitis. **A**, Clinical features, diagnosis, and treatment. **B**, Spectrum of staphylococcal infections manifesting lymphadenitis. Lymphadenitis caused by

Staphylococcus aureus may occur as a self-limited illness or may be part of another illness, as illustrated in the following section.

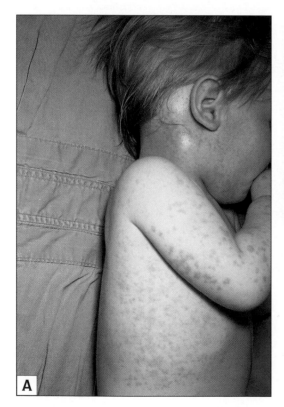

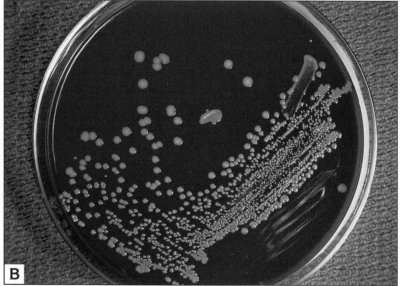

FIGURE 8-14 Lymphadenitis. **A**, Lymphadenitis with abscess due to β-hemolytic *Staphylococcus aureus* developed in a 12-month-old infant. The initial response to treatment with dicloxacillin for 2 weeks was poor. Recovery occurred after aspiration of 30 mL of pus from the abscess and 2 weeks of cephalexin therapy. **B**, A culture grew *S. aureus*.

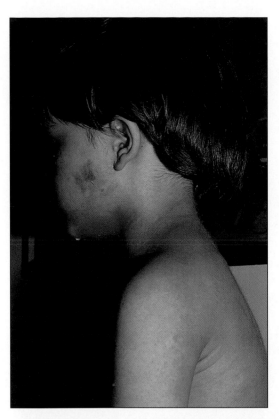

FIGURE 8-15 Staphylococcal scalded skin disease. A 6-year-old girl developed staphylococcal scalded skin disease with submental adenitis, fever, a tender generalized maculopapular exanthem with pustules, and a positive Nikolsky sign. Simultaneously, her sibling also had staphylococcal scalded skin disease, and another had staphylococcal scarlet fever, all due to the same phage type IIB *Staphylococcus aureus* strain. Oxacillin therapy was effective for all three siblings.

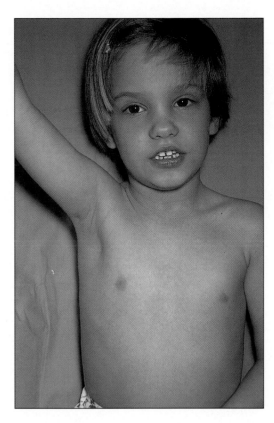

FIGURE 8-16 Staphylococcal scarlet fever. A 5-year-old girl, the sister of the girl with staphylococcal scalded skin disease in Fig. 8-15, simultaneously had staphylococcal scarlet fever due to the same phage type IIB *Staphylococcus aureus* strain. Her symptoms included fever, tonsillopharyngitis, cervical adenitis, and a fine papular scarlatiniform exanthem for 3 days, as well as characteristic Pastia's lines in the right axilla and anterior neck (also seen in streptococcal scarlet fever; *see* Fig. 8-8A). Oxacillin therapy was effective for both siblings.

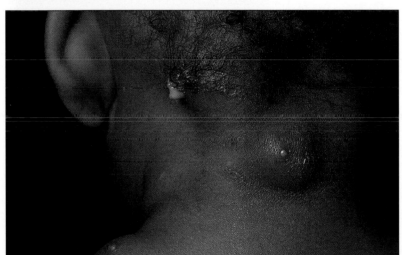

FIGURE 8-17 Furunculosis. Severe furunculosis of the posterior neck due to *Staphylococcus aureus* is seen 10 days after onset in a 17-month-old infant who had associated cervical adenopathy and fever. *S. aureus* was resistant to penicillin and ampicillin, but dicloxacillin therapy was effective.

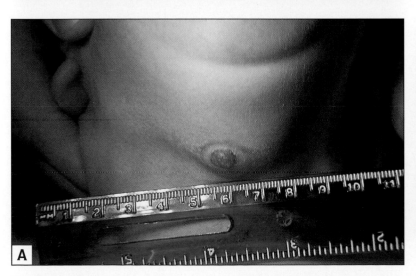

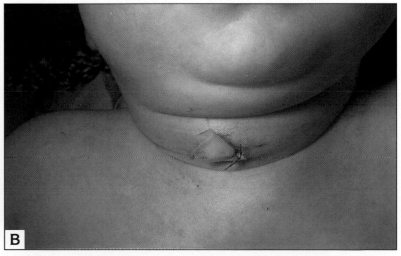

FIGURE 8-18 Thyroglossal duct cyst. Infection of the thyroid, with possible drainage tracts through the skin, is typically caused by *Staphylococcus aureus* and group A β-hemolytic streptococci. **A,** Thyroglossal duct cyst pointing is seen in a healthy 17-month-old. Surgical excision several days later was curative. **B,** In a 3-month-old infant, a thyroglossal duct cyst due to *Haemophilus influenzae* with associated cellulitis and cervical abscess was unresponsive to three antibiotics. Incision with drainage (note rubber wick) was effective, but reinfection occurred 12 days later due to *Klebsiella*.

Cat Scratch Disease

Cat scratch disease: Clinical features, diagnosis, and treatment

Etiology	*Bartonella henselae* *Afipia felis*
Onset	12 days, average (range, 7–60 days after contact with cat)
Site of adenopathy	Cervical, axillary, inguinal, or generalized
Clinical features	Fever (33% of patients) Malaise, headache, fatigue
Diagnosis	1. History of cat contact or scratches or primary lesion (95%) 2. Positive cat scratch skin test or *B. henselae* IFA 3. Negative serologies for other causes of lymphadenopathy: Negative PPD-T and PPD-Battey skin tests, PCR positive for CSD on sterile cultures of aspirated pus 4. Characteristic histopathology and/or positive Warthin-Starry stain for gram-negative bacteria in biopsy of skin, lymph node, or ocular granuloma
Treatment	Aspirate node (if painful or abscessed) TMP-SMX Rifampin Ciprofloxacin Gentamicin (intramuscularly or intravenously)

CSD—cat scratch disease; IFA—immunofluorescent antibody; PCR—polymerase chain reaction; PPD—purified protein derivative; TMP-SMX—trimethoprim-sulfamethoxazole.

FIGURE 8-19 Cat scratch disease: Clinical features, diagnosis, and treatment. The spectrum of cat scratch disease infections manifests primarily as cervical and/or axillary lymphadenitis with typical and atypical (12%) presentations, as illustrated in the following section.

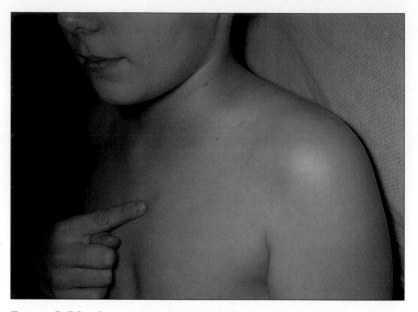

FIGURE 8-20 Cat scratch disease (CSD). An 11-year-old boy had fever, malaise, fatigue, and anorexia of 10 days' duration. A crusted primary inoculation papule due to cat scratch was seen on his sternum for 3 weeks. Tender, red masses (6 × 5 cm) on the left neck and supraclavicular region did not respond to dicloxacillin or penicillin. A CSD skin test was positive (33 mm). The lymphadenitis resolved spontaneously after 2 months. (Margileth AM: Cat scratch disease. *In* Arnoff SC, *et al.* (eds.): *Advances in Pediatric Infectious Disease*, 8th ed. St. Louis: Mosby Year Book; 1993:1–21.)

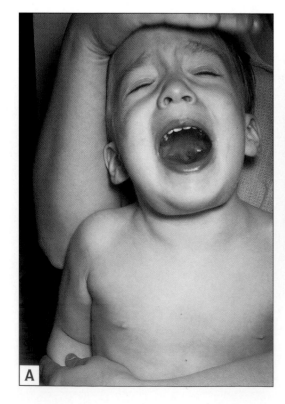

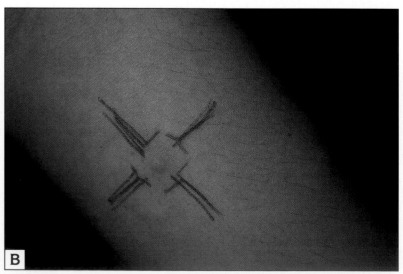

FIGURE 8-21 Cat scratch disease (CSD). A 2-year-old child had fever and bilateral submandibular lymphadenitis for 2 weeks. The patient had daily close contact with a cat but no scratches. **A,** An inoculation papule is evidence midline below his lip. Oxacillin and erythromycin were ineffective, but bilateral sterile abscesses drained spontaneously with recovery in 9 weeks. **B,** Two CSD skin tests were positive (15 mm).

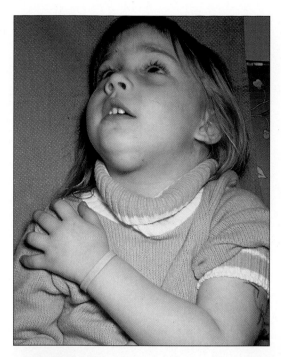

FIGURE 8-22 Submental node cat scratch disease (CSD). A healthy asymptomatic 3-year-old girl had a primary inoculation papule in the center of her chin for 3 weeks. Note the positive 28-mm CSD skin test on the left arm. The father had concurrent CSD of the inguinal nodes with cat scratches and a primary papule on his knee. Resolution occurred in 6 weeks, after application of local warm saline compresses.

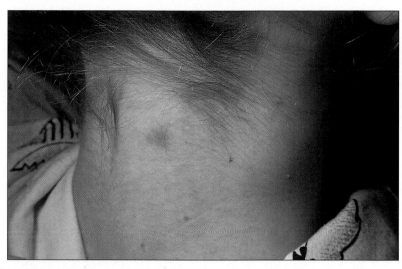

FIGURE 8-23 Cat scratch disease (CSD). A healthy asymptomatic 10-year-old had a primary posterior neck pustule for 5 weeks and three tender bilateral cervical nodes for 4 weeks. No therapy was given. A CSD skin test was positive at 24 mm, and node resolution occurred in 2 months.

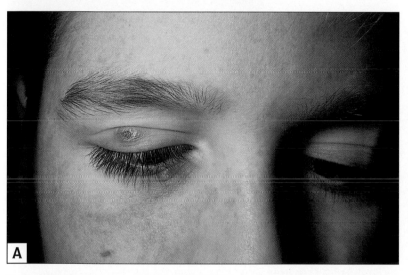

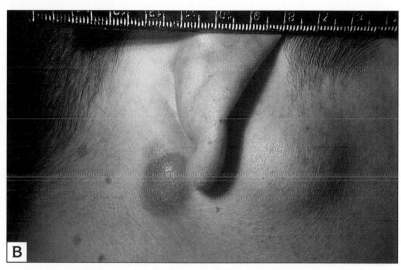

FIGURE 8-24 Cat scratch disease (CSD) postauricular abscess and "parotitis." **A,** A healthy asymptomatic 12-year-old had multiple cat scratches and two crusted primary inoculation papules on both eyelids for 3 weeks. **B,** The postauricular and parotid masses were warm, tender, discrete, and very edematous. The right Stensen's duct ostia showed clear serous drainage. A CSD skin test was positive, and spontaneous resolution of adenitis occurred in 3–4 months.

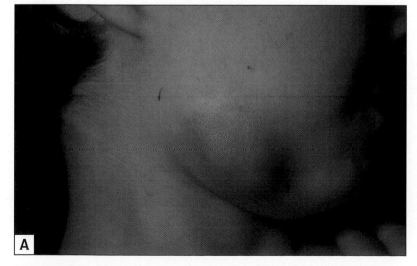

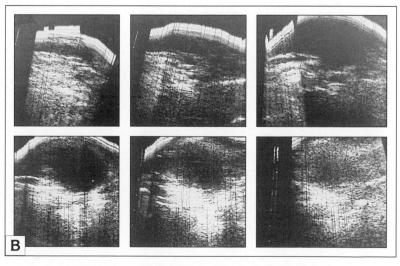

FIGURE 8-25 Cat scratch disease abscess of the right mandible. The mandibular abscess lasted for 4 weeks, with fever for 2 weeks, and there was no response to erythromycin or cefadroxil. Seven cats had scratched the child frequently on the cheek, but no inoculation lesion occurred. **A,** The patient had bit his tongue 3 weeks previously, leading to development of the 5 × 5-cm abscess. It responded to continuous warm saline compresses and an incision and drainage with resolution in 3 months. **B,** Ultrasound revealed the abscess.

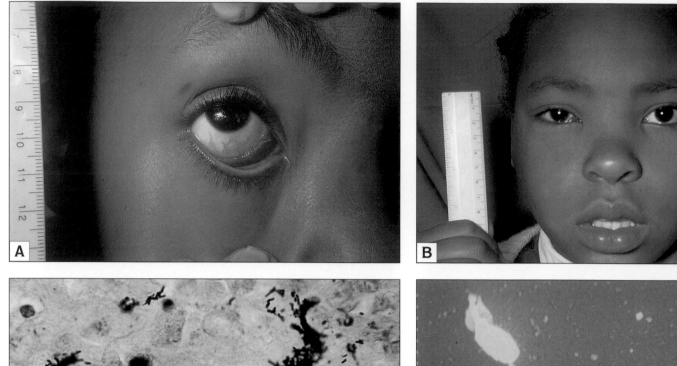

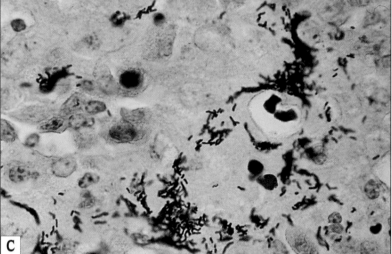

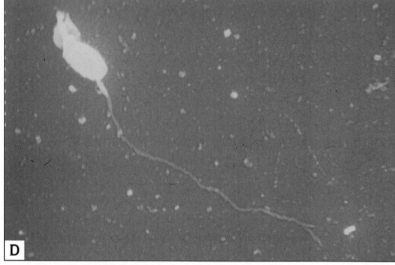

FIGURE 8-26 Cat scratch disease (CSD) due to dog licking. **A** and **B**, A healthy 8-year-old girl developed conjunctival granuloma and preauricular lymphadenitis of 2 weeks' duration. **C**, Biopsy of the ocular granuloma revealed multiple Warthin-Starry-positive bacilli of CSD. A CSD skin test was very positive. Adenopathy resolved spontaneously in 3 months. **D**, Scanning electron microscopy reveals the CSD bacillus, *Afipia felis*, with its unipolar flagellum (× 25,000). (English CK, Wear DJ, Margileth AM, Walsh GP: Cat-scratch disease: Isolation and culture of the bacterial agent. *JAMA* 1988, 259:1347-1352.) (Panel 26A *from* Margileth AM: Cervical adenitis. *Pediatr Rev* 1985, 7(Jul):16; with permission. Panel 26C *from* Wear DJ, Margileth AM, Hadfield T: Cat scratch disease, a bacterial infection? *Science* 1983, 221:1403; with permission.)

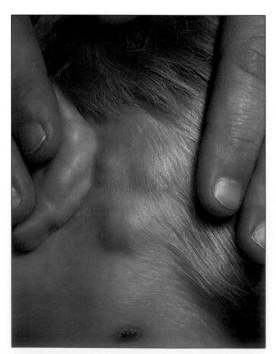

FIGURE 8-27 Cat scratch disease (CSD) with postauricular adenitis and purulent drainage. An asymptomatic 3-year-old had purulent drainage from a postauricular node for 5 weeks. She was hospitalized for 8 days for an incision and drainage of four nodes that became enlarged after 10 days' treatment with two antibiotics. A primary inoculation wound was discovered in the left scalp at the site of a cat scratch from 6 weeks previously. Spontaneous resolution of adenopathy occurred in 10–18 months. The CSD skin test was very positive. (*From* Margileth AM, Zawadsky P: Chronic lymphadenopathy in children and adolescents. *Am Fam Physician* 1985, 31:177; with permission.)

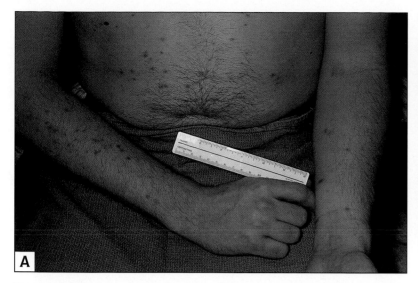

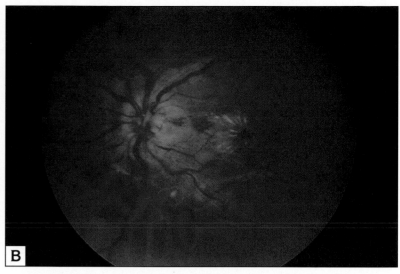

FIGURE 8-28 Cat scratch disease (CSD) neuroretinitis. **A**, A healthy 31-year-old man had flulike symptoms for 4 weeks, fever for 1 week, decreased vision in his right eye for 20 days, a papular rash on his abdomen and arms for 4 weeks secondary to flea bites and cat scratches, and submental adenopathy. **B**, The right fundus revealed optic edema with a macular star; visual acuity was 20/50. His left eye showed normal fundus and visual acuity. A CSD skin test was 35 mm. Spontaneous resolution of adenopathy and return of normal vision occurred in 3 months, and the maculopapular rash resolved in 6 months. (Panel 28B *from* Margileth AM, Hatfield T: A new look at old cat scratch. *Contemp Pediatr* 1990, 7:27; with permission.)

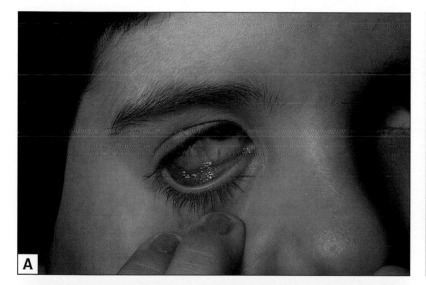

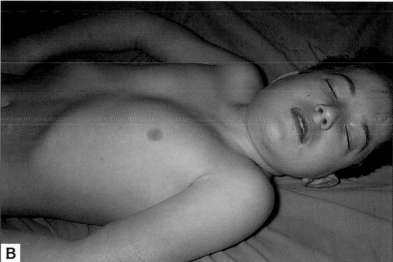

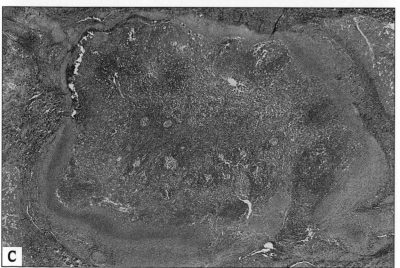

FIGURE 8-29 Cat scratch disease (CSD) oculoglandular syndrome with severe encephalitis. **A** and **B**, A 12-year-old had unilateral conjunctivitis, seizures, coma for 5 days, and preauricular and subauricular lymphadenopathy for 2 weeks. He had multiple kitten scratches. Spontaneous resolution of the adenopathy occurred in 3 months, and the patient remained well with normal development during the next 15 years. **C**, A parotid node biopsy revealed coalescing microabscesses. The CSD skin test was positive.

Mycobacterial Infections

Tuberculosis: Clinical features, diagnosis, and treatment	
Etiology	*Mycobacterium tuberculosis* (3 species)
Onset	2–7 wks
Site of adenopathy	Regional, anterior and posterior cervical, supraclavicular, rarely axillary or inguinal
Clinical features	History of TB contact
	Nontender firm node(s), matted
	Overlying skin indurated
Lab findings	CBC usually normal, anemia rare
	Sedimentation rate usually elevated
Diagnostic tests	PPD-T > 15 mm
	Chest radiograph (abnormal in 19%)
	PCR positive for TB DNA on clinical specimen
Treatment	Isoniazid and rifampin for 6–12 mos
	Excision if no response

CBC—complete blood count; PCR—polymerase chain reaction; PPD—purified protein derivative; TB—tuberculosis.

FIGURE 8-30 Tuberculosis: clinical features, diagnosis, and treatment. Although pulmonary tuberculosis is the most frequent form of tuberculosis, extrapulmonary disease due to hematogenous spread is seen within 1 year after initial lung infection in about 25% of children < 5 years old as well as in adults with immunodeficient states. Cervical lymphadenitis occurs more often than tuberculous meningitis, empyema, and osteomyelitis.

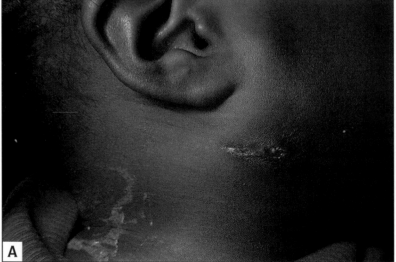

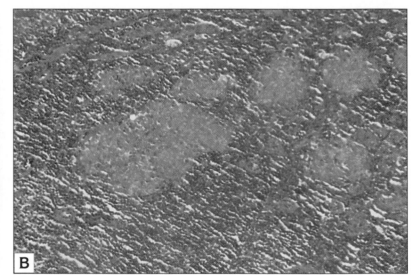

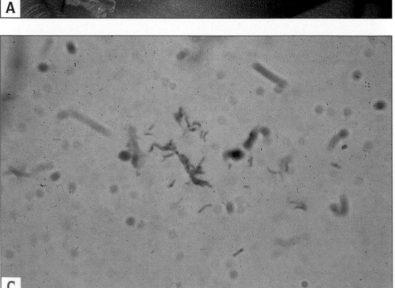

FIGURE 8-31 *Mycobacterium tuberculosis* oculoglandular syndrome. **A,** A healthy, asymptomatic, 3-year-old boy developed *M. tuberculosis* oculoglandular syndrome involving three nontender parotid nodes (2.5 × 4.5 cm) for 2 weeks. His right eye showed granular conjunctivitis, with a normal examination otherwise. The family history showed two members with active pulmonary tuberculosis. The patient's chest radiograph was normal. A PPD-T revealed a 4+ reaction with vesicles; PPD-Battey was 16 mm. **B,** Biopsy of a node revealed caseous necrosis. **C,** An acid-fast smear was positive, and a culture was positive for *M. tuberculosis*. All three nodes resolved in 4 months with isoniazid and PAS (para-aminosalicylic acid) therapy for 9 months.

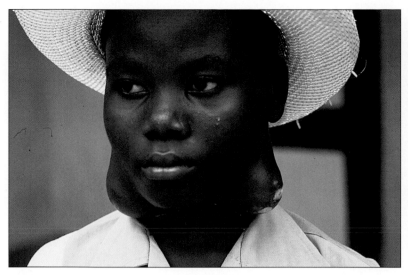

FIGURE 8-32 *Mycobacterium tuberculosis* scrofula. Extensive bilateral lymphadenopathy is seen in a 10-year-old Haitian child with a 40-mm PPD-T reaction. Isoniazid and PAS were prescribed, but the patient did not return for follow-up.

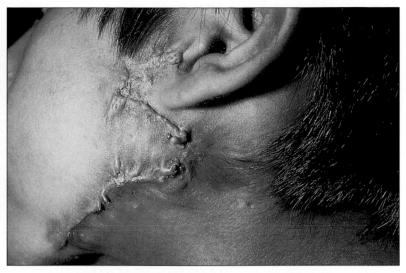

FIGURE 8-33 *Mycobacterium tuberculosis* scrofuloderma and cervical lymphadenitis. A Panamanian child had cervical lymphadenitis for many months that was not treated. Multiple healing skin ulcers and sinus tracts bridged by granulation tissue are evident. These sinus tracts are caused by discharge of necrotic material and pus channeling to the skin surface from an active focus of tuberculosis in the underlying lymph nodes.

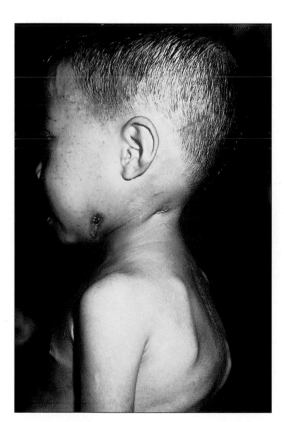

FIGURE 8-34 *Mycobacterium tuberculosis* scrofula with draining sinus tracts. Pulmonary infiltrates and Pott's disease of the spine of unknown duration were also seen in a Haitian child. Note the severe gibbus deformity of the thoracic spine, which usually occurs in the thoracolumbar region in children.

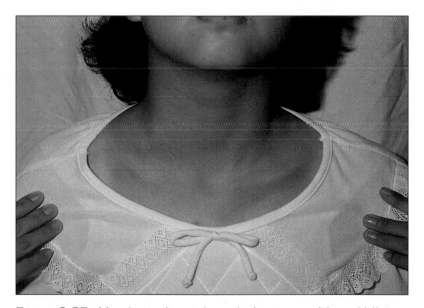

FIGURE 8-35 *Mycobacterium tuberculosis* pneumonitis and bilateral anterior cervical adenitis. The condition persisted for 4 months in the patient, a healthy 13-year-old Korean girl whose mother had *M. tuberculosis* chorioretinitis treated recently. Biopsy of her neck node was positive for acid-fast bacilli and culture yielded *M. tuberculosis*. Triple therapy (isoniazid, rifampin, and ethambutol) for 12 months was very effective.

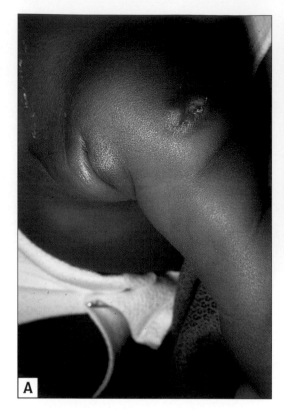

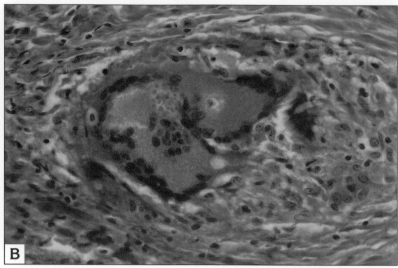

FIGURE 8-36 Bacille Calmette-Guérin (BCG)-itis. A healthy 2-month-old asymptomatic infant developed a reaction to BCG vaccine that was given subcutaneously 5 weeks previously. **A**, Axillary and supra-clavicular adenopathy developed over 5–6 days. A chest radiograph was normal. PPD-T was 15 mm. The adenopathy and skin ulceration resolved spontaneously in 7 months, leaving an atrophic scar. **B**, Histopathologic examination of a BCG vaccination site revealed a Langhans' giant cell.

Nontuberculous mycobacterial disease: Clinical features, diagnosis, and treatment

Etiology	Nontuberculous *Mycobacterium* (23 species)
Onset	2–7 wks
Site of adenopathy	Cervical, unilateral (95%)
Clinical features	No history of tuberculous contact
	Asymptomatic, healthy child < 6 yrs old
Lab findings	CBC usually normal
	Chest radiograph usually normal (95%)
Diagnostic tests	PPD-T 0–14 mm
	PPD-Battey ≥ 5 mm larger than PPD-T
	PCR positive for MAC DNA on clinical specimens
Treatment	Excisional biopsy of larger nodes
	Isoniazid and rifampin (rarely effective)

CBC—complete blood count; MAC—*Mycobacterium avium* complex; PCR—polymerase chain reaction; PPD—purified protein derivative.

FIGURE 8-37 Nontuberculous mycobacterial disease: clinical features, diagnosis, and treatment. Nontuberculous mycobacterial infections manifest primarily as cervical adenitis in children, but in patients with AIDS, the infection is often disseminated and usually due to *Mycobacterium avium* complex.

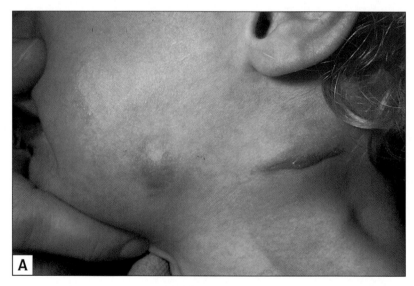

FIGURE 8-38 Nontuberculous mycobacterial lymphadenitis. **A**, A 3-year-old, healthy, asymptomatic child had lymphadenitis for several weeks. Incision and drainage produced a thick pus that grew *Mycobacterium avium-intracellulare*. (*continued*)

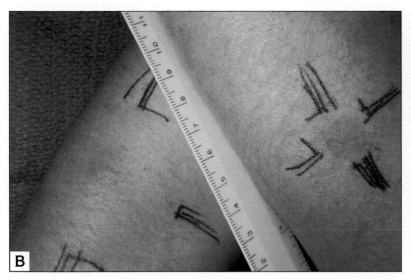

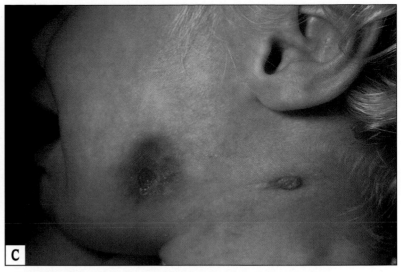

FIGURE 8-38 (*continued*) **B,** PPD-T was 16 mm; PPD-Battey was 52 mm. **C,** Spontaneous drainage of caseous material from a mandibular node occurred several weeks later. Spontaneous healing of both lesions occurred over 24 months. (Margileth AM: Nontuberculous [atypical] mycobacterial disease. *Semin Pediatr Infect Dis* 1993, 4:307–315.) (Panels 38A and 38C *from*

Margileth AM, Zawadsky P: Chronic adenopathy in children and adolescents. *Am Fam Physician* 1985, 31:178; with permission. Panel 38B *from* Longfield JM, Margileth AM: Interobserver and method variability in tuberculin skin testing. *Semin Pediatr Infect Dis* 1984, 3:323; with permission.)

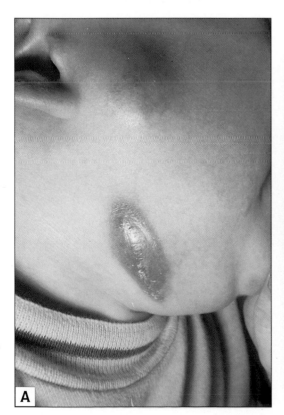

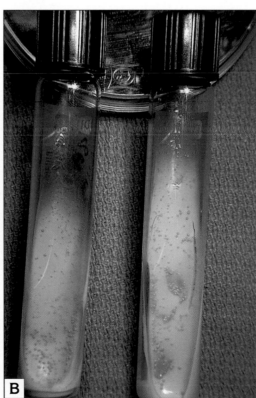

FIGURE 8-39 Nontuberculous mycobacterial lymphadenitis. **A,** A healthy 2-year-old had a tender parotid abscess and right submandibular adenitis for 5 weeks. **B,** Biopsy of the node revealed caseous necrosis and a culture grew *Mycobacterium scrofulaceum*. PPD-G was 27 mm; PPD-T was 14 mm. Isoniazid and rifampin therapies were ineffective. Spontaneous discharge of caseous matter over several weeks resulted in complete healing after 6 months. Excisional surgery is the best therapy for nontuberculous mycobacterial adenopathy.

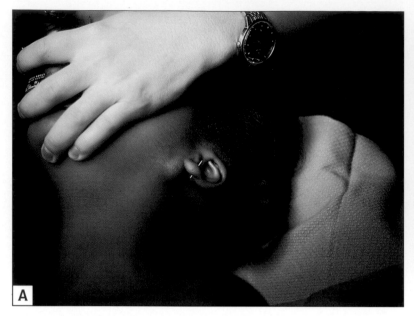

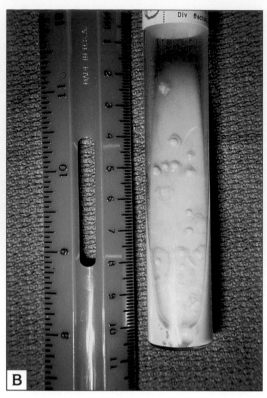

FIGURE 8-40 Nontuberculous subauricular abscess. **A**, A healthy 12-year-old developed a subauricular abscess following ear piercing. **B**, Aspiration of pus grew *Mycobacterium fortuitum* in 2 weeks on culture. Excisional surgery was very effective with minimal scar formation.

Spirochetal Infections

A. Lyme disease: Clinical features, diagnosis, and treatment	
Etiology	*Borrelia burgdorferi*
Onset	Rash occurs 3–31 days after tick bite
Site of adenopathy	Regional to ECM, generalized in 20%
Clinical features	ECM
	Regional lymphadenopathy
	Fever, chills
	Malaise, headache
	Arthralgias, myalgias, stiff neck
Lab findings	Culture of blood or skin biopsy *B. burgdorferi*
	Specific antibody titers, IFA, EIA
Diagnostic tests	History and ECM rash 5–68 cm at site of tick bite
	Isolation of *B. burgdorferi* or antibody titer rise
Treatment	Doxycycline (in patients ≥ 9 yrs old)
	Amoxicillin
	Penicillin
	Ceftriaxone (for late-stage disease)

ECM—erythema chronicum migrans; EIA—enzyme immunoassay; IFA—indirect fluorescent antibody.

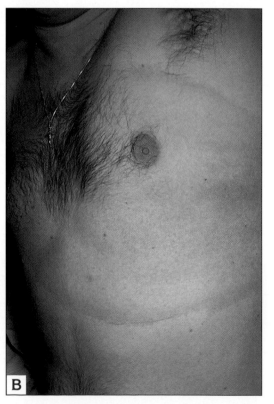

FIGURE 8-41 Lyme disease. **A**, Clinical features, diagnosis, and treatment. **B**, Erythema chronicum migrans with central punctum of 2 weeks' duration is seen in a 27-year-old man who had malaise, headache, myalgia, stiff neck, and arthralgias of multiple joints. No tick bite or fever was present, but the *Borrelia burgdorferi* titer was 1:2640 and a skin biopsy showed a perivascular lymphocytic infiltrate with inflammatory epidermal areas and central necrosis. Tetracycline therapy was effective.

A. Congenital syphilis: Clinical features, diagnosis, and treatment

Etiology	*Treponema pallidum*
Onset	At birth or asymptomatic first weeks of life
Site of adenopathy	Regional or generalized
Clinical features	"Snuffles" (rhinitis)
	Mucocutaneous lesions
	Hepatosplenomegaly, hepatitis
	Lymphadenopathy
	Pneumonitis
	Anemia, thrombocytopenia
	Osteomyelitis
	Osteitis
Lab findings	*T. pallidum* in tissue or lesion exudate on darkfield examination
	Positive direct fluorescent antibody test
Diagnostic tests	VDRL, RPR, or ART nontreponemal tests
	FTA-ABS for *Treponema*
Treatment	Penicillin for 14 days
	Benzathine penicillin G (one dose intramuscularly)

ART—automated reagin test; FTA-ABS—fluorescent treponemal antibody absorption; RPR—rapid plasma reagin; VDRL—Venereal Disease Research Laboratory.

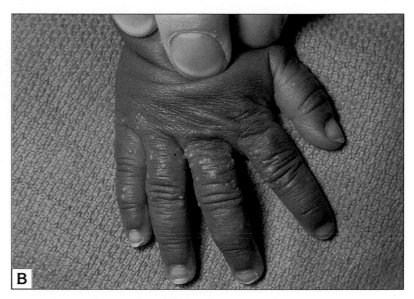

FIGURE 8-42 Congenital syphilis. **A,** Clinical features, diagnosis, and treatment. Congenital syphilis may cause stillbirth or perinatal death, as well as spontaneous abortion. **B,** Congenital syphilis, secondary stage. A pustular rash on the hand and foot of 2 weeks' duration is seen in a healthy 5-month-old child with minimal splenomegaly and with osteitis of the proximal tibiae. Aspiration of the pustule revealed many spirochetes of *Treponema pallidum* on darkfield examination. Both Venereal Disease Research Laboratory and fluorescent treponemal antibody absorption tests were positive. Penicillin therapy was effective.

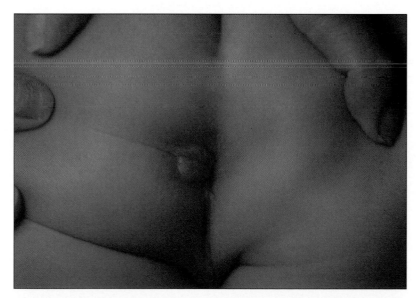

FIGURE 8-43 Congenital syphilis. Condyloma lata (2-cm diameter) of the perianal area. A healthy asymptomatic 22-month-old child with an otherwise normal physical examination had a condyloma lata of 1 month's duration. Rapid plasma reagin and fluorescent treponemal antibody absorption tests were very positive. Penicillin and benzathine penicillin G therapy were effective. The parents were also treated for syphilis.

A. Acquired syphilis: Clinical features, diagnosis, and treatment

Etiology	*Treponema pallidum*
Onset	3 wks (10–90 days) after sexual exposure
Site of adenopathy	Regional
Three clinical stages	1. Painless indurated mucocutaneous ulcers
	2. Maculopapular rash, especially of palms and soles
	Generalized lymphadenopathy
	Condyloma lata of genitalia or perianal area
	Fever, malaise, arthralgia
	Splenomegaly
	3. Neurosyphilis
	Aortitis
	Gumma of skin, bone, or viscera
Diagnostic tests	Nontreponemal tests (VDRL, RPR, or ART)
	Treponemal tests (FTA-ABS, MHA-TP) provisional
Treatment	Benzathine penicillin G (intramuscularly)
	Tetracycline (in penicillin allergy)

ART—automated reagin test; FTA-ABS—fluorescent treponemal antibody absorption; MHA-TP—microhemagglutination test–*Treponema pallidum*; RPR—rapid plasma reagin; VDRL—Veneral Disease Research Laboratory.

FIGURE 8-44 Acquired syphilis. **A,** Clinical features, diagnosis, and treatment. (*continued*)

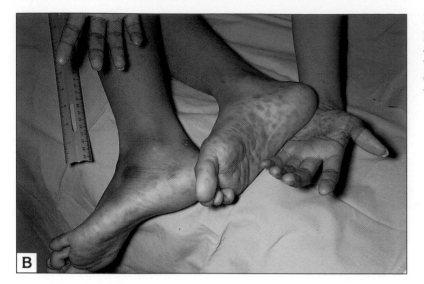

FIGURE 8-44 (*continued*) **B**, Secondary syphilitic, copper-colored papulosquamous rash of 1 week's duration was seen on the palms and soles of a healthy 9-year-old girl. Examination revealed a vaginal chancre, which showed numerous *Treponema pallidum* on darkfield examination. The Venereal Disease Research Laboratory test was positive, and penicillin therapy was effective.

Other Bacterial Infections

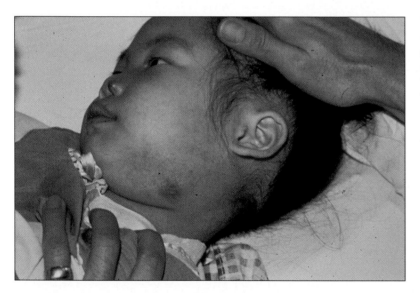

FIGURE 8-45 Cervicofacial nocardiosis. A 3-year-old child with cervicofacial nocardiosis for 7 days' duration presented with submandibular adenopathy and a draining left naris pustule that grew *Nocardia caviae* on culture. Trimethoprim-sulfamethoxazole therapy for 3 months was effective. (Lampe RL, *et al.*: Cervico-facial nocardiosis in children. *J Pediatr* 1981, 99:563–565.) (*Courtesy of* R. Lampe, MD)

A. Tularemia: Clinical features, diagnosis, and treatment

Etiology	*Francisella tularensis*
Onset	1–7 days
Site of adenopathy	Regional, 75% ulceroglandular
Clinical features	History of rabbit or squirrel contact
	Tender axillary, cervical, or preauricular nodes
	Fever, chills, headache
Lab findings	Leukocytosis
Diagnostic tests	Serum *F. tularensis* agglutinin titer
Treatment	Streptomycin intramuscularly for 6–10 days
	Tetracycline for 10 days for patients > 9 yrs old

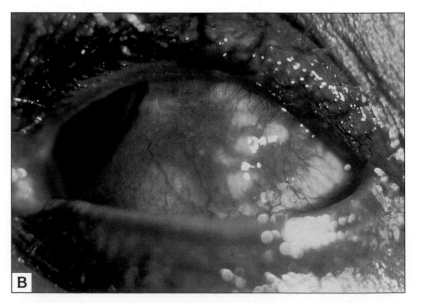

FIGURE 8-46 Tularemia. **A**, Clinical features, diagnosis, and treatment. **B**, Oculoglandular tularemia manifested by conjunctivitis with preauricular lymphadenitis developed in a healthy adult who had hunted and cleaned rabbits recently. Tetracycline therapy for 10 days was effective. A recent history of tick or insect bites or exposure to infected animals or their habitat should always be queried in suspected cases.

A. Actinomycosis: Clinical features, diagnosis, and treatment

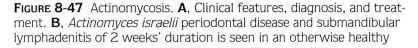

Etiology	*Actinomyces israelii*
Onset	Variable, weeks
Site of adenopathy	Cervical, unilateral
Clinical features	Tender hard nodes
	Sinus tracts
Lab findings	Normal complete blood count
	Gram-positive rods (beaded, branching) or sulfur granules in pus
Diagnostic tests	Anaerobic culture
Treatment	Penicillin for 6 mos

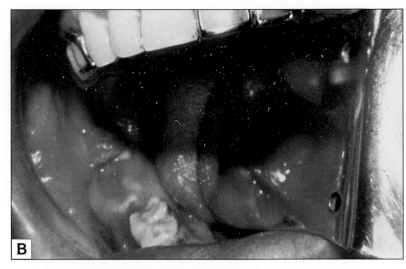

FIGURE 8-47 Actinomycosis. **A**, Clinical features, diagnosis, and treatment. **B**, *Actinomyces israelii* periodontal disease and submandibular lymphadenitis of 2 weeks' duration is seen in an otherwise healthy adult with chronic gingivitis and severe caries. Penicillin therapy for 6 months was effective. Demonstration of beaded, branched, gram-positive bacilli in aspirated pus suggests the diagnosis.

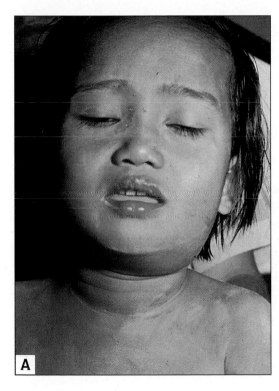

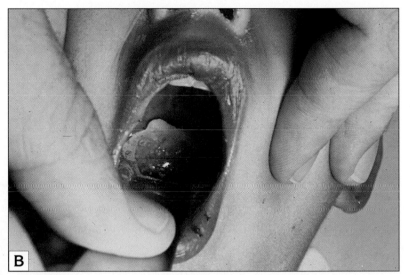

FIGURE 8-48 Nasopharyngeal diphtheria. **A** and **B**, Nasopharyngeal diphtheria with lymphadenitis (*panel 48A*) and extensive membrane formation (*panel 48B*) developed in a 4-year-old child in Thailand. Recovery occurred following treatment with penicillin G daily intramuscularly for 14 days and one dose of equine antitoxin intravenously. (*Courtesy of* R. Lampe, MD.)

Brucellosis: Clinical features, diagnosis, and treatment

Etiology	*Brucella abortus, B. melitensis*
Onset	1–7 wks to several months
Site of adenopathy	Generalized or cervical and axillary
Clinical features	History of contact with sick farm animals or ingestion of raw milk
	Afternoon fever and chills
	Sweats, malaise, headache
	Arthralgia, myalgia, backache
	Splenomegaly, rarely hepatomegaly
Lab findings	Normal or decreased WBC with lymphocytosis
	Positive cultures and serologic tests
Diagnostic tests	Blood or tissue culture
	Agglutination (SAT) test
Treatment	Tetracycline or doxycycline for 4–6 wks
	TMP-SMX in children < 9 yrs old

SAT—slide agglutination test; TMP-SMX—trimethoprim and sulfamethoxazole; WBC—white blood count.

FIGURE 8-49 Brucellosis. Clinical features, diagnosis, and treatment. Ninety percent of cases of brucellosis occur in adults who have contact with farm animals (farmers, ranchers, or veterinarians). Brucellosis in children is rare and is frequently a mild, self-limited disease if due to *Brucella abortus*; infections with *B. melitensis* can produce severe disease (meningitis, endocarditis, osteomyelitis).

Yersinia pseudotuberculosis infection: Clinical features, diagnosis, and treatment

Etiology	*Yersinia pseudotuberculosis*
Onset	1–14 days after ingestion of uncooked meat, raw milk, or contaminated water
Site of adenopathy	Cervical, mesenteric
Clinical features	Fever, rash
	Pharyngitis
	Abdominal pain
Lab findings	Throat culture positive for *Y. pseudotuberculosis*
	Leukocytosis
Diagnostic tests	Culture of blood, node aspirate, or throat swab
Treatment	Tetracycline
	Chloramphenicol
	Trimethoprim and sulfamethoxazole

FIGURE 8-50 *Yersinia pseudotuberculosis* infection. Clinical features, diagnosis, and treatment. *Yersinia* organisms cause several syndromes, most commonly fever and diarrhea in young children. *Y. pseudotuberculosis* produces a triad of fever, rash, and abdominal symptoms. Clinical features can mimic those of Kawasaki disease.

A. *Yersinia pestis* (plague): Clinical features, diagnosis, and treatment

Etiology	*Yersinia pestis*
Onset	2–8 days for bubonic form
	2–4 days for pneumonic form
Site of adenopathy	Cervical, axillary, inguinal (most often)
Clinical features	Tender, large (1–10 cm) nodes
	Fever, chills
	Weakness, headache
Lab findings	Bipolar staining of *Y. pestis* by Wayson's, Giemsa, Gram, or FA study of bubo aspirate, CSF, and blood
	Fourfold antibody titer rise in passive hemagglutination test, single >1:16
Diagnosis	Tender adenitis in patient exposed to rodents and/or flea bites in endemic area
	Stain or culture of bubo aspirate, blood, and CSF positive for *Y. pestis*
Treatment	Supportive therapy, strict isolation
	Streptomycin
	Tetracycline
	Chloramphenicol

FA—fluorescent antibody; CSF—cerebrospinal fluid.

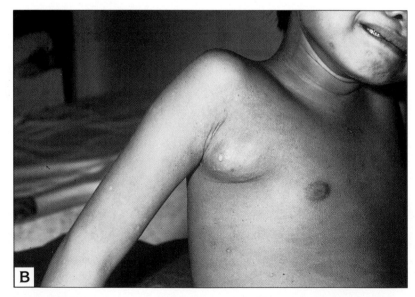

FIGURE 8-51 *Yersinia pestis* (plague). **A**, Clinical features, diagnosis, and treatment. **B**, Bubonic plague manifesting as tender, axillary adenitis in a 6-year-old Vietnamese child who had fever, malaise, and chills of 3 days' duration. Therapy with chloramphenicol was effective. Bubonic plague is caused by *Yersinia pestis*, a gram-negative bacillus, transmitted to humans by rodent fleas. In its pneumonic form, the disease is rapidly progressive and highly contagious. Pneumonic, septicemic, meningeal, and pharyngeal forms are uncommon. (*Courtesy of* F. Burkle, MD.)

VIRAL INFECTIONS

Herpes Virus Infections

Human herpesvirus infections associated with lymphadenopathy

Virus	Clinical infection
Herpes simplex 1 and 2	Herpes simplex dermatitis
	Herpes simplex dissemination (in HIV)
	Pharyngotonsillitis
	Gingivostomatitis
	Keratoconjunctivitis
	Herpetic whitlow/gladiatorum
Varicella-zoster (HHV-3)	Varicella (chickenpox)
	Herpes zoster (shingles)
Cytomegalovirus (HHV-4)	Mononucleosis syndrome
	Chorioretinitis
	Perinatal infection (CMV inclusion disease)
Epstein-Barr (HHV-5)	Infectious mononucleosis
	Burkitt's B-cell lymphoma
	Nasopharyngeal carcinoma
Herpesvirus 6	Roseola infantum
	Mononucleosis-like illness

CMV—cytomegalovirus; HHV—human herpesvirus; HSV—herpes simplex virus.

FIGURE 8-52 Human herpesvirus infections associated with lymphadenopathy. Of the seven known human herpesviruses, six produce well-described diseases manifesting as local or generalized infections that usually are self-limited in the immunocompetent patient. Severe systemic infections (encephalitis, hepatosplenomegaly, seizures, chorioretinitis) may result in serious sequelae or death.

A. Herpes simplex gingivostomatitis: Clinical features, diagnosis, and treatment

Etiology	Herpes simplex virus (usually HSV-1)
Onset	2–14 days in children < 5 yrs old
Site of adenopathy	Anterior cervical and submandibular
Clinical features	Pharyngeal and gingival erythema and edema
	Discrete vesicular and ulcerative oropharyngeal lesions
	Fever 3–5 days
	Malaise, anorexia
Lab findings	Tzanck test
Diagnostic tests	Positive viral culture in 1–3 days
Treatment	Acyclovir for serious disease

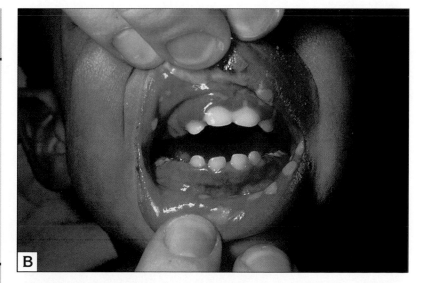

FIGURE 8-53 Herpes simplex gingivostomatitis. **A**, Clinical features, diagnosis, and treatment. **B**, A healthy 16-month-old child developed submandibular lymphadenitis and erythema multiforme due to a primary herpes simplex virus infection. Multiple superficial ulcers are evident on the mucous membranes. Spontaneous recovery occurred in 2 weeks.

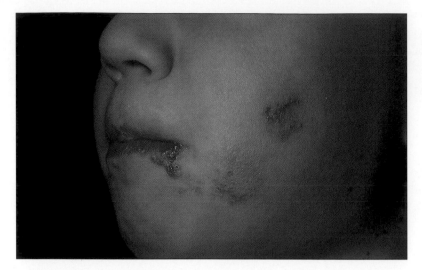

FIGURE 8-54 Recurrent herpes simplex infection showing zosteriform distribution. A healthy 8-year-old, who had 14 episodes of recurrent herpes simplex, is seen on the 10th day with spontaneously resolving vesiculopustules. Submandibular adenopathy is minimal. Immunocompromised patients and those with eczematoid dermatitis are more prone to severe local and recurrent lesions.

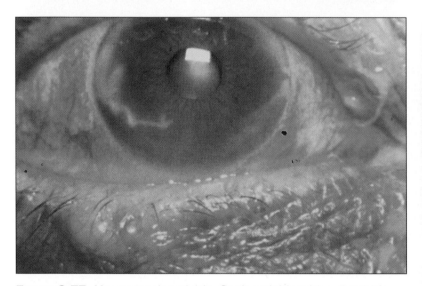

FIGURE 8-55 Herpes conjunctivitis. Conjunctivitis with a dendritic corneal ulceration due to HSV is seen in a healthy adult. Treatment of eye lesions with DNA inhibitors should be undertaken with the help of an ophthalmologist.

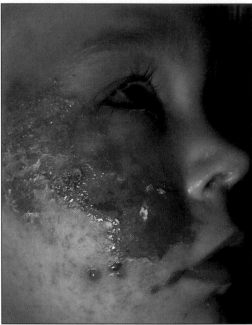

FIGURE 8-56 Streptococcal cellulitis and localized vesicular dermatitis due to herpes simplex virus (HSV). A healthy 6-year-old had fever of 40° C (104° F), local pain, conjunctivitis, and photophobia for 5 days due to coinfection with a group A, β-hemolytic streptococcus and recurrent (× 4) episodes of HSV infection on the same cheek. Penicillin therapy was effective, and the cellulitis cleared by the 12th day. Antiviral therapy was not given.

A. Herpes zoster: Clinical features, diagnosis, and treatment

Etiology	Varicella-zoster virus (HHV-3)
Onset	14–16 days
Site of adenopathy	Unilateral cervical
Clinical features	Unilateral tender nodes
	Grouped vesicles in 1 or 2 dermatomes
Lab findings	Giant cells on Tzanck smear
Diagnosis	Grouped vesicular lesions for 12–14 days
	Positive IFA membrane antigen
Treatment	Acyclovir given within < 24 hr of onset of rash, chronic skin (eczema), or respiratory disease

HHV—human herpesvirus; IFA—indirect fluorescent antibody.

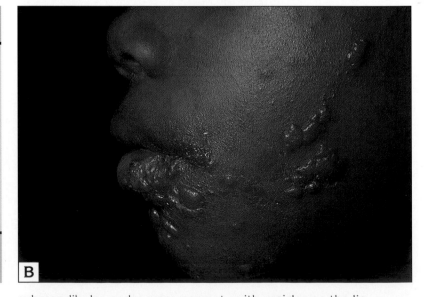

B

FIGURE 8-57 Herpes zoster. **A**, Clinical features, diagnosis, and treatment. **B**, A healthy 7-year-old girl had herpes zoster of a mandibular dermatome for 4 days. Painful cheek and enlarged submandibular nodes were present, with vesicles on the lip, tongue, and left cheek. Lesions resolved spontaneously in 12 days.

A. Varicella (chickenpox): Clinical features, diagnosis, and treatment

Etiology	Varicella-zoster virus (HHV-3)
Onset	10–21 days
Site of adenopathy	Cervical, posterior, generalized, minimal
Clinical features	Generalized pruritic, vesicular to pustular lesions crusting over at 3–5 days
	Mild fever
Lab findings	Positive Tzanck smear
Diagnostic tests	Virus isolated on vesicle culture
Treatment	Acyclovir or vidarabine intravenously for serious disease or if rash present < 24 hr

HHV—human herpesvirus.

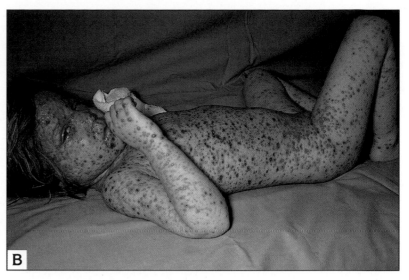

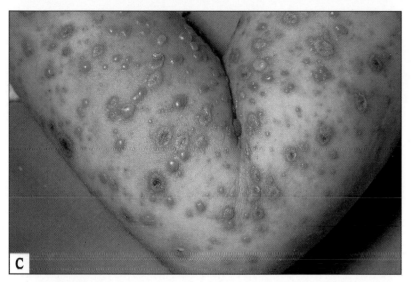

FIGURE 8-58 Varicella (chickenpox). **A**, Clinical features, diagnosis, and treatment. Primary infection with varicella-zoster virus results in chickenpox, which is usually mild in children with rare complications. However, in adults, especially immunocompromised persons, severe complications may occur, including pneumonia, encephalitis, thrombocytopenia, hepatitis, arthritis, pancreatitis, glomerulonephritis, and bacterial (group A β-hemolytic streptococcus) superinfections. **B** and **C**, Severe, prolonged chickenpox with new vesicles appearing on the 8th to 11th day is seen in a 4-year-old, otherwise healthy child. High-dose dexamethasone therapy was given for erythema multiforme due to a sulfa reaction 2 weeks previously. The patient recovered completely.

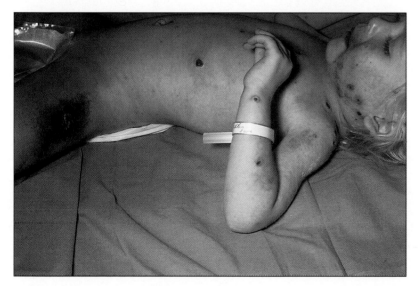

FIGURE 8-59 Hemorrhagic chickenpox. A 3-year-old girl with hemorrhagic chickenpox developed purpura fulminans due to group A β-hemolytic streptococcal septicemia. Her leukocyte count was 50,000/μL and the platelet count was 50,000/μL, with a hemoglobin of 6 g/dL. Recovery was complete following penicillin therapy.

A. Cytomegalovirus mononucleosis: Clinical features, diagnosis, and treatment

Etiology	CMV (HHV-4)
Onset	1–2 wks
	3–12 wks after blood transfusion
Site of adenopathy	Generalized or cervical
Clinical features	Fever, malaise, fatigue
	Occasional hepatosplenomegaly
	Pneumonia in infants
	Mild hepatitis in adults
Lab findings	Lymphocytosis
	Atypical lymphocytes > 15%
Diagnostic tests	Virus isolation in urine, leukocytes, pharynx, body fluids
	Anti-CMV IgM
Treatment	Reassure; follow-up for hepatic or CNS sequelae
	Ganciclovir for retinitis
	Foscarnet for retinitis in HIV patients

CMV—cytomegalovirus; CNS—central nervous system; HHV—human herpesvirus.

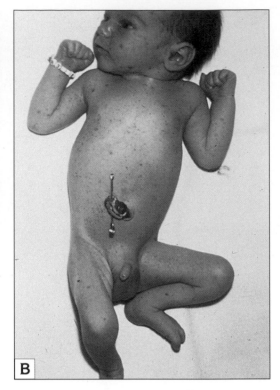

B

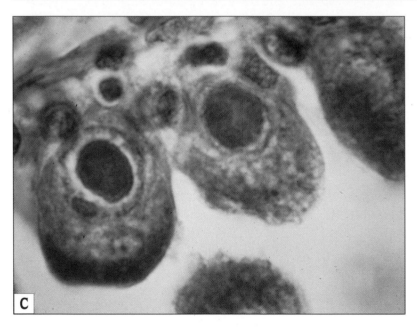

C

FIGURE 8-60 Cytomegalovirus (CMV) mononucleosis. **A**, Clinical features, diagnosis, and treatment. Asymptomatic CMV infections are most common. Congenital infection (resulting in jaundice, purpura, hepatosplenomegaly, microcephaly, chorioretinitis, growth and mental retardation) occurs in about 4% of patients with CMV infection. An infectious mononucleosis-like syndrome (prolonged fever, hepatitis, negative heterophil antibody test) may occur in adults and older children. **B**, Congenital CMV infection in a 3-day-old, small-for-date infant with jaundice, purpura, hepatosplenomegaly, microcephaly, and thrombocytopenia. **C**, Numerous giant inclusion cells are seen in urine sediment. Severe mental retardation persisted in this child during 15 years' follow-up.

A. Infectious mononucleosis: Clinical features, diagnosis, and treatment

Etiology	EBV (HHV-5)
Onset	1–2 wks (after incubation of 30–50 days)
Site of adenopathy	Anterior or posterior cervical, generalized
Clinical features	Tonsillopharyngitis, exudative
	Splenomegaly (> 50%)
	Fever, malaise, fatigue
Lab findings	Atypical lymphocytosis
	Positive Monospot (90% sensitive in persons > 4 yrs old)
	Positive EBV titers
Diagnostic tests	Anti-VCA IgM, early antigen
Treatment	Symptomatic

EBV—Epstein-Barr virus; HHV—human herpesvirus;
VCA—viral capsid antigen.

FIGURE 8-61 Infectious mononucleosis. **A**, Clinical features, diagnosis, and treatment. (*continued*)

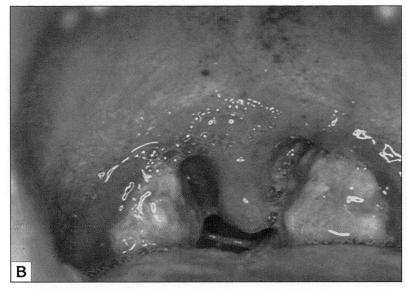

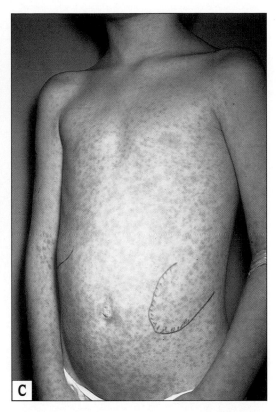

FIGURE 8-61 (*continued*) **B** and **C.** A healthy 7-year-old developed fever, exudative tonsillopharyngitis, tender cervical nodes (*panel 61B*), and splenomegaly for 3 days due to Epstein-Barr virus infection (*panel 61C*). A generalized maculopapular exanthem developed after 3 days of ampicillin therapy, which is a very common occurrence. Atypical lymphocytes (22%) were seen on a blood smear; a Monospot test was positive on the 10th day.

A. Roseola infantum: Clinical features, diagnosis, and treatment

Etiology	HHV-6
Onset	9 days (range, 5–15); usually in infants 6–24 mos old
Site of adenopathy	Occipital, postauricular
Clinical features	Fever to 40° C (104° F) for 3–7 days
	Pink maculopapular rash for 1–3 days postfever
Lab findings	CBC normal
Diagnostic tests	None (clinical course)
Treatment	Supportive

CBC—complete blood count; HHV–human herpesvirus.

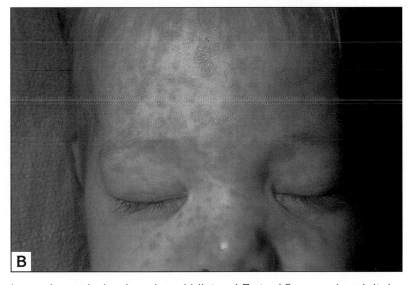

FIGURE 8-62 Roseola infantum. **A,** Clinical features, diagnosis, and treatment. **B,** A healthy 7-month-old child had fever of 40° C (104° F) for 3 days, irritability, and normal findings on physical examination. On the 4th day, an extensive, generalized, macu-lopapular rash developed, and bilateral 5- to 10-mm suboccipital nodes were palpated. The patient was afebrile. The rash faded over 36–48 hours with complete recovery. Sixth disease (exanthem subitum) is caused by human herpesvirus 6.

Other Viral Infections

A. Adenovirus infection: Clinical features, diagnosis, and treatment

Etiology	Adenovirus DNA (47 distinct serotypes)
Onset	2–14 days
Site of adenopathy	Anterior cervical or preauricular
Clinical features	Nonspecific pharyngeal inflammation
	Tonsillar exudate
	Conjunctivitis
Lab findings	Positive viral culture of pharyngeal secretions
Diagnostic tests	Pharyngeal isolate
	IFA, EIA antibody tests
Treatment	Supportive

EIA—enzyme immunoassay; IFA—indirect fluorescent antibody.

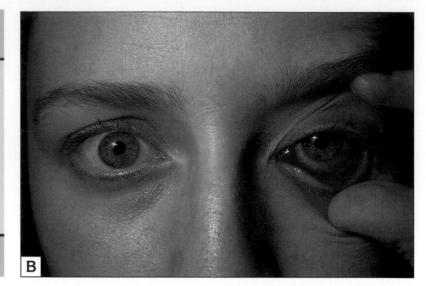

FIGURE 8-63 Adenovirus. **A,** Clinical features, diagnosis, and treatment. **B,** Adenovirus keratoconjunctivitis. A healthy medical student developed photophobia, local pain, and clear ocular discharge, with a tender 9-mm preauricular node on her left side. An adenovirus was isolated. Spontaneous resolution occurred in 10 days.

A. Coxsackievirus herpangina: Clinical features, diagnosis, and treatment

Etiology	Coxsackievirus RNA (23 group A, 6 group B serotypes)
Onset	3–6 days
Site of adenopathy	Anterior cervical
Clinical features	Discrete ulcers on labial mucosa, gingiva, tongue, or tonsillar pillars
Lab findings	Positive viral throat culture
Diagnostic tests	Fourfold rise in serum antibody titer
Treatment	Supportive

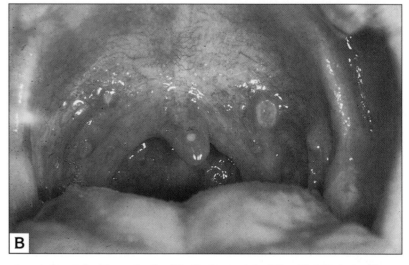

FIGURE 8-64 Coxsackievirus herpangina. **A,** Clinical features, diagnosis, and treatment. **B,** Herpangina due to coxsackievirus type A. A healthy 10-year-old had fever, severe sore throat with dysphagia, and cervical lymphadenitis that persisted for 7–10 days. Two courses of antibiotics were ineffective. Recovery developed slowly in 2 weeks. No specific therapy exists for enteroviral infections.

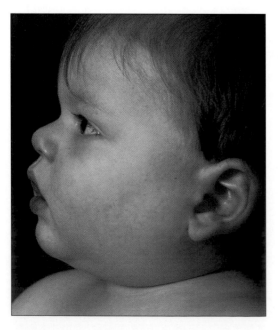

FIGURE 8-65
Mumps. Mumps in a healthy 9-month-old infant. Bilateral, tender, doughy, enlarged salivary parotid glands resolved without therapy in 7 days. Mumps, caused by a paramyxovirus, is a systemic disease that after puberty can cause severe orchitis and encephalitis or pancreatitis.

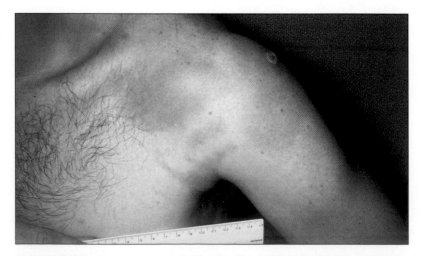

FIGURE 8-66 Postvaccinal lymphadenitis. A lymphadenitis involving the supraclavicular and axillary nodes developed with fever in a healthy medical student who was vaccinated 9 days previously with smallpox vaccine. Spontaneous resolution occurred in 6–10 days with a residual eschar only on the 24th day.

A. Rubella (German measles): Clinical features, diagnosis, and treatment

Etiology	Rubella virus (Togaviridae)
Onset	14–21 days
Site of adenopathy	Postauricular, suboccipital, cervical
Clinical features	Fine, discrete maculopapular rash lasts 3 days
	Forscheimer spots on palate
	Minimal fever
Lab findings	Positive rubella titer by EIA, IFA, or IgM antibody
	Positive tissue culture of nasal swab
Diagnosis	Clinical course
Treatment	Supportive

EIA—enzyme immunoassay; IFA—indirect fluorescent antibody.

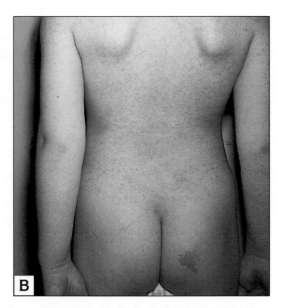

FIGURE 8-67 Rubella (German measles). **A**, Clinical features, diagnosis, and treatment. Rubella is a mild disease, characterized by an erythematous, maculopapular rash lasting 3 days, lymphadenopathy, minimal fever, and rarely, transient polyarthralgias, especially in adolescent girls and adult women. Encephalitis and thrombocytopenia are very rare complications. **B**, Uncomplicated rubella in a healthy 6-year-old girl, who had fever and rash for 3 days. Bilateral suboccipital (> 1 cm) adenopathy was present.

A. HIV lymphadenopathy: Clinical features, diagnosis, and treatment

Etiology	HIV
Onset	3–6 wks (acute HIV syndrome) followed by variable latent phase (approximately 10–15 yrs)
Site of adenopathy	Generalized, persistent
Clinical features	Acute syndrome:
	Acute mononucleosis-like syndrome lasting 1–2 wks
	Symptomatic phase:
	Oral thrush, hairy leukoplakia, aphthous ulcers
	Persistent or recurrent bacterial infections
	Opportunistic infections and cancers
Lab findings	Lymphopenia
	↓ CD4+T-lymphocyte count
	Thrombocytopenia
Diagnostic tests	ELISA or EIA
	Western blot or IFA to confirm
	PCR for HIV-DNA in children
	HIV p24 antigen in children
Treatment	Antiretroviral agents
	Specific treatment and/or prophylaxis for secondary infections and cancers

EIA—enzyme immunoassay; ELISA—enzyme-linked immunosorbent assay; IFA—indirect fluorescent antibody; PCR—polymerase chain reaction.

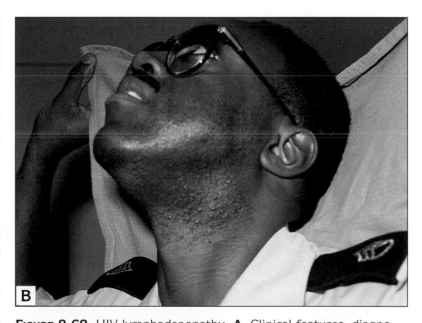

FIGURE 8-68 HIV lymphadenopathy. **A**, Clinical features, diagnosis, and treatment. HIV infection in children and adults causes a broad spectrum of disease and a variable clinical course over many months to years (10–15 yrs). Opportunistic infections caused by candida, herpes, mycobacteria, cryptococci, cryptosporidia, toxoplasma, pneumocystis, and other unusual pathogens are common. **B**, A 31-year-old man, positive for HIV infection for 2 years, shows generalized lymphadenopathy (at least 10 nodes) in the neck, axillae, and epitrochlear areas. The patient is otherwise healthy and asymptomatic; results of tests for other diseases were as follows: cat scratch disease, negative; purified protein derivative (PPD-Battey), 14 mm; PPD-T, 5 mm.

OTHER INFECTIONS

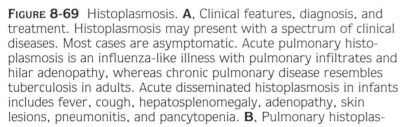

A. Histoplasmosis: Clinical features, diagnosis, and treatment

Etiology	*Histoplasma capsulatum*
Onset	Few weeks
Site of adenopathy	Cervical
Clinical features	Fever, cough
	Usually asymptomatic
Lab findings	Positive skin test
	Fourfold rise in yeast-phase titer
Diagnostic tests	Node biopsy and culture
	Gomori methenamine silver stain
	Detection of *H. capsulatum* antigen in urine or serum
Treatment	Symptomatic in most patients
	Amphotericin B
	Itraconazole or ketoconazole

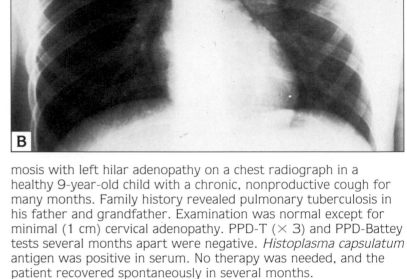

B

FIGURE 8-69 Histoplasmosis. **A**, Clinical features, diagnosis, and treatment. Histoplasmosis may present with a spectrum of clinical diseases. Most cases are asymptomatic. Acute pulmonary histoplasmosis is an influenza-like illness with pulmonary infiltrates and hilar adenopathy, whereas chronic pulmonary disease resembles tuberculosis in adults. Acute disseminated histoplasmosis in infants includes fever, cough, hepatosplenomegaly, adenopathy, skin lesions, pneumonitis, and pancytopenia. **B**, Pulmonary histoplasmosis with left hilar adenopathy on a chest radiograph in a healthy 9-year-old child with a chronic, nonproductive cough for many months. Family history revealed pulmonary tuberculosis in his father and grandfather. Examination was normal except for minimal (1 cm) cervical adenopathy. PPD-T ($\times$ 3) and PPD-Battey tests several months apart were negative. *Histoplasma capsulatum* antigen was positive in serum. No therapy was needed, and the patient recovered spontaneously in several months.

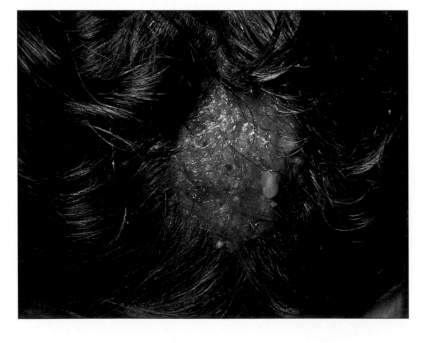

FIGURE 8-70 Celsus' kerion. Tinea kerion due to *Microsporum audouinii* and *Staphylococcus aureus* developed in a healthy 4-year-old, resulting in alopecia of 1 month's duration and occipital lymphadenitis. Griseofulvin therapy for 2 months was effective. In the absence of an inflammatory reaction, alopecia with multiple black dots and broken hairs strongly suggests tinea capitis infection.

A. Toxoplasmosis: Clinical features, diagnosis, and treatment

Etiology	*Toxoplasma gondii*
Onset	4–21 days (after ingestion of poorly cooked meat or exposure to cat feces)
Site of adenopathy	Posterior cervical, generalized
Clinical features	Usually asymptomatic
	Myalgias, fatigue, fever
	Occasional hepatosplenomegaly
	Maculopapular, nonpruritic rash
Lab findings	IFA IgM > 1:1000
	Atypical lymphocytosis
	> Fourfold rise in serum titer of IgG-specific antibody
Diagnostic tests	Serologic tests
Treatment	Reassure; if ill, pyrimethamine plus sulfadiazine or trisulfapyrimidine

IFA—indirect fluorescent antibody.

FIGURE 8-71 Toxoplasmosis. **A**, Clinical features, diagnosis, and treatment. **B**, Toxoplasmosis lymphadenopathy. Lympha-

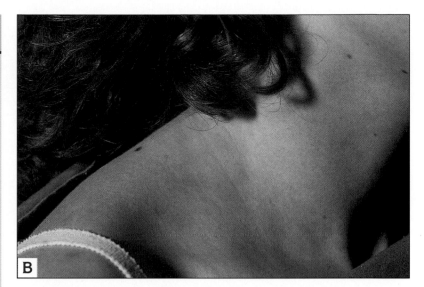

denopathy of the right posterior cervical triangle persisting for 10 months was seen in a healthy 14-year-old girl. Her *Toxoplasma* IgM–specific antibody titer was 1:2048. Skin tests for tuberculosis, nontuberculous mycobacteria, and cat scratch disease were negative. The patient had daily contact with a cat. The adenopathy resolved spontaneously in 17 months.

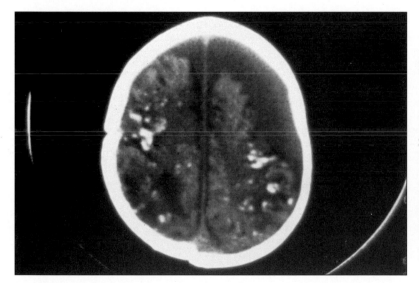

FIGURE 8-72 Congenital toxoplasmosis. An infant with AIDS developed hepatosplenomegaly, lymphadenopathy, and cerebral calcifications, which were seen on a computed tomography scan of the brain. The infant was retarded with moderate hydrocephalus.

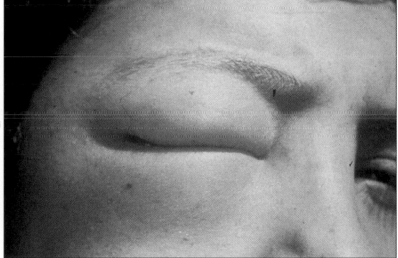

FIGURE 8-73 Trypanosomiasis. Trypanosomiasis is a chronic disease of tropical areas caused by the protozoan *Trypanosoma* spp. African sleeping sickness, caused by *T. brucei*, is spread by the tsetse fly and is characterized by fever, headache, malaise, myalgias, and generalized lymphadenopathy that progresses to meningoencephalopathy and death. Chagas' disease, or American trypanosomiasis, is a mild febrile illness seen predominantly in young children in Central and South America. It is caused by *T. cruzi*, transmitted by the reduviid bug, and produces a characteristic facial or orbital edema (Romaña's sign). (*Courtesy of* E. Kuschnir, MD.)

A. Kawasaki disease: Clinical features, diagnosis, and treatment

Etiology	Unknown
Onset	Abrupt onset of fever (12 days) and rash in children < 5 yrs old
Site of adenopathy	Cervical
Clinical features	Nodes > 1.5 cm diameter
	Fever, rash, red lips
	Conjunctival bulbar injection
	Red mouth and pharynx, strawberry tongue
	Hand/feet erythema and induration
Lab findings	Elevated sedimentation rate
	Elevated platelet count > 450,000/mm³
Diagnostic tests	Clinical criteria, exclusion of other diseases
Treatment	Aspirin (high dose initially, then low dose)
	High-dose immunoglobulin intravenously

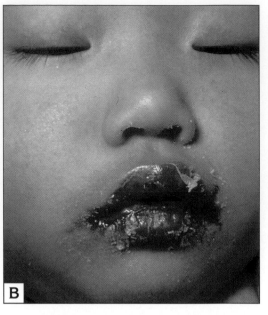

B

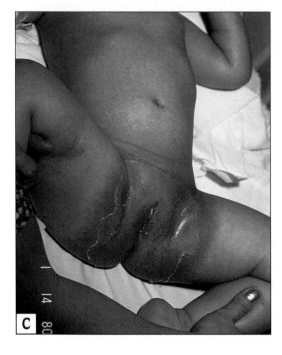

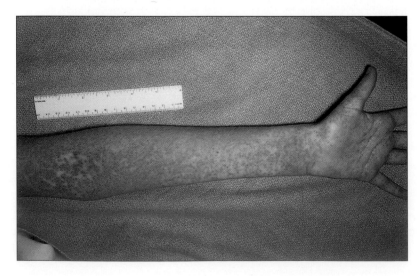

FIGURE 8-74 Kawasaki disease. **A**, Clinical features, diagnosis, and treatment. **B**, A previously healthy 2-year-old child presented with fever, scarlatiniform rash, conjunctival injection, pharyngitis, cervical adenitis, edema of the hands and feet, and red, cracked lips with a white strawberry tongue persisting for 4–7 days' duration. **C**, Desquamation of fingertips and an extensive diaper rash resolved in 18 days. No sequela occurred during a 7-year follow-up.

NONINFECTIOUS DISEASES ASSOCIATED WITH LYMPHADENOPATHY

FIGURE 8-75 Serum sickness due to phenytoin. One month after starting phenytoin therapy for temporal lobe seizures, an 11-year-old child developed a pruritic, generalized rash and lymphadenopathy that persisted for 2–3 weeks. She had fever, sore throat with oral mucosal ulcerations, a maculopapular rash with petechiae, arthralgia, hepatosplenomegaly, and severe malaise for 10–20 days. Leukocytosis of 23,000/µL with atypical lymphocytosis of 43% were present. Complete, spontaneous recovery followed.

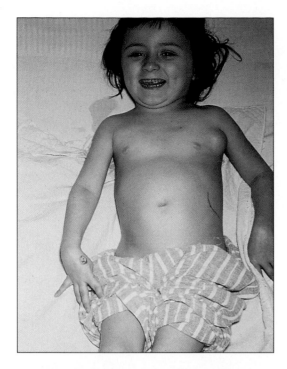

FIGURE 8-76
Hodgkin's disease. A 6-year-old child with Hodgkin's disease of several months' duration shows prominent axillary adenopathy. Antimetabolite and radiotherapy were effective, with complete resolution of generalized lymphadenopathy.

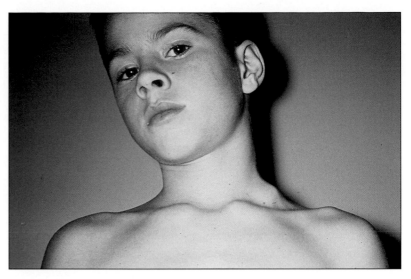

FIGURE 8-77 Neurofibroma. A healthy 11-year-old boy presented with a nontender, hard, immobile neck mass (6 × 7 cm) of several weeks' duration that appeared following cat scratches on the left cheek. A cat scratch skin test was negative. Biopsy of the mass revealed a neurofibroma of the left brachial plexus.

FIGURE 8-78 Benign cystic hygroma. A healthy, asymptomatic, 7-year-old girl developed a rapidly enlarging neck mass over several weeks. The mass transilluminated very well. Skin tests were negative for tuberculosis and cat scratch disease. Excisional biopsy revealed a benign cystic hygroma.

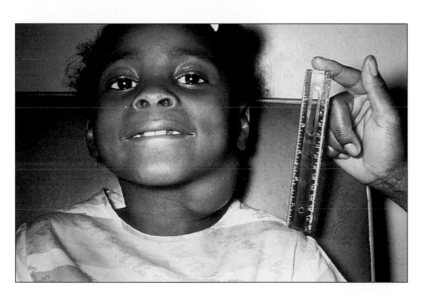

SELECTED BIBLIOGRAPHY

Baker CJ: Cervical lymphadenitis. *In* Feigen RD, Cherry JD (eds.): *Textbook of Pediatric Infectious Diseases*, 3rd ed. Philadelphia: W.B. Saunders Co.; 1992:220–230.

Faller DV: Diseases of the lymph nodes and spleen. *In* Wyngaarden JB, Smith LH Jr, Bennett JC (eds.): *Cecil Textbook of Medicine*, 19th ed. Philadelphia: W.B. Saunders Co.; 1991:978–981.

Margileth AM: Cat scratch disease. *In* Arnoff SC, *et al.* (eds.): *Advances in Pediatric Infectious Diseases*, 8th ed. St. Louis: Mosby Year-Book; 1993:1–21.

Margileth AM: Sorting out the causes of lymphadenopathy. *Contemp Pediatr* 1995, 12:23–40.

Mazur PM, Kornberg AE: Lymphadenopathy. *In* Fleisher GR, Ludwig S (eds.): *Textbook of Pediatric Emergency Medicine*, 3rd ed. Baltimore: Williams & Wilkins; 1993:310–317.

CHAPTER 9

Parotitis and Thyroiditis

Stephen G. Baum
Moses Nussbaum

PAROTITIS

Causes of parotitis

Viral infection
  Mumps virus
  Cytomegalovirus
  HIV (with lymphoproliferation)

Bacterial infection
  Staphylococcus aureus (most common)
  Mixed oral anaerobes
  Streptococcus pneumoniae
  Viridans streptococci
  Streptococcus pyogenes, Pseudomonas spp., *Rochalimaea henselae, Haemophilus influenzae,* others (rarely)

Collagen-vascular diseases
  Sjögren's syndrome

Granulomatous diseases
  Sarcoidosis
  Mycobacterium tuberculosis infection

Drug-related conditions
  Phenothiazines
  Iodides

FIGURE 9-1 Causes of parotitis. Inflammation of the parotid glands (parotitis) can occur as a manifestation of many diverse conditions. These conditions include viral infection (mumps virus and cytomegalovirus), bacterial infection (*Staphylococcus aureus, Rochalimaea henselae,* and mixed anaerobes), collagen-vascular conditions such as Sjögren's syndrome, granulomatous diseases such as sarcoidosis, and chemical insult with agents such as the phenothiazines and iodides. The hallmark of parotitis is enlargement of the parotid gland, either unilaterally or bilaterally, often accompanied by inflammation of Stensen's duct in the mouth with or without discharge. Identification of the site of facial swelling as the parotid gland depends on the findings of obliteration of the angle of the mandible and a forward tilting of the earlobe. Determination of the cause of parotitis, and therefore the treatment, usually depends on assessment of the factors in the clinical status of the patient, such as age, vaccination history, presence of severe dehydration, immune status, presence of infection with HIV, presence of other underlying diseases, or medication history.

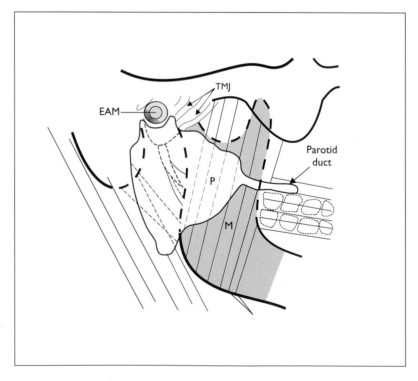

FIGURE 9-2 Anatomy of the parotid gland and neck. An anatomical diagram of the neck shows the relationship of the parotid gland (P) to the external auditory meatus (EAM) and temporomandibular joint (TMJ). The parotid (Stensen's) duct pierces the masseter muscle (M) and empties into the mouth next to the upper second molar. Swelling of the parotid will obscure the angle of the jaw to palpation. (*Adapted from* Paff GH: *Anatomy of the Head and Neck.* Philadelphia: W.B. Saunders; 1973:49, with permission.)

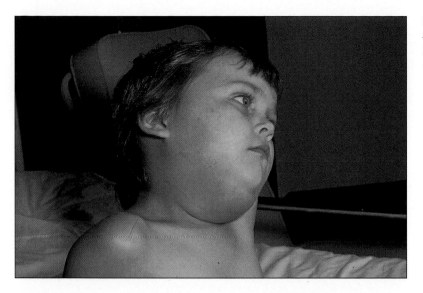

FIGURE 9-3 Unilateral parotitis due to mumps virus infection in a 4-year-old girl. The angle of the jaw is obliterated, and the earlobe is tilted forward, hallmark findings of parotitis. (*Courtesy of* the Centers for Disease Control and Prevention.)

Clinical features, diagnosis, and treatment of mumps

Etiology	Mumps virus (paramyxovirus)
Onset	14–21 days after exposure
Involved sites	Parotids, usually bilateral
	Testes, unilateral
	Lymph nodes in neck
Clinical features	Preauricular and submandibular swelling
	Orchitis
	Meningoencephalitis (rare)
Lab findings	Leukocytosis, elevated amylase
Diagnostic tests	Amylase, IgM antibodies
Treatment	Supportive
Prevention	Vaccine (MMR in childhood, mumps vaccine alone in adults)

MMR—measles, mumps, and rubella.

FIGURE 9-4 Clinical features, diagnosis, and treatment of mumps. Swelling of the parotid gland occurs rapidly after an incubation period of 2 to 3 weeks, and parotitis is unilateral in less than 50% of cases. The incidence of mumps in children has decreased dramatically since the introduction of a live virus vaccine in 1967. However, because of the rapid decrease in occurrence of natural mumps at that time many children escaped natural infection, and their parents did not have them vaccinated because the threat seemed to be gone. These people, now in their 20s, are susceptible to natural mumps infection, which has lead to outbreaks at colleges in the last few years. These outbreaks carry with them the danger of orchitis (usually unilateral), which occurs in about 20% to 30% of adult men infected, and meningitis, which although rare, also has an increased incidence in men. Other viruses that can cause parotitis include influenza A virus, parainfluenza virus type 3, coxsackievirus and, in the immunocompromised patient, cytomegalovirus.

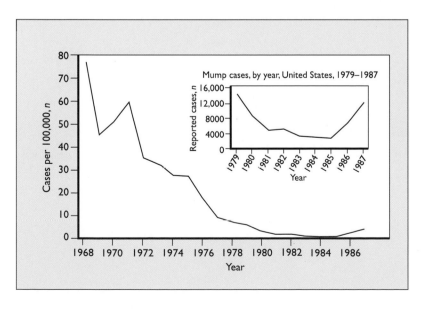

FIGURE 9-5 Annual incidence of mumps in the United States from 1968 to 1987. The yearly incidence of mumps is shown, starting with the year after the mumps vaccine was licensed in the United States. The resurgence of mumps beginning in 1986 occurred in a population of young adults who, as children, had not been vaccinated and had escaped natural infection because of the decreased risk of exposure from a largely vaccinated population. (*From* Cocchi SL, Preblud SR, Orenstein WA: Perspectives on the relative resurgence of mumps in the United States. *Am J Dis Child* 1988, 142:499–507; with permission.)

Suppurative Parotitis

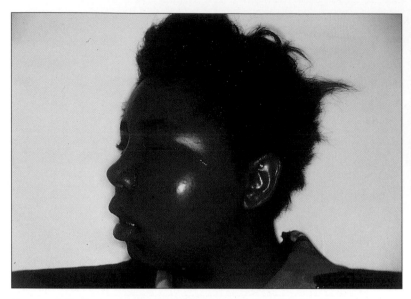

FIGURE 9-6 Suppurative parotitis. A female patient had become dehydrated and developed suppurative parotitis. The area around the angle of the jaw and extending up to the ear was red, swollen, rock hard, and exquisitely tender. Inspissated secretions had produced inflammation in Stensen's duct. *Staphylococcus aureus* was isolated from the pus in Stensen's duct. (*Courtesy of* A.M. Schwimmer, DDS.)

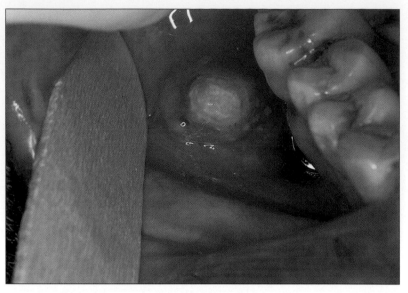

FIGURE 9-7 Stensen's duct showing inflammation and purulent discharge. (*Courtesy of* C.E. Barr, DDS.)

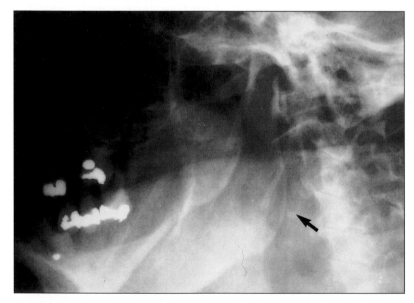

FIGURE 9-8 Sialogram showing a stone in Stensen's duct (*arrow*). (*Courtesy of* B.A. Zeifer, MD.)

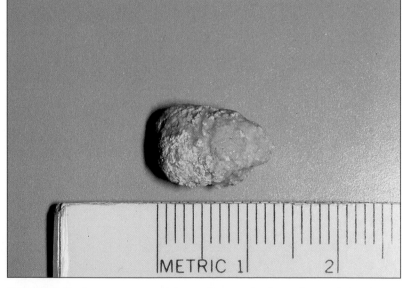

FIGURE 9-9 Stone removed from Stensen's duct. Bacterial culture of the stone and of the purulent drainage (shown in Fig. 9-7) grew *Staphylococcus aureus*. (*Courtesy of* C.E. Barr, DDS.)

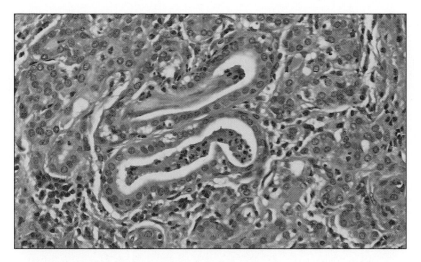

FIGURE 9-10 Histopathology of suppurative parotitis after stone removal showing acute and chronic sialadenitis. Ducts contain polymorphonuclear leukocytes, and an acinus is infiltrated with plasma cells. (Magnification, × 200.) (*Courtesy of* J. Sarlin, MD.)

Clinical features, diagnosis, and treatment of suppurative parotitis

Etiology	Bacterial infection, usually *Staphylococcus aureus*
Predisposing factors	Dehydration, stone formation
Involved sites	Parotid, usually unilateral
Clinical features	Rock hard, very tender preauricular swelling
	Dehydration, obtundation, and high fever
Lab findings	Leukocytosis
Diagnostic tests	Elevated amylase, culture positive for *S. aureus*
Treatment	Antibiotics (β-lactamase–resistant penicillin, first-generation cephalosporin, or vancomycin) and rehydration, stone removal, drainage of abscess (if present), occasional parotidectomy

FIGURE 9-11 Clinical features, diagnosis, and treatment of suppurative parotitis. It is not clear why *Staphylococcus aureus* is by far the most common etiologic agent in suppurative parotitis, because staphylococci are not the predominant organisms in the oral flora. Personal unpublished experiments to test whether parotid secretions selectively enhance the growth of staphylococci over other organisms did not confirm this theory. Infection due to oral anaerobes, including peptostreptococci and *Bacteroides* species, and aerobes, such as *Haemophilus influenzae* and *Escherichia coli*, have been reported. Suppurative parotitis usually responds to hydration and antibiotic treatment, although mortality rates in debilitated patients are high. (Brook I, Frazier EH, Thompson DH: Aerobic and anaerobic microbiology of acute suppurative parotitis. *Laryngoscope* 1991, 101:170–172.)

Parotitis in HIV Infection

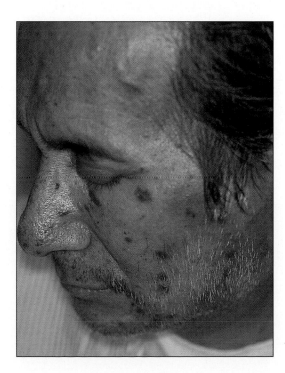

FIGURE 9-12 Left parotid swelling in an HIV-positive man. A 59-year-old man with HIV infection had a 2-week history of progressive left parotid swelling and left upper eyelid swelling associated with fever. The parotid mass measured 5 cm in diameter and was warm but minimally tender. There was no evidence of dehydration. Because of the patient's HIV-positive status, infection with cytomegalovirus was suspected. The red lesions on the face were proven by biopsy to be Kaposi's sarcoma. (*Courtesy of* S.R. Yancovitz, MD, and L.M. Laya, MD.)

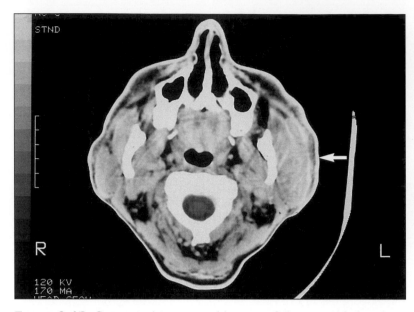

FIGURE 9-13 Computed tomographic scan of the parotid showing a well-circumscribed mass on the left (*arrow*). This mass, in the patient shown in Figure 9-12, underwent biopsy and yielded primarily red blood cells. The skin over the parotid underwent biopsy, and the specimen is shown in Figure 9-14. (*Courtesy of* S.R. Yancovitz, MD, and L.M. Laya, MD.)

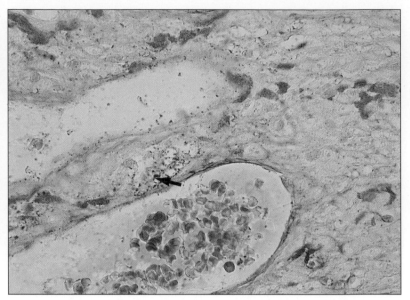

FIGURE 9-14 Skin biopsy specimen from an HIV-positive patient with left parotid swelling. On Warthin-Starry stain, a specimen from the patient seen in Figure 9-12 shows the presence of aggregated short rods (*arrow*) typical of *Rochalimaea henselae*, the causative organism of bacillary angiomatosis. The patient was treated with erythromycin and developed a Jarisch-Herxheimer reaction, consisting of high fever and chills with transient swelling of the parotid area. After 2 days, the entire parotid lesion resolved, confirming that the gland had been infected with *R. henselae*. The parotid glands have also been the site of benign lymphocytic infiltration in patients infected with HIV. Disseminated *Pneumocystis carinii* infection can also affect this organ. (Rubin MM, Ford HC, Sadoff RS: Bilateral parotid gland enlargement in a patient with AIDS. *J Oral Maxillofac Surg* 1991, 49:529–531.) (*Courtesy of* S.R. Yancovitz, MD, and L.M. Laya, MD.)

THYROIDITIS

Types of thyroiditis	
Acute	
Infection	Rare
Bacterial	*Staphylococcus aureus, Streptococcus pyogenes, Escherichia coli, Haemophilus influenzae*
Others	*Pneumocystis carinii,* fungi
Subacute	
Granulomatous (De Quervain's)	Painful, may have viral etiology
Lymphocytic	Painless, may be autoimmune, sporadic, or postpartum
Chronic	
Lymphocytic (Hashimoto's)	Most common form of thyroiditis
Fibrous replacement (Riedel's)	Rare

FIGURE 9-15 Types of thyroiditis. Inflammation of the thyroid gland is not uncommon, but acute bacterial infection of this gland is a very rare occurrence. Direct involvement by viruses occurs in the course of a number of viral infections. It is possible that some so-called autoimmune thyroiditidies are the indirect result of viral infection, but this hypothesis remains to be proven. When bacterial infection does occur, it may be as a result of trauma to the anterior neck that carries the infecting organism directly into the gland; local spread from the trachea, esophagus, or other adjacent area of the neck; or hematogenous spread from other organs. When direct trauma is the preceding event, *Staphylococcus aureus* is the most common etiologic agent, whereas infection from adjacent structures is often caused by *Streptococcus pneumoniae* or *S. pyogenes.*

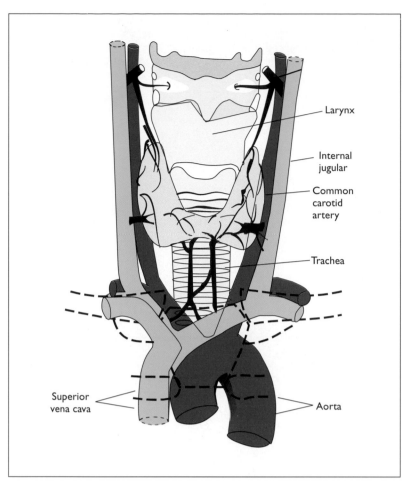

FIGURE 9-16 Anatomy of the thyroid gland and neck. An anatomical diagram of the neck shows the relationship of the thyroid gland to the trachea, larynx, internal jugular vein, aorta, superior vena cava, and common carotid artery. (*Adapted from* Paff GH: *Anatomy of the Head and Neck*. Philadelphia: W.B. Saunders; 1973:33; with permission.)

Labels in figure: Larynx; Internal jugular; Common carotid artery; Trachea; Superior vena cava; Aorta

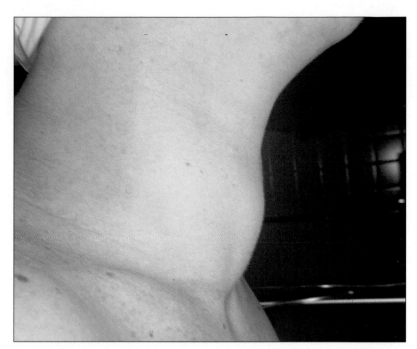

FIGURE 9-17 Subacute thyroiditis in a 40-year-old woman. This episode was the second bout of thyroiditis in this patient, and it was thought that the swelling was a thyroid tumor until biopsy revealed Hashimoto's thyroiditis.

Differentiation of acute and subacute thyroiditis

	Acute	Subacute
Onset	Abrupt	Gradual after "viral" prodrome
Gender	M=F	80% female
Haplotype	None known	HLA-Bw 35
Pain	Severe	Mild to severe
Swelling	Unilateral	Unilateral
Fever	High	Low grade
Leukocytosis	Present	Present
Thyroid function	Euthyroid	Hyperthyroid → euthyroid → hypothyroid
Radioiodine uptake	Normal	Depressed
Scan	"Cold" over swelling	"Cold"
Treatment	Antibiotics	Corticosteroids

FIGURE 9-18 Differentiation of acute and subacute thyroiditis. Acute suppurative thyroiditis presents with the sudden onset of severe pain, fever, neck swelling, and dysphagia or dysphonia. The gland is usually very tender. Subacute (De Quervain's) thyroiditis is thought to be of viral etiology; the onset is more insidious and is accompanied by a syndrome of malaise, myalgia, and fatigue. There have been reports of localized unexplained outbreaks of this syndrome as well as outbreaks during mumps epidemics. Other agents, including the enteroviruses, measles virus, influenza virus, and adenovirus, have been implicated in this condition. (deBruin TW, Riekoff FP, deBoer JJ: An outbreak of thyrotoxicosis due to atypical subacute thyroiditis. *J Clin Endocrinol Metab* 1990, 70:396–402. Eylan E, Zmucky R, Sheba C: Mumps virus and subacute thyroiditis. *Lancet* 1990, 1:1062–1063.)

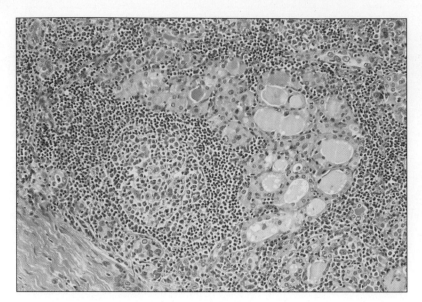

FIGURE 9-19 Histopathology of Hashimoto's thyroiditis showing chronic inflammation. A germinal center shows oncocytic changes of the follicular epithelium. The presence of some fibrosis indicates the subacute nature of the process. (Magnification, × 100.) (*Courtesy of* J. Sarlin, MD.)

SELECTED BIBLIOGRAPHY

Baum SG, Litman N: Mumps virus. *In* Mandell GL, Bennett JE, Dolin R (eds.): *Principles and Practice of Infectious Diseases*, 4th ed. New York: Churchill Livingstone; 1994:1496–1501.

Brook I: Diagnosis and management of parotitis. *Arch Otolaryngol Head Neck Surg* 1992, 118:469–471.

Singer PA: Thyroiditis. *Med Clin North Am* 1991, 75:61–77.

Tomer Y, Davies T: Infection, thyroid disease and autoimmunity. *Endocrine Rev* 1993, 14:107–120.

CHAPTER 10

Deep Neck Infections and Postoperative Infections

James N. Endicott
Janet Seper

DEEP NECK INFECTIONS

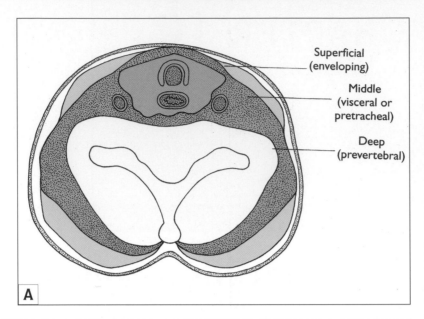

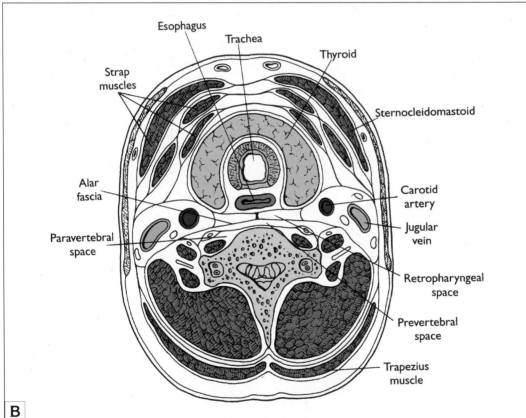

FIGURE 10-1 Anatomy of the neck. Deep neck infections, although uncommon, may have life-threatening sequelae despite antibiotic therapy. An understanding of the anatomic relationships of the fascial planes and potential spaces of the neck is essential for the surgical management required for most deep neck infections. **A**, The "tube within the tube" concept helps one to visualize the three layers of the deep cervical fascia. **B**, Cross-section of the neck at the mid-thyroid level reveals the contents of the three fascial layers. As the superficial layer of the deep cervical fascia passes through the neck, it attaches to the bony and cartilaginous structures, the clavicle, mandible, mastoid, pterygoid, and skull, thereby forming potential spaces. The "rule of twos" describes the muscles (sternocleidomastoid and trapezius), spaces (posterior triangle and Burns' suprasternal space), and glands (parotid and submandibular) incorporated in this fascia. The strap muscles are also incorporated into this fascia. The middle or visceral layer of deep cervical fascia surrounds the esophagus, trachea, larynx, and thyroid. The deep layer surrounds the paraspinous muscles of the neck. Each of the three layers contributes to the carotid sheath as it courses through the neck. (Panel 1B *adapted from* Endicott J: Infections of the deep fascial spaces of the head and neck: Update of diagnosis and management. *In* Johnson JT, *et al.* (eds.): *AAO-HNS Instructional Courses*, vol 3. St. Louis: Mosby Year-Book; 1990; with permission.)

FIGURE 10-2 The fascial layers of the neck (sagittal view). A fascial plane represents a condensation of connective tissue lying between adjacent structures. Fascial spaces are the potential spaces between these connective tissue planes. When an abscess forms in a space, spread to other spaces occurs along planes of least resistance because of the interrelationship and continuity of all the deep cervical fascia and potential spaces. The fascial layers and space relationships through the length of the neck are shown. The alar fascia is a portion of the deep layer, extending inferiorly from the skull base and attaching to the transverse processes of the vertebrae as it descends to the level of the tracheal bifurcation at T2. This fascial layer separates the retropharyngeal space from the prevertebral space. (*From* Endicott J: Infections of the deep fascial spaces of the head and neck: Update of diagnosis and management. *In* Johnson JT, *et al.* (eds.): *AAO-HNS Instructional Courses*, vol 3. St. Louis: Mosby Year-Book; 1990; with permission.)

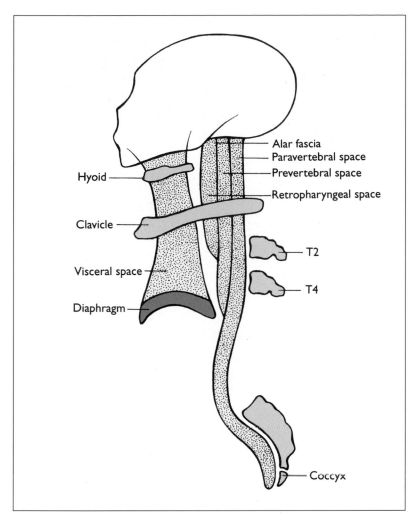

Clinically important potential neck spaces

Spaces involving the entire length of the neck
  Retropharyngeal space (posterior visceral space, retrovisceral space, retroesophageal space)
  Prevertebral ("danger" space)
  Paravertebral space
  Visceral vascular space (within the carotid sheath)
Spaces above the hyoid bone
  Submandibular space
    Sublingual (medial)
    Submaxillary (lateral)
  Lateral pharyngeal (pharyngomaxillary space, parapharyngeal space)
  Masticator space
  Parotid space
  Peritonsillar space
Spaces below the hyoid bone (anterior only)
  Anterior visceral (pretracheal space)

FIGURE 10-3 Clinically important potential neck spaces. The spaces of the neck are divided into those that run the length of the neck and those that are anterior and isolated above or below the hyoid bone. It is because of these fasciae and the musculofascial planes anteriorly that infections 1) tend to be held within the neck, 2) gravitate to the mediastinum, and 3) cause asphyxiation and dysphagia from the resulting pressure, pain, and swelling. The primary sources of deep space infections of the head and neck are isolated nodal abscesses and dental, tonsillar, or pharyngeal infections. (Brook I: Microbiology of abscesses of the head and neck in children. *Ann Otol Rhinol Laryngol* 1987, 96:429–433.) (*From* Endicott J: Infections of the deep fascial spaces of the head and neck: Update of diagnosis and management. *In* Johnson JT, *et al.* (eds.): *AAO-HNS Instructional Courses*, vol 3. St. Louis: Mosby Year-Book; 1990; with permission.)

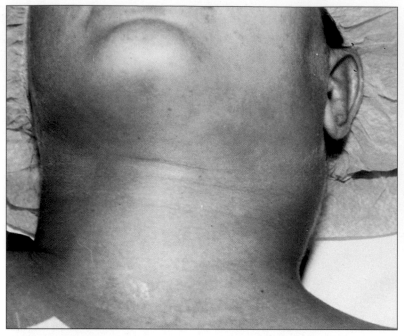

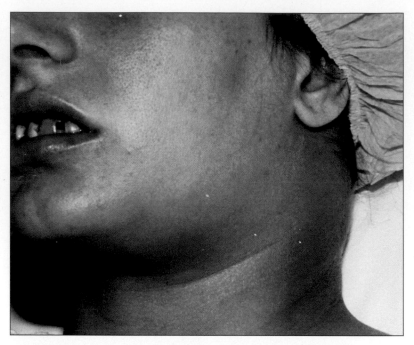

FIGURE 10-4 Parapharyngeal space abscess. The infection in this patient presented as a rapidly growing unilateral tender neck mass obliterating the angle of the mandible. Such a patient with a deep neck abscess may have an elevated temperature. Sepsis may be present. The most common organisms are *Staphylococcus aureus*, *Streptococcus* sp., and anaerobic bacteria. The patient should be treated with maximum therapeutic doses of intravenous antibiotics after blood is drawn for culture. High-dose aqueous penicillin G plus clindamycin is the recommended antibiotic treatment for a deep neck abscess. However, β-lactamase–producing aerobic and anaerobic organisms were found in almost one half of head and neck abscesses in children, suggesting that penicillin may no longer be the drug of choice. Clindamycin, chloramphenicol, metronidazole, cefoxitin, imipenem, and the combination of a penicillin (*ie*, amoxicillin or ticarcillin) plus a β-lactamase inhibitor (clavulanic acid) are more appropriate antibiotics for these infections. Surgical drainage is an important adjuvant treatment to antibiotic coverage. (Brook I: Microbiology of abscesses of the head and neck in children. *Ann Otol Rhinol Laryngol* 1987, 96:429–433.)

FIGURE 10-5 Parapharyngeal space abscess. The lateral view of the same patient in Fig. 10-4 suggests involvement of the parotid and submaxillary regions. The patient is unable to open her mouth (trismus) and has poor dentition, the most likely source of the infection. Intubation for the necessary surgical drainage would be difficult and even hazardous, mandating that the patient have a preliminary tracheostomy under local anesthesia without muscle relaxants or drying agents. A deep neck abscess has no fluctuance but has pitting edema of the skin. Rarely will such an abscess drain spontaneously, but it can progress to other spaces in the neck.

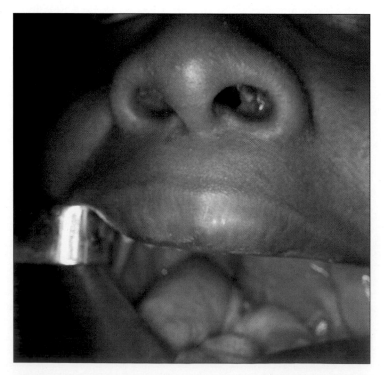

FIGURE 10-6 Parapharyngeal space abscess. This patient has a characteristic swelling of the palate and lateral pharyngeal wall behind the tonsillar pillars, which may occlude the upper airway. The plum color of the swollen oral mucosa is a sign of submucosal hemorrhage, suggesting arterial erosion. Despite the prominence of the lateral pharyngeal wall, perioral incision is contraindicated because of the risk to the great vessels. Systemic diseases such as diabetes, nephritis, tuberculosis, or AIDS are often associated with deep neck infections, and unless they are diagnosed and managed properly, the patient's outcome may be poor.

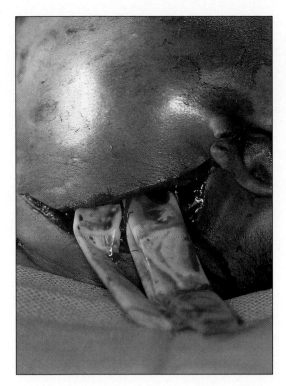

FIGURE 10-7 Surgical drainage of the left parapharyngeal space abscess. The same patient in Fig. 10-6 is seen immediately after surgical drainage. The proper time for surgical drainage depends of the stage of infection, which can be monitored effectively by computed tomography with contrast. Rarely will an abscess rupture spontaneously and drain externally; instead, it should be drained surgically, even when no complications have occurred. However, no drainage attempts should be made during the stage of phlegmon formation (cellulitis), when antibiotics alone may suffice. A week may be required for abscess formation, although some patients progress very rapidly. A 48-hour period of antibiotic coverage and careful observation and monitoring in an intensive care unit should be allowed when the airway is at risk. A surgical approach through the neck should be made at a point where vessel ligation can be performed if necessary during the drainage operation. Surgical drainage of the lateral pharyngeal space by the submaxillary approach can be accomplished by a modification of the Mosher T-shaped incision.

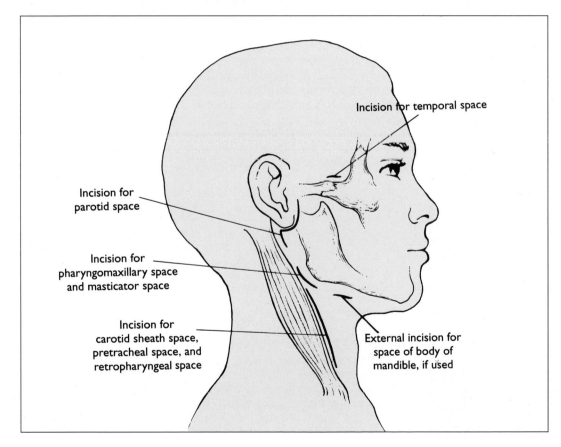

FIGURE 10-8 Incision sites for deep space abscesses. After cultures for aerobic and anaerobic bacteria are taken and sensitivity and Gram stains are obtained, copious irrigation of the incision with saline then is followed by the insertion of several well-placed Penrose drains, sutured to the wound edge to avoid accidental displacement during dressing change. The drains are advanced over several days and removed when local and general signs of inflammation and sepsis have disappeared. The method of drainage varies according to the location of the deep space infection. The offending tooth should be extracted if one is identified as the source of infection. Drainage is not a cosmetic procedure; one should use large incisions with well-loosened and retracted neck flaps, taking precautions to avoid cranial nerve injury. Immediate surgical intervention is necessary in the presence of sepsis, respiratory distress, or hemorrhage from the pharynx or ear. Repeated hemorrhage of small amounts of blood into the pharynx or ear indicates vessel erosion. Erosion of the walls of the jugular vein may be accompanied by only thrombus formation and may be reflected by repeated chills with spiking temperatures, indicating bacteremia. (Endicott JN: Deep neck infections. *In* Gates GA (ed.): *Current Therapy in Otolaryngology–Head and Neck Surgery, 1982–1983.* Toronto: BC Decker; 1982.)

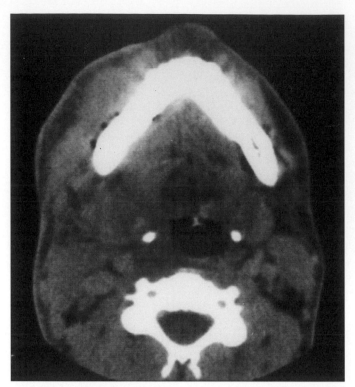

FIGURE 10-9 Masseteric space abscess. A computed tomography (CT) scan shows a swollen masseter and air adjacent to the right side of the mandible. A masticator space infection is a subperiosteal abscess and cellulitis of the mandible and soft tissue and may involve the fascial sling containing the muscles of mastication (*ie*, masseter, pterygoid, and temporalis muscles). There is a brawny induration over the area of the angle and body of the mandible externally, which may resemble the swelling of a lateral pharyngeal space abscess. Trismus is marked. The oral cavity and oropharynx are swollen with displacement of the tonsil, although the lateral pharyngeal wall is not swollen. This abscess can be differentiated from a parapharyngeal abscess by CT, which will demonstrate the site and whether both spaces are involved. The fat planes of the parapharyngeal space are obscured when this abscess is present. An intraoral incision is indicated for a masticator space abscess. (Endicott JN, Nelson RJ, Saraceno CA: Diagnosis and management decisions in infections of the deep fascial spaces of the head and neck utilizing computerized tomography. *Laryngoscope* 1986, 96:751–757.)

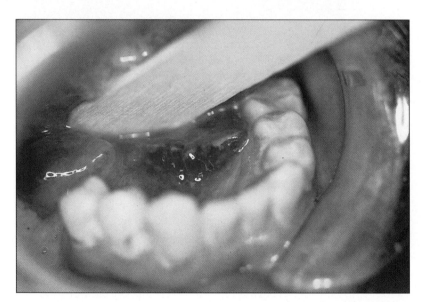

FIGURE 10-10 Ludwig's angina with bilateral sublingual space infection. A sublingual space abscess responds to intraoral drainage, but when it progresses to the submandibular space followed by a crossover to the opposite side and involvement of similar compartments, Ludwig's angina has developed. This highly virulent infection is a cellulitis and not a true abscess and can cause rapid death from upper airway obstruction or mediastinitis if it descends past the hyoid. Most abscesses in these spaces are of dental origin. A computed tomography scan for this abscess is not helpful in management decisions.

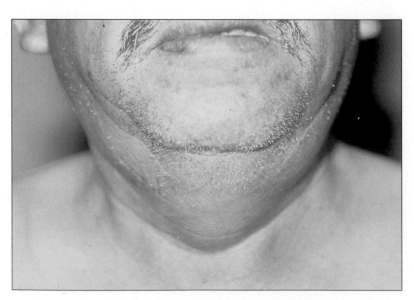

FIGURE 10-11 Tender bilateral suprahyoid swelling in Ludwig's angina. Originally described by Ludwig in 1836, Ludwig's angina is characterized by a patient in acute distress with the following findings: 1) all the tissues of the floor of the mouth are greatly swollen and extremely inflamed, 2) displacement of the tongue upward and backward toward the palatal vault, 3) woodenlike induration at first confined to the submandibular compartment, 4) trismus, and 5) hoarseness and dyspnea. (*From* Endicott J: Infections of the deep fascial spaces of the head and neck: Update of diagnosis and management. *In* Johnson JT, *et al.* (eds.): *AAO-HNS Instructional Courses*, vol 3. St. Louis: Mosby Year-Book; 1990; with permission.)

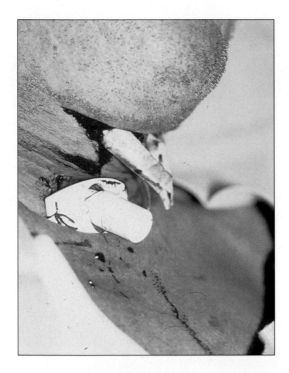

FIGURE 10-12 Wide surgical drainage and tracheostomy in Ludwig's angina. The airway may become obstructed by displacement of the tongue into the pharynx or by edema of the larynx, as manifested by hoarseness and dyspnea. A tracheostomy is indicated under local anesthesia, often through edematous anterior neck tissue. Trismus and hypopharyngeal mucosal edema contraindicate preliminary intubation. (*From* Endicott J: Infections of the deep fascial spaces of the head and neck: Update of diagnosis and management. *In* Johnson JT, *et al.* (eds.): *AAO-HNS Instructional Courses*, vol 3. St. Louis: Mosby Year-Book; 1990; with permission.)

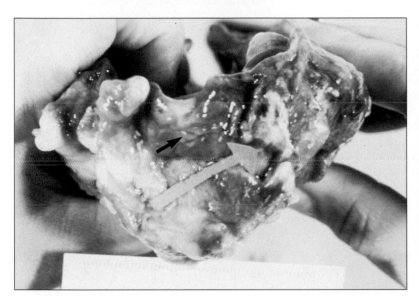

FIGURE 10-13 Larynx in Ludwig's angina. An autopsy specimen with open larynx demonstrates swelling of the perilaryngeal tissues and edema in the preepiglottic space (*small arrow*). The *large arrow* points to the large-bore needle track from the unsuccessful attempt to obtain an airway by needle cannulation. Tracheostomy under local anesthesia with the patient in a sitting position is the treatment of choice. (*From* Endicott J: Infections of the deep fascial spaces of the head and neck: Update of diagnosis and management. *In* Johnson JT, *et al.* (eds.): *AAO-HNS Instructional Courses*, vol 3. St. Louis: Mosby Year-Book; 1990; with permission.)

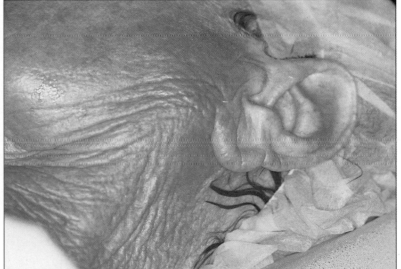

FIGURE 10-14 Parotid space abscess. The parotid space formed by the superficial layer of the deep cervical fascia is not a true anatomical space; many fascial septa run vertically through it. A parotid space abscess is actually an infection of the gland with loculated miniabscesses. The proximity of the parotid space to the parapharyngeal space inferomedially and to the submaxillary space anteromedially explains the mode of spread of the infection through the neck. The common pathogenic organism is *Staphylococcus*. This patient has erythematous skin and a swollen parotid. The patient usually has a temperature of ≥ 38.3° C (101° F) with pain. There is tenderness but no trismus or swelling of the lateral pharyngeal wall. Stenson's duct usually reveals a purulent flow on massage. Parotid space infection classically occurs in dehydrated postoperative patients as a result of stasis of salivary flow or duct obstruction. Surgical drainage may be necessary when antibiotic treatment is unsuccessful.

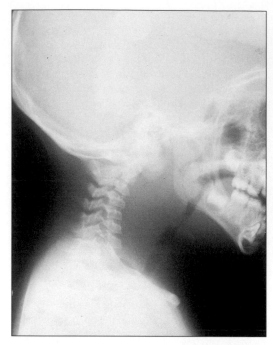

FIGURE 10-15 Retropharyngeal abscess. Retropharyngeal tissue on this lateral plain film is equal to the width of the body of C_2 in this small child. Normally, it should be no more than one third the width of C_2. Air in the retropharyngeal soft tissues or widening of the prevertebral retropharyngeal soft tissues may also be noted. Although no mass is palpable, this abscess may threaten the airway. Abscesses localized above the hyoid are more common in children under age 4 years secondary to suppurative retropharyngeal nodes, which drain the posterior two thirds of the nose, paranasal sinuses, pharynx, and eustachian tube. A midline fascia divides the retropharyngeal space, restricting abscesses to a position lateral to the midline. The classical appearance of the retropharyngeal abscess is a unilateral swelling of the posterior pharyngeal wall, which may push the palate forward.

Clinical symptoms and signs of retropharyngeal abscess

Drooling
Low-grade fever
Neck rigidity
Muffled ("hot potato") voice
Noisy breathing (with partial obstruction)
Torticollis (late sign)

FIGURE 10-16 Clinical symptoms and signs of retropharyngeal abscess. Infants and children may not complain of pain but may have drooling from dysphagia and refuse to eat. Torticollis with the neck tilted toward the uninvolved side is a late sign. No trismus is present. Palpation and aspiration of the mass with an 18-gauge spinal needle are valuable in examination and diagnosis. A lateral neck radiograph in a cooperative patient is useful. A preliminary tracheostomy under local anesthesia is necessary to avoid asphyxia during throat examinations or manipulation when stridor is too great to allow the patient to lie supine. Management is by perioral drainage under general or local anesthesia. The patient's head should be in a Rose position, and suction should be available to prevent aspiration of purulent material.

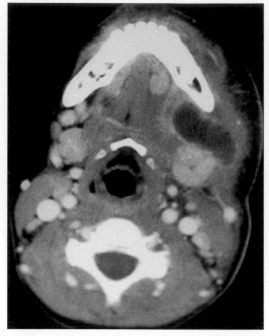

FIGURE 10-17 Submasseteric space abscess. A computed tomography (CT) scan shows a left submasseteric space abscess in a child. CT can generally differentiate between cellulitis of the neck tissues and an abscess that displaces the adjacent structures. CT defines differences in soft tissue density, contributing to the indirect assessment of the site and extent of infection, and may identify complications such as venous thrombosis. Follow-up CT examination may indicate the need for initial surgery or reoperation when there is progression of disease. CT requires minimal positioning of the patient and allows examination of the critically ill patient. (Endicott JN, Nelson RJ, Saraceno CA: Diagnosis and management decisions in infections of the deep fascial spaces of the head and neck utilizing computerized tomography. *Laryngoscope* 1986, 96:751–757.)

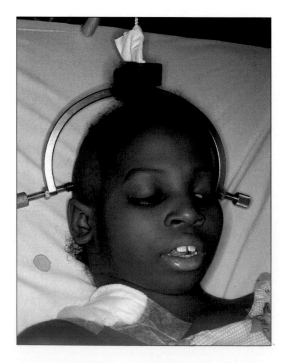

FIGURE 10-18 Subluxation of vertebrae as a complication of deep neck abscess. This 12-year-old child has a subluxation of C_1 on C_2 secondary to actinomycosis (of dental origin) with deep neck infection of the retropharyngeal and prevertebral spaces. A drainage site through the lateral neck is used for the retropharyngeal space and mediastinum, and neurosurgical tongs are used for cervical stabilization. The patient recovered and later had a surgical fusion of the vertebrae. Quadriplegia or subluxation of vertebrae may result from osteomyelitis of the cervical spine. A prevertebral space abscess may cause diaphragmatic and abdominal abscess. A paravertebral space abscess may result in a psoas muscle sheath abscess.

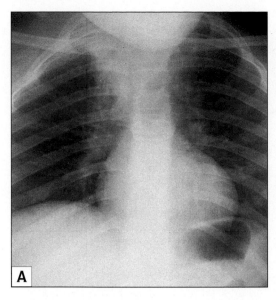

B. Complications of deep space abscess

Osteomyelitis (subluxation of vertebrae)
Mediastinitis
Horner's syndrome
Hoarseness
Unilateral tongue paralysis
Dysphagia
Thrombophlebitis
Erosion of arteries or veins
Airway loss
Septicemia

deep neck abscess depend on the site of abscess. Lateral pharyngeal space abscess may cause Horner's syndrome, hoarseness, unilateral tongue paralysis, dysphagia, thrombophlebitis of the internal jugular vein, and erosion of the carotid artery. The airway may be at risk with a deep neck abscess. Ludwig's angina may result in loss of airway or mediastinitis when the abscess breaks past the hyoid barrier. Septicemia may result in shock, pericarditis, or embolic abscess to the lung or brain. Instrumentation of pharyngeal abscesses without airway control may result in aspiration, lung abscess, pneumonia, empyema, and acute respiratory distress syndrome. Carotid artery erosion requires ligation of the common carotid artery. A preliminary arteriogram may localize the site of erosion to a branch of the external carotid in a few cases. (Rabuzzi DD, Johnson JT: *Diagnosis and Management of Deep Neck Infections.* Arlington, VA: American Academy of Ophthalmology and Otolaryngology; 1978.)

FIGURE 10-19 Complications of deep space abscesses. **A**, Widening of the mediastinum is seen on a chest radiograph of the patient in Fig. 10-18. Mediastinitis may occur as a result of abscesses in the spaces running the length of the neck and has a mortality of 35%. Mediastinal abscess below T4 requires transthoracic drainage. **B**, Other complications of

POSTOPERATIVE INFECTIONS

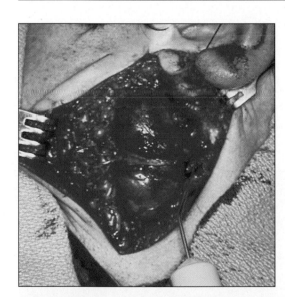

FIGURE 10-20 Clean surgical procedures. Infection is a potential sequelae of all surgical procedures. Clean surgical procedures are defined as those in which no infection exists prior to the procedure. Sterility of the wound is maintained during the surgery and following closure of the wound; the wound is never again exposed to direct contact with bacteria. Examples of such procedures include parotidectomy (shown here), thyroidectomy, submandibular gland excision, and neck dissection.

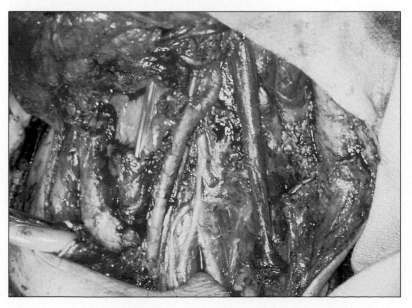

FIGURE 10-21 Clean-contaminated surgical procedures. Clean-contaminated procedures are those performed without a preexisting established focus of infection, but during the course of the surgical procedure, the wound is contaminated by bodily secretions containing microorganisms. Many head and neck surgical procedures involve incisions through mucous membranes, which are colonized by oropharyngeal flora including aerobic and anaerobic organisms, inherently predisposing patients to greater infection risk. In the radical neck dissection and laryngectomy illustrated here, mucosal exposure in the center of the surgical field is a source of wound contamination. In patients undergoing major head and neck surgery, infection rates of 28% to 87% have been reported. The efficacy of perioperative antibiotic administration is well established in these cases. Cefazolin, clindamycin, cefuroxime, cefaperazone, cefotaxime, moxalactam, and the combination clindamycin-gentamicin are effective in preventing postoperative wound infection, reducing the incidence to < 10%. One-day perioperative coverage is as effective as 5-day postoperative coverage. (Johnson J, *et al.*: Antibiotic prophylaxis in high-risk head and neck surgery: One-day vs five-day therapy. *Otolaryngol Head Neck Surg* 1986, 95:554–557.)

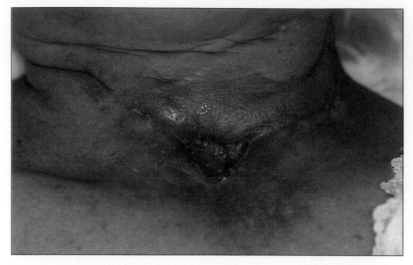

FIGURE 10-22 Pharyngocutaneous fistula. This alcoholic patient, shown postoperatively after laryngopharyngectomy and neck dissection, had failed radiation therapy for a squamous cell carcinoma involving the tonsils, tongue base, larynx, and neck. On the 15th postoperative day, he developed an oral or pharyngocutaneous fistula, which is the most common postoperative complication after laryngectomy or pharyngectomy.

Risk factors for postoperative oropharyngocutaneous fistula

Infection by salivary contamination
Large tumor size (large tissue resection)
Radiation therapy
Poor nutrition
Systemic or metabolic diseases
Residual tumor at suture line

FIGURE 10-23 Risk factors for postoperative oropharyngocutaneous fistula. The development of oropharyngocutaneous fistulas after resection for head and neck carcinoma leads to prolonged hospitalization, significant patient morbidity, and occasional mortality. The incidence of fistula formation ranges from 6% for oral resection to 38% for laryngectomy. Many factors have been implicated in their development. A lack of watertight seal may allow salivary contamination with resultant infection, leading to wound breakdown and fistulization. A larger tumor size results in a larger tissue resection, placing suture lines under tension with the possible development of ischemia, necrosis, and fistula. Systemic or metabolic disease, including diabetes, arteriosclerosis, chronic obstructive pulmonary disease, hypothyroidism, residual tumor, and renal failure, has also been implicated.

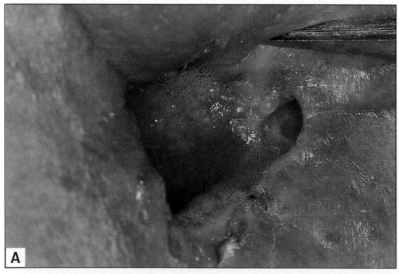

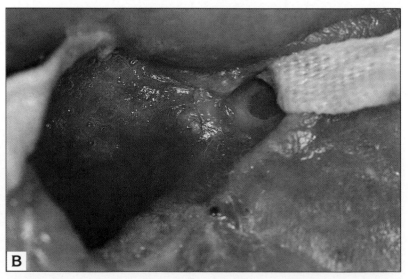

FIGURE 10-24 Management of oropharyngocutaneous fistula. As seen in a close-up of the patient's wound in Fig. 10-22, the fistula tract is kept clean by placing the patient on no oral intake. Treatment is by local wound care. **A** and **B**, Initial irrigation of the wound with saline (*panel 24A*) followed by packing the fistula sites with sterile 1/2- or 1/4-inch plain packing strip soaked in 0.25% acetic acid solution (*panel 24B*) is our preferred method of management. The most common pathogen in the fistula tract is *Pseudomonas*. Surgical closure may be necessary if the fistula does not show gradual diminished output by 1 week of observation. Surgical closure or diversion of the fistula to the midline is indicated if the fistula crosses the carotid artery.

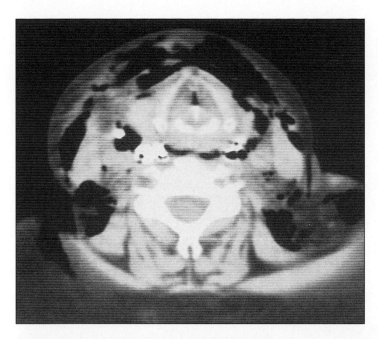

FIGURE 10-25 Esophageal perforation during diagnostic endoscopy. Instrumentation of the esophagus or hypopharynx by rigid or flexible scopes or bougies may result in perforation of the upper digestive tract, with contamination of the neck or mediastinum and potential life-threatening complications. A computed tomography (CT) scan of the neck shows air and contrast in the retropharyngeal space and circumferential compromise of the tracheal air column. The airway is compromised from swelling. Tracheostomy and surgical drainage are indicated. Observation and administration of high-dose broad-spectrum antibiotics may be tried, but a rapid development of deep neck abscess may occur, requiring surgical drainage. CT is useful for monitoring the patient's response to antibiotics and for deciding when to intervene surgically.

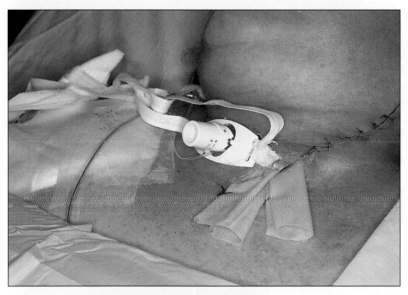

FIGURE 10-26 Management and repair of esophageal perforation. In the same patient, the retropharyngeal space abscess is drained through the lateral neck and upper mediastinum. The lateral oblique incision is used to open the retropharyngeal abscess, as well as for abscesses of the prevertebral, paravertebral, pretracheal, and visceral vascular spaces. Computed tomography scanning of the neck, correlated with clinical symptoms, helps to localize the site of abscess. Bilateral drainage may be required. The space is irrigated, and Penrose drains are left in place. This abscess is below the hyoid bone or middle constrictor muscle and thus requires external drainage. If the infection has spread below the clavicle into the chest and posterior mediastinum to the level of T4, drainage by external thoracotomy is also necessary. If possible, a viscus perforation should be covered with soft tissue. A feeding jejunostomy or gastrostomy tube is necessary until the perforation has healed. Specimens for aerobic and anaerobic culture and Gram's stain are obtained intraoperatively. Foreign bodies, gunshot wounds, or endoscopic trauma are the common causes of this abscess.

FIGURE 10-27 Intraoperative rhinoplasty. Infections following nasal surgery, including septorhinoplasty and endoscopic sinus surgery, occur infrequently. However, reports have noted the possible development of septal abscess, meningitis, toxic shock syndrome, and cavernous sinus thrombosis.

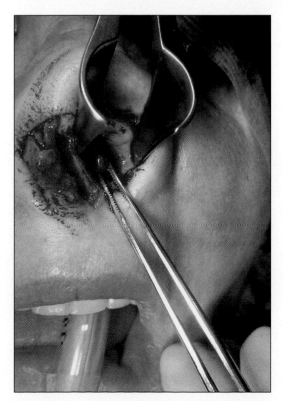

Organ system involvement in toxic shock syndrome	
Muscular	Severe myalgias or > fivefold increase in creatine phosphokinase
Mucous membranes (pharynx, conjunctiva, vagina)	Frank hyperemia
Gastrointestinal	Vomiting, profuse diarrhea
Renal	Renal insufficiency (blood urea nitrogen or creatinine at least 2 × ULN with pyuria in the absence of urinary tract infection)
Liver	Hepatitis (bilirubin and alanine and aspartate aminotransferases at least 2 × ULN)
Blood	Thrombocytopenia < 100,000/mL
Central nervous system	Disorientation without focal neurologic signs

ULN—upper limit of normal.

FIGURE 10-28 Toxic shock syndrome. Toxic shock syndrome is an acute multisystem disease that can occur as a complication of various operative procedures. It has been reported in multiple cases following septorhinoplasty. The mechanism of infection in septorhinoplasty is uncertain, but packing inserted after septoplasty and septorhinoplasty following trauma to the mucous membranes perhaps facilitates growth of toxin-producing *Staphylococcus aureus* and subsequent entry of toxin into the body. Toxic shock syndrome is diagnosed by the following criteria: 1) systolic blood pressure < 90 mm Hg; 2) temperature > 38.9° C; 3) rash with desquamation focused on the palms and soles; 4) negative results in serologic tests for Rocky Mountain spotted fever, leptospirosis, and measles; and 5) involvement of three or more of the organ systems listed in the figure.

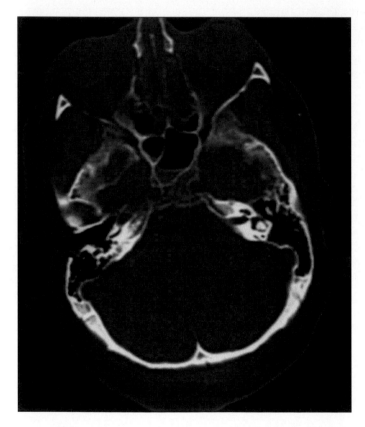

FIGURE 10-29 Meningitis following endoscopic sinus surgery. A patient with chronic sinusitis underwent bilateral middle meatal antrostomies and anterior ethmoidectomies. During the procedure, while work was proceeding in the ethmoid area, a leak of cerebrospinal fluid (CSF) was noted. This leak was repaired using a mucosal flap. The patient received one dose of clindamycin preoperatively and every 8 hours postoperatively. She initially did well but complained of headaches 10 hours postoperatively and began to exhibit mental status changes 24 hours postoperatively. A computed tomography scan reveals nasal packing in place bilaterally and is otherwise unremarkable without obvious bony dehiscence or intracranial air. A lumbar puncture revealed a CSF leukocyte count of 13,020/mL, erythrocyte count of 5565/mL, glucose of 69 mg/dL, and protein of 1002 mg/dL; culture grew no organisms. The patient responded to vancomycin, ceftazidime, and clindamycin within 3 days. A CSF leak with resultant meningitis represents one of the severe complications of endoscopic sinus surgery. Temporary blindness secondary to postoperative infection has also been reported.

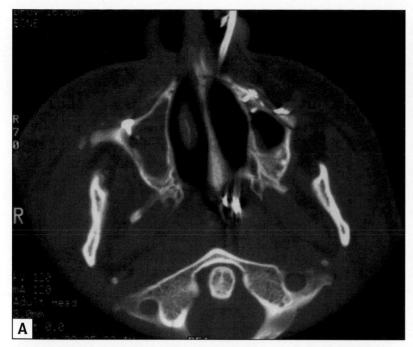 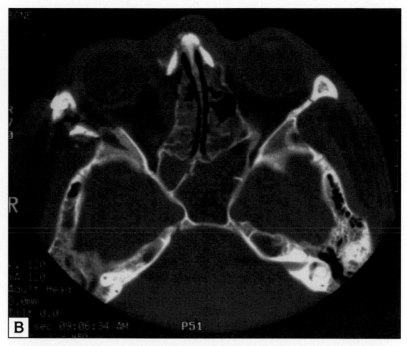

FIGURE 10-30 Sinusitis due to nasogastric intubation. Nasal intubation with an endotracheal and/or nasogastric tube is commonly encountered in intensive care unit and postoperative patients. Blockage of sinus outflow secondary to obstruction of the natural ostia occurs with resultant sinusitis. A young man involved in a motor vehicle accident underwent open reduction and internal fixation of his facial fractures. Postoperatively, he remained febrile, despite broad-spectrum antibiotics. **A**, A computed tomography scan of the sinuses reveals opacification of his right maxillary sinus, which was fractured during the accident. The nasogastric tube is seen in the left side of his nose. **B**, Opacification of both ethmoid and sphenoid sinuses is seen. Maxillary aspiration revealed multiple aerobic gram-positive and -negative organisms that had been cultured from his sputum as well. The patient underwent open gastrostomy tube placement with removal of his nasogastric tube. Imipenem, vancomycin, ciprofloxacin, and fluconazole were continued with resolution of his sinusitis. Nosocomial sinusitis is a common disease, though seldom is it the sole source of fever or the cause of major febrile illness. Most patients respond to nonoperative management, with removal of the nasal tubes being the most important step in treatment.

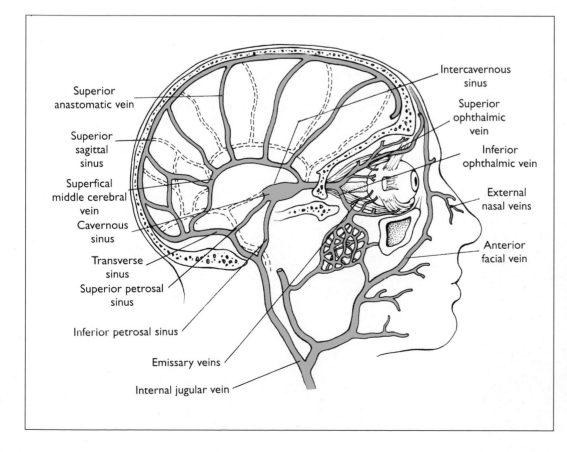

FIGURE 10-31 Cavernous sinus thrombosis. The cavernous sinuses are two intercommunicating spongy structures situated on each side of the sella turcica. They drain the face, nose, and sinuses directly via the ophthalmic veins and indirectly by the pterygoid plexus via emissary veins. These different vessels of the cavernous sinus are valveless. This venous junction is crossed by the internal carotid artery, the IIIrd, IVth, and VIth cranial nerves, and the first two branches of the Vth cranial nerve. Postoperative infections of the nose, paranasal sinuses, and orbits may spread readily to the cavernous sinus. Clinical signs include bilateral orbital involvement, rapidly progressive severe chemosis, ophthalmoplegia, retinal engorgement, and fever. Detection of thrombus by radiographic means is difficult but can be suggested by magnetic resonance imaging. Treatment includes intravenous antibiotics directed against gram-positive and anaerobic organisms, drainage of any abscess, orbital decompression if visual acuity declines, and heparinization to minimize the progression of thrombus.

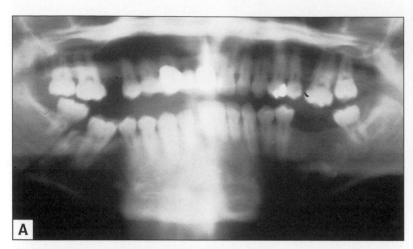

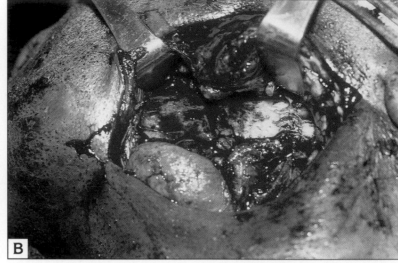

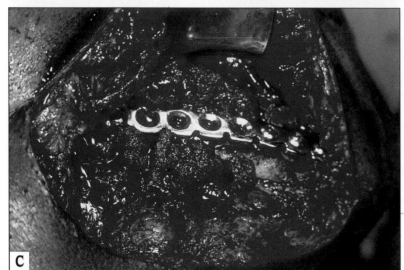

FIGURE 10-32 Osteomyelitis following mandibular fracture. One complication of facial fracture repair is infection, which can subsequently result in malunion or nonunion. **A**, A Panorex taken in a young man following 6 weeks of intermaxillary fixation to treat bilateral parasymphyseal fractures suffered in an altercation reveals malunion of the bone with evidence of bony destruction on the left. **B** and **C**, On operation, the bone in the area was debrided (*panel 32B*) and a reconstruction plate with iliac crest bone graft was placed (*panel 32C*). The patient was successfully treated with 6 weeks of intravenous antibiotics. Traumatic wounds that fail to heal or break down after initial healing may do so because of the presence of a foreign body. In this case, glass was embedded at the time of the trauma, but fragments of tooth or gum that have become devitalized over time, as well as materials implanted at the time of repair including plates, wires, or Silastic, may also subsequently become infected.

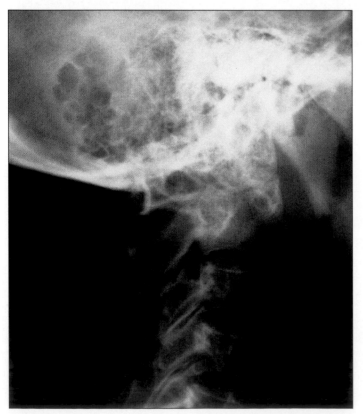

FIGURE 10-33 Alantoaxial subluxation. Tonsillectomy and adenoidectomy may be complicated by infection, including local infection, otitis media, meningitis, brain abscess, cavernous sinus thrombosis, and, rarely, alantoaxial subluxation. Following adenoidectomy, postoperative hyperemia and infection result in decalcification of the vertebrae and laxity of the anterior transverse ligament between the atlas and axis, as illustrated here. Destruction of the vertebral bodies of C_1 and C_2 is seen with anterior subluxation of C_1 over C_2. The patient will have severe neck pain with limitation of range of motion. A low-grade fever, high erythrocyte sedimentation rate, and increased leukocyte count exist. Prompt antibiotic therapy is necessary.

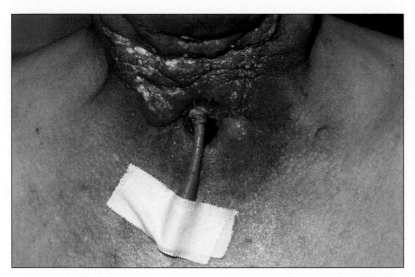

FIGURE 10-34 Cellulitis after tracheoesophageal puncture. Tracheoesophageal puncture is a major advance in the vocal rehabilitation of laryngectomy patients. The procedure involves the creation of a tracheal-esophageal fistula for placement of a one-way valve prosthesis. Though the procedure is not complex, significant infectious complications are possible. Cellulitis around the puncture site, as illustrated, may occur, requiring postoperative antibiotic coverage for gram-positive organisms and anaerobes. Mediastinitis may occur secondary to puncture of the posterior wall of the esophagus. Pneumonia may result from aspiration of saliva into the trachea secondary to leakage around the prosthesis.

SELECTED BIBLIOGRAPHY

Endicott J: Infections of the deep fascial spaces of the head and neck: Update of diagnosis and management. *In* Johnson JT, Blitzer A, Ossoff R, Thomas JR (eds.): *AAO-HNS Instructional Courses*, vol 3. St. Louis: Mosby Year-Book; 1990.

Endicott JN, Nelson RJ, Saraceno CA: Diagnosis and management decisions in infections of the deep fascial spaces of the head and neck utilizing computerized tomography. *Laryngoscope* 1986, 96:751–757.

Johnson J, *et al.*: Antibiotic prophylaxis in high-risk head and neck surgery: One-day vs five-day therapy. *Otolaryngol Head Neck Surg* 1986, 95:554–557.

INDEX